Common Complications in Orthopedics

Editors

JAMES H. CALANDRUCCIO
BENJAMIN J. GREAR
BENJAMIN M. MAUCK
JEFFREY R. SAWYER
PATRICK C. TOY
JOHN C. WEINLEIN

ORTHOPEDIC CLINICS OF NORTH AMERICA

www.orthopedic.theclinics.com

April 2016 • Volume 47 • Number 2

ELSEVIER

1600 John F. Kennedy Boulevard • Suite 1800 • Philadelphia, Pennsylvania, 19103-2899.

http://www.orthopedic.theclinics.com

ORTHOPEDIC CLINICS OF NORTH AMERICA Volume 47, Number 2
April 2016 ISSN 0030-5898, ISBN-13: 978-0-323-41761-7

Editor: Jennifer Flynn-Briggs
Developmental Editor: Kristen Helm

Orthopedic Clinics of North America (ISSN 0030-5898) is published quarterly by Elsevier Inc., 360 Park Avenue South, New York, NY 10010-1710. Months of issue are January, April, July, and October. Business and Editorial Offices: 1600 John F. Kennedy Blvd., Suite 1800, Philadelphia, PA 19103-2899. Customer Service Office: 3251 Riverport Lane, Maryland Heights, MO 63043. Periodicals postage paid at New York, NY and additional mailing offices. Subscription prices are $310.00 per year for (US individuals), $653.00 per year for (US institutions), $365.00 per year (Canadian individuals), $797.00 per year (Canadian institutions), $450.00 per year (international individuals), $797.00 per year (international institutions), $100.00 per year (US students), $220.00 per year (Canadian and international students). Foreign air speed delivery is included in all *Clinics* subscription prices. All prices are subject to change without notice. **POSTMASTER:** Send change of address to *Orthopedic Clinics of North America*, **Elsevier Health Sciences Division, Subscription Customer Service, 3251 Riverport Lane, Maryland Heights, MO 63043. Customer Service (orders, claims, online, change of address): Elsevier Health Sciences Division, Subscription Customer Service, 3251 Riverport Lane, Maryland Heights, MO 63043. Tel: 1-800-654-2452 (U.S. and Canada); 314-447-8871 (outside U.S. and Canada). Fax: 314-447-8029. E-mail:** journalscustomerservice-usa@elsevier. com **(for print support);** journalsonlinesupport-usa@elsevier.com **(for online support).**

Reprints. For copies of 100 or more, of articles in this publication, please contact the Commercial Reprints Department, Elsevier Inc., 360 Park Avenue South, New York, NY 10010-1710. Tel.: 212-633-3874; Fax: 212-633-3820; E-mail: reprints@elsevier. com.

Orthopedic Clinics of North America is covered in *MEDLINE/PubMed (Index Medicus), Cinahl, Excerpta Medica,* and *Cumulative Index to Nursing and Allied Health Literature.*

PROGRAM OBJECTIVE
Orthopedic Clinics of North America offers clinical review articles on the most cutting-edge technologies and techniques in the field, including adult reconstruction, the upper extremity, pediatrics, trauma, oncology, and sports medicine.

TARGET AUDIENCE
Practicing orthopedic surgeons, orthopedic residents, and other healthcare professionals who specialize in orthopedic technologies and techniques for adult reconstruction, the upper extremity, pediatrics, trauma, oncology, and sports medicine.

LEARNING OBJECTIVES
Upon completion of this activity, participants will be able to:
1. Review possible complications following pediatric orthopedic procedures such as spine surgery and scoliosis treatment.
2. Discuss complications following upper extremity injuries such as distal radius fractures and distal biceps tears.
3. Recognize potential proprioceptive and stability insufficiencies following adult reconstructive surgeries.

ACCREDITATION
The Elsevier Office of Continuing Medical Education (EOCME) is accredited by the Accreditation Council for Continuing Medical Education (ACCME) to provide continuing medical education for physicians.

The EOCME designates this enduring material for a maximum of 15 *AMA PRA Category 1 Credit*(s)™. Physicians should claim only the credit commensurate with the extent of their participation in the activity.

All other health care professionals requesting continuing education credit for this enduring material will be issued a certificate of participation.

DISCLOSURE OF CONFLICTS OF INTEREST
The EOCME assesses conflict of interest with its instructors, faculty, planners, and other individuals who are in a position to control the content of CME activities. All relevant conflicts of interest that are identified are thoroughly vetted by EOCME for fair balance, scientific objectivity, and patient care recommendations. EOCME is committed to providing its learners with CME activities that promote improvements or quality in healthcare and not a specific proprietary business or a commercial interest.

The planning committee, staff, authors and editors listed below have identified no financial relationships or relationships to products or devices they or their spouse/life partner have with commercial interest related to the content of this CME activity:

Matthew P. Abdel, MD; Anthony Bell, MD; John Chao, MD; Umberto Cottino, MD; Lorena V. Floccari, MD; Jennifer Flynn-Briggs; Anjali Fortna; Stephanie M. Gancarczyk, MD; Mark Tyson Garon, MD; Capt Brad T. Hyatt, MD; A. Alex Jahangir, MD, MMHC; Matthew Karam, MD; John W. Karl, MD, MPH; Dennis S. Lee, MD; Hongchao Liu, MD; Ian McAlister, MD; Mitchell McDowell, DO; Rodrigo Góes Medéa de Mendonça, MD; Todd A. Milbrandt, MD; Keith M. Nord, BS; Santha Priya; Andrew Park, MD; Michael Lucius Pomerantz, MD; John Roaten, MD; Maj Jeremy K. Rush, MD; Maj Matthew R. Schmitz, MD; Peter K. Sculco, MD; Megan Suermann; David D. Spence, MD; Robert J. Strauch, MD; Colin W. Swigler, MD; Patrick C. Toy, MD; Douglas R. Weikert, MD; Paul S. Whiting, MD; Michael Willey, MD; Andrew J. Wodowski, MD.

The planning committee, staff, authors and editors listed below have identified financial relationships or relationships to products or devices they or their spouse/life partner have with commercial interest related to the content of this CME activity:

Tad L. Gerlinger, MD is on the speakers' bureau for, and consultant/advisor for, Smith & Nephew.
Jeffrey A. Greenberg, MD, MS is a consultant/advisor for Stryker; Acumed; Biomedical Enterprises, Inc.; and AxoGen, Inc., and stock ownership in AxoGen, Inc.
Derek M. Kelly, MD receives royalties/patents from Elsevier Inc.
William M. Mihalko, MD, PhD is on the speakers' bureau for Aesculap, Inc. and Medtronic, is a consultant/advisor for Aesculap, Inc.; Medtronic; and Panoramic Healthcare Communications, has research support from Aesculap, Inc.; Microport Scientific Corporation; and U.S. Department of Defense, and receives royalties/patents from Aesculap, Inc. and Elsevier Inc.
Jeffrey R. Sawyer, MD is a consultant/advisor for DePuy Synthes, has research support from Medicrea, and receives royalties/patents from Elsevier Inc.
Stephen Andrew Sems, MD receives royalties/patents from Biomet, Inc.
Rafael J. Sierra, MD is a consultant/advisor for, with research support from, and royalties/patents from Biomet, Inc.
David Templeman, MD is on the speakers' bureau for Stryker; Orthofix Holdings, Inc.; and Naroflex Corporation, is a consultant/advisor for Zimmer Inc.; Stryker; Orthofix Holdings, Inc., and has stock ownership in Naroflex Corporation.
John C. Weinlein, MD receives royalties/patents from Elsevier Inc.

UNAPPROVED/OFF-LABEL USE DISCLOSURE
The EOCME requires CME faculty to disclose to the participants
1. When products or procedures being discussed are off-label, unlabelled, experimental, and/or investigational (not US Food and Drug Administration [FDA] approved); and

2. Any limitations on the information presented, such as data that are preliminary or that represent ongoing research, interim analyses, and/or unsupported opinions. Faculty may discuss information about pharmaceutical agents that is outside of FDA-approved labelling. This information is intended solely for CME and is not intended to promote off-label use of these medications. If you have any questions, contact the medical affairs department of the manufacturer for the most recent prescribing information.

TO ENROLL
To enroll in the *Orthopedic Clinics of North America* Continuing Medical Education program, call customer service at 1-800-654-2452 or sign up online at http://www.theclinics.com/home/cme. The CME program is available to subscribers for an additional annual fee of USD 215.

METHOD OF PARTICIPATION
In order to claim credit, participants must complete the following:
1. Complete enrolment as indicated above.
2. Read the activity.
3. Complete the CME Test and Evaluation. Participants must achieve a score of 70% on the test. All CME Tests and Evaluations must be completed online.

CME INQUIRIES/SPECIAL NEEDS
For all CME inquiries or special needs, please contact elsevierCME@elsevier.com.

Editorial Board

Contributors

AUTHORS

MATTHEW P. ABDEL, MD
Assistant Professor, Department of Orthopedic
Surgery, Mayo Clinic, Rochester, Minnesota

ANTHONY BELL, MD
Assistant Professor, Department of
Orthopaedics and Rehabilitation, Ambulatory
Care Center, University of Florida College of
Medicine-Jacksonville, Jacksonville, Florida

JOHN CHAO, MD
Peachtree Orthopaedic Clinic; Faculty, Foot
and Ankle Division, Orthopedic Surgery
Residency, Atlanta Medical Center, Atlanta,
Georgia

UMBERTO COTTINO, MD
Adult Reconstruction Research Fellow,
Department of Orthopedic Surgery, Mayo
Clinic, Rochester, Minnesota

**RODRIGO GÓES MEDÉA DE MENDONÇA,
MD**
Santa Casa de Sao Paulo Hospital Central Sao
Paulo, Rua Dr Cesario Motta Jr, Sao Paulo,
Brasil

LORENA V. FLOCCARI, MD
Department of Orthopedic Surgery, Mayo
Clinic, Rochester, Minnesota

STEPHANIE M. GANCARCZYK, MD
Resident Physician, Department of
Orthopaedic Surgery, Columbia University
Medical Center, New York, New York

MARK TYSON GARON, MD
Fellow, Indiana Hand to Shoulder Center,
Indianapolis, Indiana

TAD L. GERLINGER, MD
Assistant Professor, Rush University, Midwest
Orthopaedics at Rush, Chicago, Illinois;
Associate Professor of Surgery, Uniformed

Services University of the Health Sciences,
Bethesda, Maryland

JEFFREY A. GREENBERG, MD, MS
Physician, Indiana Hand to Shoulder Center,
Indianapolis, Indiana

Capt BRAD T. HYATT, MD
Department of Orthopaedics and
Rehabilitation, San Antonio Military Medical
Center, Fort Sam Houston, Texas

A. ALEX JAHANGIR, MD, MMHC
Associate Professor, Department of
Orthopaedics and Rehabilitation, Vanderbilt
University Medical Center, Nashville,
Tennessee

MATTHEW KARAM, MD
Clinical Assistant Professor, Department of
Orthopaedic Surgery and Rehabilitation,
University of Iowa Hospitals and Clinics, Iowa
City, Iowa

JOHN W. KARL, MD, MPH
Resident Physician, Department of
Orthopaedic Surgery, Columbia University
Medical Center, New York, New York

DEREK M. KELLY, MD
Associate Professor, University of
Tennessee-Campbell Clinic, Department of
Orthopaedic Surgery and Biomedical
Engineering, Le Bonheur Children's Hospital,
Memphis, Tennessee

DENNIS S. LEE, MD
Resident, Orthopaedic Surgery and
Rehabilitation, Vanderbilt University Medical
Center, Nashville, Tennessee

HONGCHAO LIU, MD
Attending Surgeon, The First Hospital, Qiqihar,
China

IAN McALISTER, MD
Department of Orthopaedic Surgery, Mayo Clinic, Rochester, Minnesota

MITCHELL McDOWELL, DO
Kaiser Permanente Riverside Medical Center, Riverside, California

WILLIAM M. MIHALKO, MD, PhD
Professor and J.R. Hyde Chair, Department of Orthopaedic Surgery and Biomedical Engineering, University of Tennesse-Campbell Clinic, Memphis, Tennessee

TODD A. MILBRANDT, MD
Department of Orthopedic Surgery, Mayo Clinic, Rochester, Minnesota

KEITH M. NORD, BS
University of Tennessee Health Science Center Medical School, Memphis, Tennessee

ANDREW PARK, MD
Midwest Orthopaedics at Rush, Chicago, Illinois

MICHAEL LUCIUS POMERANTZ, MD
Synergy Specialists Medical Group, Orthopaedic Surgery, Hand/Upper Extremity Sub-specialization, Chula Vista, California

JOHN ROATEN, MD
Pediatric Orthopaedic Fellow, University of Tennessee-Campbell Clinic, Department of Orthopaedic Surgery and Biomedical Engineering, Memphis, Tennessee

Maj JEREMY K. RUSH, MD
Department of Orthopaedics and Rehabilitation, San Antonio Military Medical Center, Fort Sam Houston, Texas

JEFFREY R. SAWYER, MD
Professor of Orthopaedic Surgery; Director, Pediatric Orthopaedic Fellowship, University of Tennessee-Campbell Clinic, Memphis, Tennessee

Maj MATTHEW R. SCHMITZ, MD
Department of Orthopaedics and Rehabilitation, San Antonio Military Medical Center, Fort Sam Houston, Texas

PETER K. SCULCO, MD
Adult Reconstruction Clinical Fellow, Department of Orthopedic Surgery, Mayo Clinic, Rochester, Minnesota

STEPHEN ANDREW SEMS, MD
Department of Orthopaedic Surgery, Mayo Clinic, Rochester, Minnesota

RAFAEL J. SIERRA, MD
Professor, Department of Orthopedic Surgery, Mayo Clinic, Rochester, Minnesota

DAVID D. SPENCE, MD
Assistant Professor, University of Tennessee-Campbell Clinic, Department of Orthopaedic Surgery and Biomedical Engineering, Memphis, Tennessee

ROBERT J. STRAUCH, MD
Professor, Department of Orthopaedic Surgery; Hand, Elbow and Microvascular Surgery, Columbia University Medical Center, New York, New York

COLIN W. SWIGLER, MD
Orthopedic Resident, Department of Orthopaedic Surgery and Biomedical Engineering, University of Tennesse-Campbell Clinic, Memphis, Tennessee

DAVID TEMPLEMAN, MD
Hennepin County Medical Center; Professor, Department of Orthopaedic Surgery, University of Minnesota, Minneapolis, Minnesota

PATRICK C. TOY, MD
Assistant Professor, Department of Orthopaedic Surgery and Biomedical Engineering, University of Tennesse-Campbell Clinic, Memphis, Tennessee

DOUGLAS R. WEIKERT, MD
Associate Professor, Orthopaedic Surgery and Rehabilitation, Hand and Upper Extremity Center, Vanderbilt University Medical Center, Nashville, Tennessee

JOHN C. WEINLEIN, MD
Assistant Professor, University of
Tennessee-Campbell Clinic, Memphis, Elvis
Presley Memorial Trauma Center, Regional
One Health, Tennessee

PAUL S. WHITING, MD
Assistant Professor, Department of
Orthopaedics and Rehabilitation, University of
Wisconsin, Madison, Wisconsin

MICHAEL WILLEY, MD
Clinical Assistant Professor, Department of
Orthopaedic Surgery and Rehabilitation,
University of Iowa Hospitals and Clinics, Iowa
City, Iowa

ANDREW J. WODOWSKI, MD
Orthopaedic Surgery Resident, Department of
Orthopaedic Surgery and Biomedical
Engineering, University of Tennesse-Campbell
Clinic, Memphis, Tennessee

Contents

Adult Reconstruction

Patrick C. Toy

Andrew J. Wodowski, Colin W. Swigler, Hongchao Liu, Keith M. Nord, Patrick C. Toy, and William M. Mihalko

Proprioceptive mechanoreceptors provide neural feedback for position in space and are critical for three-dimensional interaction. Proprioception is decreased with osteoarthritis of the knees, which leads to increased risk of falling. As the prevalence of osteoarthritis increases, so does the need for total knee arthroplasty (TKA), and knowing the effect of TKA on proprioception is essential. This article reviews the literature regarding proprioception and its relationship to balance, aging, osteoarthritis, and the effect of TKA on proprioception. Knee arthroplasty involving retention of the cruciate ligaments is also reviewed, as well as the evidence of proprioception in the posterior cruciate ligament after TKA.

Umberto Cottino, Peter K. Sculco, Rafael J. Sierra, and Matthew P. Abdel

Instability is one of the most common causes of failure after total knee arthroplasty. Although there are several contributing causes, surgical error and poor implant design selection contribute. For this reason, an accurate diagnosis is fundamental and is largely based on a thorough history and physical examination. In general, tibiofemoral instability can be classified into 3 different patterns: flexion instability, genu recurvatum, and extension instability. In this article, these 3 patterns are reviewed in greater depth.

Mitchell McDowell, Andrew Park, and Tad L. Gerlinger

There are many causes of residual pain after total knee arthroplasty (TKA). Evaluation and management begins with a comprehensive history and physical examination, followed by radiographic evaluation of the replaced and adjacent joints, as well as previous films of the replaced joint. Further workup includes laboratory analysis, along with a synovial fluid aspirate to evaluate the white blood cell count with differential as well as culture. Advanced imaging modalities may be beneficial when the diagnosis remains unclear. Revision surgery is not advisable without a clear diagnosis, as it may be associated with poor results.

Peter K. Sculco, Umberto Cottino, Matthew P. Abdel, and Rafael J. Sierra

Instability and limb length discrepancy are two common complications after total hip arthroplasty (THA) and the most common cause for revision surgery. Maximizing impingement-free range of motion, recreating appropriate offset, and equalizing limb lengths and producing a pain-free and dynamically stable THA is the ultimate goal of a successful THA. In this article, patient risk factors for hip instability and limb length discrepancy are reviewed along with, key elements of the preoperative template, the anatomic landmarks for accurate component placement, device options, the leg positions for soft tissue stability testing, and the management of postoperative instability.

Trauma

John C. Weinlein

Paul S. Whiting and A. Alex Jahangir

Orthopedic trauma results in systemic physiologic changes that predispose patients to venous thromboembolism (VTE). In the absence of prophylaxis, VTE incidence may be as high as 60%. Mechanical and pharmacologic thromboprophylaxis are effective in decreasing rates of VTE. Combined mechanical and pharmacologic thromboprophylaxis is more efficacious for decreasing VTE incidence than either regimen independently. If pharmacologic thromboprophylaxis is contraindicated, mechanical prophylaxis should be used. Patients with isolated lower extremity fractures who are ambulatory, or those with isolated upper extremity trauma, do not require pharmacologic prophylaxis in the absence of other VTE risk factors.

Ian McAlister and Stephen Andrew Sems

Arthrofibrosis after periarticular fractures can create clinically significant impairments in both the upper and lower extremities. The shoulder, elbow, and knee are particularly susceptible to the condition. Many risk factors for the development of arthrofibrosis cannot be controlled by the patient or surgeon. Early postoperative motion should be promoted whenever possible. Manipulations under anesthesia are effective for a period of time in certain fracture patterns, and open or arthroscopic surgical debridements should be reserved for the patient for whom nonoperative modalities fail and who has a clinically significant deficit.

Michael Willey and Matthew Karam

Surgical site infection can be a devastating complication that results in significant morbidity in patients who undergo operative fixation of fractures. Reducing the rate of infection and wound complications in high-risk trauma patients by giving early effective antibiotics, improving soft tissue management, and using antiseptic techniques is a common topic of discussion. Despite heightened awareness, there has not been a significant reduction in surgical site infection over the past 40 years. Patients should be treated aggressively to eliminate or suppress the infection, heal the fracture if there is a nonunion, and maintain the function of the patient.

Nonunion of the Femur and Tibia: An Update

Anthony Bell, David Templeman, and John C. Weinlein

Delayed union and nonunion of tibial and femoral shaft fractures are common orthopedic problems. Numerous publications address lower extremity long bone nonunions. This review presents current trends and recent literature on the evaluation and treatment of nonunions of the tibia and femur. New studies focused on tibial nonunion and femoral nonunion are reviewed. A section summarizing recent treatment of atypical femoral fractures associated with bisphosphonate therapy is also included.

Pediatrics

Jeffrey R. Sawyer

Complications of Pediatric Elbow Fractures

Brad T. Hyatt, Matthew R. Schmitz, and Jeremy K. Rush

Fractures about the elbow in children are common and varied. Both diagnosis and treatment can be challenging, and optimal treatment protocols continue to evolve with new research data. This article reviews common complications related to pediatric elbow fractures and presents recent literature to help guide treatment.

Surgical Site Infections After Pediatric Spine Surgery

Lorena V. Floccari and Todd A. Milbrandt

Surgical site infection (SSI) after spinal deformity surgery is a complication in the pediatric population resulting in high morbidity and cost. Despite modern surgical techniques and preventative strategies, the incidence remains substantial, especially in the neuromuscular population. This review focuses on recent advancements in identification of risk factors, prevention, diagnosis, and treatment strategies for acute and delayed pediatric spine infections. It reviews recent literature, including the best practice guidelines for infection prevention in high-risk patients. Targets of additional research are highlighted to assess efficacy of current practices to further reduce risk of SSI in pediatric patients with spinal deformity.

Complications After Surgical Treatment of Adolescent Idiopathic Scoliosis

Rodrigo Góes Medéa de Mendonça, Jeffrey R. Sawyer, and Derek M. Kelly

Even with current techniques and instrumentation, complications can occur after operative treatment of adolescent idiopathic scoliosis. The most dreaded complications—neurologic deficits—are relatively infrequent, occurring in 1% or less of patients. Nonneurologic deficits, such as infection, pseudarthrosis, curve progression, and proximal junctional kyphosis, are more frequent, but are much less likely to require reoperation or to cause poor functional outcomes. Understanding the potential complications of surgical treatment of pediatric spinal deformity is essential for surgical decision-making.

John Roaten and David D. Spence

Slipped capital femoral epiphysis (SCFE) is a condition of the immature hip in which mechanical overload of the proximal femoral physis results in anterior and superior displacement of the femoral metaphysis relative to the epiphysis. The treatment of SCFE is surgical, as the natural history of nonsurgical treatment is slip progression and early arthritis. Despite advances in treatment, much controversy exists regarding the best treatment, and complication rates remain high. Complications include osteonecrosis, chondrolysis, SCFE-induced impingement, and related articular degeneration, fixation failure and deformity progression, growth disturbance of the proximal femur, and development of bilateral disease.

Upper Extremity

Benjamin M. Mauck and James H. Calandruccio

Dennis S. Lee and Douglas R. Weikert

Complications following any form of distal radius fixation remain prevalent. With an armamentarium of fixation options available to practicing surgeons, familiarity with the risks of newer plate technology as it compares with other conventional methods is crucial to optimizing surgical outcome and managing patient expectations. This article presents an updated review on complications following various forms of distal radius fixation.

John W. Karl, Stephanie M. Gancarczyk, and Robert J. Strauch

Carpal tunnel release for compression of the median nerve at the wrist is one of the most common and successful procedures in hand surgery. Complications, though rare, are potentially devastating and may include intraoperative technical errors, postoperative infection and pain, and persistent or recurrent symptoms. Patients with continued complaints after carpal tunnel release should be carefully evaluated with detailed history and physical examination in addition to electrodiagnostic testing. For those with persistent or recurrent symptoms, a course of nonoperative management including splinting, injections, occupational therapy, and desensitization should be considered prior to revision surgery.

Mark Tyson Garon and Jeffrey A. Greenberg

Modern techniques to repair the distal biceps tendon include one-incision and 2-incision techniques that use transosseous sutures, suture anchors, interference screws, and/or cortical buttons to achieve a strong repair of the distal biceps brachii. Repair using these techniques has led to improved functional outcomes when compared with nonoperative treatment. Most complications consist of neurapraxic injuries to the lateral antebrachial cutaneous nerve, posterior interosseous nerve, stiffness and weakness with forearm rotation, heterotopic ossification, and wound infections. Although complications certainly affect outcomes, patients with distal biceps repairs report a high satisfaction rate after repair.

Foot and Ankle

Benjamin J. Grear

ORTHOPEDIC CLINICS OF NORTH AMERICA

FORTHCOMING ISSUES

July 2016
Orthopedic Urgencies and Emergencies
James H. Calandruccio, Benjamin J. Grear,
Benjamin M. Mauck, Jeffrey R. Sawyer,
Patrick C. Toy, and John C. Weinlein, *Editors*

October 2016
Sports-Related Injuries in Orthopedics
James H. Calandruccio, Benjamin J. Grear,
Benjamin M. Mauck, Jeffrey R. Sawyer,
Patrick C. Toy, and John C. Weinlein, *Editors*

January 2017
Controversies in Fracture Care
James H. Calandruccio, Benjamin J. Grear,
Benjamin M. Mauck, Jeffrey R. Sawyer,
Patrick C. Toy, and John C. Weinlein, *Editors*

THE CLINICS ARE AVAILABLE ONLINE!
Access your subscription at:
www.theclinics.com

Note from the Publisher

Elsevier would like to welcome the new Editorial Board for the *Orthopedic Clinics*, a talented team of staff physicians from the Campbell Clinic in Memphis, Tennessee, a world leader in orthopedic surgery. The Editorial Board includes:

James H. Calandruccio
    Upper Extremity

Benjamin J. Grear
    Foot and Ankle

Benjamin M. Mauck
    Upper Extremity

Jeffrey R. Sawyer
    Pediatrics

Patrick C. Toy
    Adult Reconstruction

John C. Weinlein
    Trauma

Elsevier is proud to publish *Campbell's Operative Orthopaedics*, which is authored by staff physicians at the Campbell Clinic. Now in its 12th edition, it is widely regarded as the preeminent international reference in orthopedic surgery. We are thrilled to extend this knowledge and expertise to the *Orthopedic Clinics*.

Based upon feedback from our subscribers and the new Editorial Board, the *Orthopedic Clinics* will revert to a single-topic focus for each issue. Future topics include "Orthopedic Urgencies and Emergencies," "Sports-Related Injuries in Orthopedics," and "Controversies in Fracture Care."

We very much appreciate your continued readership. Please feel free to contact me with any further feedback.

Jennifer Flynn-Briggs
Senior Clinics Editor, Elsevier

E-mail address:
j.flynn-briggs@elsevier.com

Orthop Clin N Am 47 (2016) xvii
http://dx.doi.org/10.1016/j.ocl.2015.12.002
0030-5898/16/$ – see front matter © 2016 Published by Elsevier Inc.

Preface

Common Complications in Orthopedics

The majority of patients do not encounter problems after orthopedic surgery; however, as with any surgery, there are potential risks. This issue includes articles on some of the most common complications in orthopedic surgery.

The authors of these sections have provided much useful information on this topic that can help surgeons avoid some of these complications. All of these articles contain much information from experienced surgeons in orthopedics, and we are most appreciative of their willingness to share their knowledge.

Articles in the Adult Reconstruction Section focus on the loss of proprioception after primary TKA, hip instability and leg length discrepancy after THA, instability after TKA, and the painful total knee arthroplasty.

Articles in the Trauma Section focus on thromboembolic disease after orthopaedic trauma, arthrofibrosis after periarticular fracture fixation, impact of infection on fracture fixation, and nonunion.

Articles in the Pediatric Section focus on complications of pediatric elbow fractures, infections after pediatric spine surgery, complicatons after adolescent idiopathic spine surgery, and complications of slipped capital femoral epiphysis.

Articles in the Upper Extremity Section focus on complications of distal radius fixation, complications of carpal tunnel release, complications of distal biceps repair, and complications of lateral epicondylar release.

Articles in the Foot and Ankle Section focus on DVT in foot and ankle surgery.

I hope that our readers will find the material useful in their practices.

Jennifer Flynn-Briggs
Senior Clinics Editor, Elsevier

E-mail address:
j.flynn-briggs@elsevier.com

Orthop Clin N Am 47 (2016) xix
http://dx.doi.org/10.1016/j.ocl.2015.12.001
0030-5898/16/$ – see front matter © 2016 Published by Elsevier Inc.

orthopedic.theclinics.com

Adult Reconstruction

Proprioception and Knee Arthroplasty
A Literature Review

Andrew J. Wodowski, MD[a], Colin W. Swigler, MD[a],
Hongchao Liu, MD[b], Keith M. Nord, BS[c], Patrick C. Toy, MD[a],
William M. Mihalko, MD, PhD[a],*

KEYWORDS

- Proprioception • Knee • Arthroplasty • Mechanoreceptor • Balance • Cruciate

KEY POINTS

- Retention of the posterior cruciate ligament in total knee arthroplasty (TKA) may benefit proprioception.
- The anterior cruciate ligament has been shown to play a significant role in proprioception, and it commonly is sacrificed in TKA. Evidence suggests that unicompartmental TKA that is cruciate sparing may result in improved proprioception compared with standard TKA.
- Patients who are candidates for TKA are likely to already have decreased proprioception.
- The overall effect of TKA on proprioception is debated, but many studies show evidence that it improves proprioception in appropriate surgical candidates.
- Proper gap balancing and surgical technique are crucial to proprioception after TKA.

INTRODUCTION

The standard definition of proprioception is "the reception of stimuli produced in (an) organism."[1] More colloquial use in orthopedic surgery has resulted in a general definition of proprioception as the ability to sense position of a joint in space. It provides crucial and fundamental somatosensory input for everyday functioning and is called on for the simple task of standing to more complex activities such as walking, running, and navigating unstable ground. Proprioceptive mechanoreceptors provide feedback for position in space and are, therefore, a critical asset for interacting with the surrounding three-dimensional world. Previous research has shown that proprioception is decreased with osteoarthritis (OA) of the knee, leading to an increased risk of falling.[2–5] As the prevalence of OA increases with an aging population, so does the need for total knee arthroplasty (TKA), and knowing the effect of TKA on proprioception is essential. The purpose of this article is to review the relevant literature regarding proprioception and its relationship to balance, aging, and the effect of TKA.

BASIC SCIENCE OF PROPRIOCEPTION

Proprioception is made possible by length-sensing muscle spindle units in skeletal muscle, stretch receptors in the fibrous joint capsule, and

Disclosures: Dr W.M. Mihalko is a consultant for Aesculap/B.Braun, Medtronic, and Panoramic Health Care and is the recipient of research support from Microport, Smith & Nephew, and Stryker; he receives speaker fees from Aesculap/B.Braun and publishing royalties from Elsevier. Dr P.C. Toy receives publishing royalties from Elsevier. The other authors have no conflicts to disclose.
[a] University of Tennessee-Campbell Clinic, Department of Orthopaedic Surgery & Biomedical Engineering, 1211 Union Avenue, Memphis, TN 38104, USA; [b] The First Hospital, Qiqihar, China; [c] University of Tennessee Health Science Center Medical School, 910 Madison Avenue, Memphis, TN 38163, USA
* Corresponding author. University of Tennessee-Campbell Clinic, Department of Orthopaedic Surgery & Biomedical Engineering, 1211 Union Avenue, Suite 510, Memphis, TN 38104.
E-mail address: wmihalko@campbellclinic.com

Golgi organs in tendons and ligaments. The inputs from these various receptors are processed in the brain and integrated with visual and vestibular information to generate a sense of position and movement through space.[6] A major component of proprioception is joint position sense, which can be examined by having patients determine the position of a limb or joint without use of their eyes or vestibular system. A commonly used method of quantifying proprioception is called joint position matching, during which a patient's limb is held at a specific angle for a moment, then returned to the neutral position before asking the patient to recreate the angle.[7] It is normal to have a slight and gradual decrease in proprioception as part of the aging process; however, sudden or gross decreases in proprioceptive abilities should be considered pathologic and investigated.[8]

MECHANORECEPTORS

OA of the knee is accompanied by restricted mobility because of pain, altered joint mechanics, and muscle atrophy. These changes cause deficits in balance, which have been demonstrated to be important requirements for the independent and safe performance of the activities of daily life and in the prevention of falls. During TKA many intra-articular structures of the knee joint known to contribute to proprioception are resected. The menisci, cruciates, and other soft tissues about the knee have important functions in load transmission, gliding movements, nutrition of the articular cartilage, and stability of the knee joint. The population of nerve fibers and receptors within a meniscus provides the central nervous system with information related to mechanical stimulation, including motion and excessive loading, and may be related to protective reflexes. Mechanoreceptors are neural elements that mediate tactile and position sense. They convert stimuli into neural impulses, which are then deciphered and interpreted by the central nervous system. Although considerable controversy still exists about the types and exact locations of mechanoreceptors in human ligaments, it has been shown that they receive sensory input and mediate a response that regulates muscle tone and, therefore, coordination.[9–11]

EFFECT OF THE POSTERIOR CRUCIATE LIGAMENT

A suggestion of the proprioceptive role of the posterior cruciate ligament (PCL) is supported by the presence of varied mechanoreceptors found in aging and normal PCLs. One study demonstrated a large array of mechanoreceptors in the PCL, even in arthritic knees.[10] In addition, because comparable clinical results have been demonstrated with either PCL retention or sacrifice, it may be desirable to consider retention to preserve its proprioceptive role to the knee, although it is unclear if mechanoreceptors persist after a PCL-retaining TKA.[10,11] One analysis of the effect of the PCL on the biomechanics of TKA demonstrated no evidence of posterior edge loading on the medial aspect of the polyethylene insert, but edge loading was evident on the lateral side of the insert. This forward pattern of wear on the medial side of the polyethylene insert helps confirm that the PCL is involved in proper coronal balance of the knee and suggests that maintenance of the mechanoreceptors in a PCL-retaining knee may benefit the physiology and mechanics of the knee.[12]

QUADRICEPS AND PATELLAR TENDON

The quadriceps extensor mechanism of the knee is a major structure that contributes to knee stability. Proprioceptive information is transmitted to the nervous system via muscle spindles in the quadriceps. Researchers have reported that elderly individuals had less quadriceps muscle strength and a higher error in reproduction of joint position sense compared with young or middle-aged individuals; no correlation between quadriceps strength and knee proprioception was found.[13] However, a study of the effects of patellar strap use showed slight improvements in proprioception, suggesting that the knee extensors indeed play a role in proprioception.[14]

BALANCE, AGING, AND TOTAL KNEE ARTHROPLASTY

Balance requires the central integration of proprioceptive, somatosensory, visual, and vestibular inputs linked to appropriate musculoskeletal output for postural responses. Just as proprioception declines with age and/or OA, vestibular and visual inputs may also decline, resulting in an overall reduction in sensory input required for balance.[15–17] A study by Teasdale and colleagues[18] showed that disturbance of just 1 of these inputs was not of substantial significance. Because of an increased reliance on other inputs, however, disturbance of more than 1 is likely in the aging population. Therefore, after a TKA in this population, the negative effects on balance were far greater. The risk of falling before TKA is correlated with risk after TKA and, therefore, preoperative assessment of balance is an important consideration in postoperative rehabilitation.[19]

As the human body ages, muscle mass declines to an extent of up to 20% to 40% by the seventh decade.[20] This correlates with a loss of corrective postural musculature strength needed to maintain adequate balance. Postural musculature responds to cortical input via anticipatory postural adjustments (APA) and compensatory postural adjustments (CPA), which in combination aim to maintain center of mass or center of pressure over base support. Kanekar and Aruin[21] demonstrated delays in APA with resultant increase in CPA in the elderly compared with younger controls, suggesting decreased control of posture and increased risk of falls. The risk of falling should not be confused with the fear of falling, which is often increased with multiple sensory deficits. Fear of falling affects up to 30% of community-dwelling geriatric adults. This can be as debilitating as an injury sustained in a fall and can lead to decline in physical and social function, depression, loss of independence, and decreased quality of life.[22,23] Swinkels and colleagues[19] demonstrated an overall improvement in balance confidence and reduction in depression symptomology after TKA in people who had not fallen preoperatively, but these results were not demonstrated in those who had fallen preoperatively. Furthermore, multiple studies have shown improvement in proprioception after TKA,[9,12,24,25] whereas contradicting studies exist that argue decreased proprioception and balance after TKA could result in increased risk of falling.[26–28] This topic is discussed in later sections. Although studies have shown balance strategies of TKA patients approach those of normal controls, they continue to remain asymmetric.[29]

Introduction of an artificial joint disrupts the native proprioceptive system of the knee; however, this must be weighed against the inability of an anatomically deformed, painful, and weak knee to execute the necessary motor and functional demands required to maintain balance. In the native knee, intracapsular mechanoreceptors exist within structures such as the cruciate ligaments and menisci to provide proprioceptive information. In addition, performance of the knee has been shown to be related to the integrity of the anterior cruciate ligament (ACL).[30] Often, the cruciates are resected in TKA, and this can contribute to alterations in proprioception after TKA. The proprioceptive input of extracapsular structures such as the collateral ligaments and surrounding musculature are not fully known,[12,31] but integrity of these structures can be altered by deformities associated with severe OA. The exact relevance of the knee as a primary proprioceptive input is in doubt because of the suggestion that better

balance performance in static and dynamic situations is typically seen with the use of anticipatory strategies using signals from the ankle rather than the hip/core.[32] Studies using electromyography (EMG) have demonstrated hip/core proprioceptive signals to be the primary source of autonomic proprioceptive input, with the knee being supplemental for recruiting the gastrocnemius-soleus complex.[33] The ambiguities in lower extremity proprioceptive systems are not entirely understood, but nonetheless remain an important link in dynamic balance control.

A recent study by Gauchard and colleagues[34] used dynamic platform posturography in an attempt to independently analyze proprioception, vestibular, and proprioceptive inputs in patients who had recently undergone TKA and in age-matched controls. Their study demonstrated that patients with a recent TKA approached the performance of age-matched controls once they reached sufficient rehabilitation 34 and 41 days postoperatively; however, those in the early perioperative period between 17 and 20 days showed substantial deficits. Hip/core dominance was found in the early perioperative group, suggesting that early rehabilitation was insufficient for both motor strength and adaptive proprioceptive strategies. Of key interest is the result of altering proprioceptive input with the primary determinant of balance being vision, vestibular, or integration of vestibular with altered visual inputs. There was no significant difference between controls and rehabilitated patients, suggesting that any or all loss of articular proprioception may be compensated by an increase in muscular or alternate joint (hip, ankle) proprioception after appropriate rehabilitation.[34] One limitation, however, was that the degree of OA was not evaluated in the age-matched controls. Overall, proprioceptive abilities are a result of many peripheral and central structures. Aging certainly plays a role in the ability of these structures to function properly and, as a result, balance can be affected.

PROPRIOCEPTION, OSTEOARTHRITIS, AND TOTAL KNEE ARTHROPLASTY

Normal bony, capsular, ligamentous, and muscular structures about the knee are vital for native knee proprioception, and alterations in these structures bring variations in proprioceptive abilities. OA of the knee leads to physiologic changes about the knee resulting in a cycle of pain, disuse, body weight imbalance, muscle atrophy, and ultimately loss of proprioception.[35,36] Numerous studies have shown a definitive link between OA and proprioceptive loss. Loss of joint space, an essential component of OA, has been associated with decreased joint position sense.[37] Barrett and colleagues[25] described decreased joint position sense in 45 patients with knee OA compared with nonarthritic controls. Other studies have described loss of joint position sense (measured by various techniques) in patients with osteoarthritic knees. Not only does loss of proprioceptive mechanisms about the knee lead to OA, the inverse also can be true: OA can cause loss of proprioception.[26,38,39]

The human body is remarkable in its ability to compensate for physiologic stresses. Loss of major joint proprioception may result in a compensatory attempt to maintain balance. In their review, Pua and colleagues[40] described the importance of skeletal muscle about the knee. As OA leads to pain and, therefore, decreased conscious use of the knee joint, the body may increase swaying on that knee as an attempt by the central nervous system to "ensure an adequate level of sensory input." This swaying recruits skeletal muscles about the knee and the result is a greater excursion distance in the center of pressure of the knee. Pua and colleagues[40] noted that increased sway was associated with better physical function in patients with OA of the knee. This is further supported by other studies showing that OA leading to knee joint instability may induce recruitment of additional dynamic stabilizers about the knee.[41,42] Other contrasting instability-reducing strategies also have been postulated. Reduction in the excursion of the center of pressure resulting in a "postural stiffening gait" has been described as a different strategy of the central nervous system to combat knee instability caused by OA.[40]

PROPRIOCEPTION AND TOTAL KNEE ARTHROPLASTY

Knee arthroplasty continues to be the gold standard for definitive treatment of knee arthritis. Pain relief, improved knee range of motion, and increased mobility are generally the results of this procedure; however, maintenance of fine balance and proprioception has been questioned. This continues to be studied across multiple specialties, including orthopedics, gerontology, and physical therapy. Multiple sources have shown that TKA significantly restores the ability to maintain upright balance.[2,9] Single-leg standing balance was improved after TKA when compared with patients with high tibial osteotomy. This suggests that restoration of joint space and not simply mechanical realignment of the knee plays an important role in proprioception and balance.[37] Another study evaluated 11 patients who had

TKA and found that standing balance was improved as measured by a 59% decrement in postural sway.[43] When Ishii and colleagues[44] looked at the effect of unilateral and staged bilateral TKAs, both groups had a benefit from the operation with regard to balance. In the unilateral group, the center of balance remained on the operative extremity, which may offload the contralateral extremity. In patients with staged bilateral TKAs, improved balance was found after the second TKA. Joint position sense improvement after TKA is further supported by a study in which 21 TKA knees were compared with normal, control knees, and osteoarthritic knees. The group undergoing TKA showed improved postoperative joint position sense. Another study revealed an improvement in recruiting the quadriceps muscles after TKA, which may contribute to improved proprioception.[45] However, decreased EMG amplitudes in the vastus lateralis and biceps femoris have been found in patients with TKA compared with control patients with OA.[46] This suggests that certain dynamic knee stabilizers may be over-recruited, whereas others are under-recruited after TKA. This may explain the postural stiffening gait sometimes seen early after TKA.

Other studies have shown no difference in proprioception between knees with TKA and knees with OA. Barrack and colleagues[38] and Skinner and colleagues[39] compared TKA knees with age-matched controls and with a group of younger control patients. They noted no improvement of proprioception in any group as measured by the ability to detect passive motion or to reproduce knee flexion angles. They stated that loss of proprioception after TKA may be implicated in some TKA failures because of increased stress placed on the implanted components. In a similar study, 28 TKA knees were compared with controls and similar physical tests were performed; no difference was found between the 2 groups overall, but a significant decrease in proprioceptive ability of the TKA knees was identified at 60° of flexion.[26]

STRATEGIES FOR MAINTAINING PROPRIOCEPTION AFTER TOTAL KNEE ARTHROPLASTY
Physical Therapy

After TKA it is customary to prescribe outpatient physical therapy for several visits in an attempt to maintain range of motion and prevent arthrofibrosis of the affected joint. The benefits of postoperative physical therapy are numerous. Postoperative training in the immediate and early (3–6 months) postoperative periods results in a measurable improvement in motor coordination, and postoperative therapy should be a vital component in the rehabilitation of a TKA patient.[47] Postoperative balance exercise programs have been shown to have beneficial effects on ipsilateral lower extremity function. In their study, Piva and colleagues[48] found improvements in gait speed, single-leg stance, and stiffness in a group of patients undergoing proprioceptive balance activities as part of their rehabilitation. Thewlis and colleagues,[36] in a recent paper, described a critical time for proprioceptive loss in the early postoperative period. In their study, they identified a decrease in balance at 6 weeks postoperatively and suggested that this time may be a transition point between proprioceptive loss and early adaptations to new, learned motor patterns and recommended that postoperative rehabilitation protocols include motor re-learning principles in an attempt to train the body to recognize a new pattern of knee load distribution.

Postoperative rehabilitation may not be the only way to combat proprioceptive loss after TKA. The effect of a preoperative training program on proprioception has also been explored and was found to result in improved balance and gait speed after surgery, as well as subjective function scores.[35]

Surgical Factors

The importance of the surgical procedure itself in maintaining proprioception cannot be overstated. Numerous papers have assessed certain factors regarding the surgical procedure and their effect on postoperative proprioception. Gstoettner and colleagues[35] stated that numerous tissues around the knee that remain after TKA contribute to proprioception. This suggests that the influence of proper gap balancing during the surgical procedure plays a large role in proprioception and may influence patient outcomes after TKA. A review by Wada and colleagues[12] noted that "proper ligament balance may partly contribute to better proprioception after TKA." This is supported by an additional study of the effect of gap balancing on proprioception in which the investigators found that well-balanced TKAs had significantly better proprioceptive function than those with residual imbalance.[4] Another surgical factor is the presence of bilateral knee OA. Performing a TKA on both extremities in a staged fashion may be beneficial to balance. One study found improved balance in patients with bilateral TKAs compared with those with unilateral TKA. During the postoperative period, the position of the center of gravity became more centralized in those with bilateral TKAs, whereas in the unilateral TKA group it remained on the operative extremity.[44] This important finding may help surgeons offset some of the proprioceptive losses after unilateral TKA, especially in patients with bilateral knee OA.

A final surgical factor is the decision to resect or retain the PCL. Proponents of PCL retention cite improved tibiofemoral biomechanics and equivalent subjective knee rating scores; these results have been well documented.[49] Numerous investigators have also studied the clinical role of the PCL in proprioception with varying results. One study found that patients with PCL excision had better proprioception in their knees than those with PCL retention up to 6 months postoperatively. The investigators suggested that this could be because of a feedback mechanism involving the collateral ligaments. In patients with PCL resection, there may be more stability imparted by tension in the collaterals and other soft tissues. This may be perceived as a varus or valgus moment (in the knee), and an antagonistic and corrective action from the hamstring and quadriceps muscles may be produced, resulting in improved proprioception.[4]

Most studies comparing PCL-sacrificing to PCL-retaining implants have found equivalent results, both clinically and with respect to proprioception. One retrospective study analyzed 27 PCL-retaining and 18 posterior-stabilized TKAs and found no clinical differences in subjective scores. Proprioception, as measured by balance and posture using the Balance Master system (Natus Medical, Inc, Pleaston, CA), was not significantly different between the 2 groups.[50] Using balance as a surrogate for proprioceptive abilities after TKA, Swanik and colleagues[9] found no significant difference in balance between the 2 groups of posterior-stabilized and cruciate-retaining knees. Although there was high variability in the method of reporting results and in the quality of the studies included overall, the differences between the 2 types of implants were not significantly different.[9] In patients with a more severe preoperative deformity, it is reasonable to assume that posterior-stabilized TKA would result in superior outcomes over a PCL-retaining implant with a possibly attenuated ligament. Some studies have shown posterior-stabilized implants to have an advantage over cruciate-retaining implants. Cho and colleagues[43] evaluated balance after posterior-stabilized TKA, they found an improved standing balance in those with a posterior-stabilized implant. In a similar study, improvements in range of motion, patient satisfaction, and posterior knee pain were found for posterior-stabilized knees.[51] It is not known, however, whether this perceived benefit is because of correction of the typically greater preoperative deformity of knees that demand the increased constraint that posterior-stabilized knees provide.

SPECIAL TYPES OF KNEE ARTHROPLASTY

Various special types of arthroplasty in use today include unicompartmental knee arthroplasty (UKA), a design that retains the ACL and PCL and only resurfaces either the lateral or (more commonly) the medial compartment of the knee on both the femoral and tibial sides, and bicruciate-retaining TKA, which is similar to a standard PCL-retaining TKA with the exception that the ACL is retained as well.

Anterior Cruciate Ligament Retention

Preservation of the ACL in addition to retention of the PCL may offer additional benefit. There is no doubt that the ACL confers proprioceptive information to the central nervous system.[52,53] Mechanical instability and diminished proprioception after ACL injury have been well described.[54] Studies of the effects of ACL reconstruction after injury have shown significant improvement in proprioceptive reaction times for knee extension and flexion, with reductions of 20.2% and 43.2%, respectively $(P<.01)$.[55] Intraoperatively, the ACL has been found to be deficient in 13% to 23% of OA knees, and deficient in up to 39% by MRI examination.[56,57] These results are consistent with another study that demonstrated the ACL to be intact in 60% of patients undergoing TKA.[58]

Unicompartmental Arthroplasty

Medial UKA has been in use for at least the last 50 years. Its proponents cite improved proprioception and preservation of bone stock, but both cruciate ligaments must be functional for optimal results.[59] Its minimally invasive approach does not involve as extensive soft-tissue dissection as standard TKA, which may be a reason for improved proprioception.[60] If indicated, a UKA may be better at preserving more native proprioception characteristics of a knee than a TKA. A prospective study analyzed this effect in 34 patients, half of whom had UKA and half had TKA. Joint position sense and knee scores were measured. Both groups had similar improvements in subjective scoring scales and in proprioception overall, but the amount of postural sway in the UKA group was significantly less. This suggests that the proprioceptive capabilities may be better retained after UKA than after TKA.[37] Another study comparing UKA with TKA reported an interesting finding: "A higher number of patients with UKA felt that they had forgotten they had a prosthetic

knee in situ compared to the TKA group." This finding suggests that UKA retains near-native proprioceptive characteristics postoperatively.[61] In addition, published results for UKA are generally positive and the procedure is regaining popularity.[62]

Bicruciate-Retaining Total Knee Arthroplasty

Bicruciate-retaining TKA was developed to promote minimal bone resection with less constraint in an effort to maintain normal knee kinematics. Reports of the results of bicruciate-retaining TKA are limited, and there are no studies that directly evaluate the effect on proprioception. However, bicruciate-retaining TKA may lead to improved proprioception and therefore function because of the retention of both cruciate ligaments. Komistek and colleagues[63] suggested that a bicruciate-retaining TKA maintains the "four-bar linkage" system of the knee, which leads to more normal kinematic patterns during gait resulting in improved proprioceptive abilities and a more "natural feeling" knee. Another study suggested that the improved mechanics after bicruciate-retaining TKA make posterior condylar contact less likely and, therefore, wear mechanics and ultimately longevity may be improved over conventional TKA implants.[64]

In a study of 489 bicruciate-retaining knees by Pritchett,[58] an 89% survivorship was noted at 23-year follow-up. Patients showed significant improvements in subjective scoring scales and range of motion; only 1 late ACL rupture occurred, and the main reason for revision was polyethylene wear. The investigator emphasized that gap balancing is of vital importance in this particular procedure because any imbalance can lead to an ACL rupture or the tibial eminence may fracture; however, the investigator did not consider a macroscopically degenerated ACL to be a contraindication to bicruciate-retaining TKA if it was clinically functional. In a similar series of 163 patients described by Sabouret and colleagues,[65] the 22-year survival rate was 82%, and polyethylene wear was again the most common cause for revision. These investigators confirmed the finding of Pritchett that when the ACL is functional, as measured by normal anterior drawer and Lachman tests, it will provide sufficient stability for good long-term results. Christen and colleagues[66] evaluated short-term function and satisfaction after bicruciate-retaining TKA and noted good results in function and subjective scores at 1-year follow-up, but a higher complication and revision rate when compared with other total knee systems. They cautioned that experience is necessary for good outcomes with this operation. Another smaller series looked at the clinical function and risk of prosthetic loosening after bicruciate-retaining TKA compared with posterior-stabilized TKA. In 41 knees with bicruciate-retaining TKA, there was a higher incidence of pain and limited mobility than in the posterior-stabilized group, but no difference in loosening was noted between the groups. These investigators again emphasized the attention to detail that the bicruciate retaining TKA demands during the surgical procedure.[67] Overall, bicruciate-retaining TKA preserves knee bone stock and vital proprioceptive structures that may lead to a knee that is similar biomechanically to a native knee. Acceptable outcomes can be expected if the practitioner is experienced with the procedure.

REFERENCES

1. Available at: www.merriam-webster.com/dictionary/proprioception. Accessed August 5, 2015.
2. Wegener L, Kisner C, Nichols D. Static and dynamic balance responses in persons with bilateral knee osteoarthritis. J Orthop Sports Phys Ther 1997;25: 13–8.
3. Lipsitz LA, Josson PV, Kelley MM, et al. Causes and correlates of recurrent falls in ambulatory frail elderly. J Gerontol 1991;46:M114–22.
4. Attfield SF, Wilton TJ, Pratt DJ, et al. Soft-tissue balance and recovery of proprioception after total knee replacement. J Bone Joint Surg Br 1996;78:540–5.
5. Sharma L, Pai YC. Impaired proprioception and osteoarthritis. Curr Opin Rheumatol 1997;9:253–8.
6. Sahin N, Bianco A, Patti A, et al. Evaluation of knee joint proprioception and balance of young female volleyball players: a pilot study. J Phys Ther Sci 2015;27:437–40.
7. Goble DJ. Proprioceptive acuity assessment via joint position matching: from basic science to general practice. Phys Ther 2010;90:1176–84.
8. Boisgontier MP, Olivier I, Chenu O, et al. Presbypropria: the effects of physiological ageing on proprioceptive control. Age 2012;34:1179–94.
9. Swanik CB, Lephart SM, Rubash HE. Proprioception, kinesthesia, and balance after total knee arthroplasty with cruciate-retaining and posterior stabilized prostheses. J Bone Joint Surg Am 2004; 86:328–34.
10. Mihalko WM, Creek AT, Mary MN, et al. Mechanoreceptors found in a posterior cruciate ligament from a well-functioning knee arthroplasty retrieval. J Arthroplasty 2011;26:e504–509.
11. Zhang K, Mihalko WM. Posterior cruciate mechanoreceptors in osteoarthritic and cruciate-retaining TKA retrievals: a pilot study. Clin Orthop Relat Res 2012;470:1855–9.
12. Wada M, Kawahara H, Shimada S, et al. Joint proprioception before and after total knee arthroplasty. Clin Orthop Relat Res 2002;403:161–7.
13. Liao CD, Liou TH, Huang YY, et al. Effects of balance training on functional outcome after total knee replacement in patients with knee osteoarthritis: a randomized controlled trial. Clin Rehabil 2013;27: 697–709.
14. de Vries AJ, van den Akker-Scheek I, Diercks RL, et al. The effect of a patellar strap on knee joint proprioception in healthy participants and athletes with patellar tendiopathy. J Sci Med Sport 2015. [Epub ahead of print].
15. Baloh RW, Jacobson KM, Socotch TM. The effect of aging on visual-vestibuloocular responses. Exp Brain Res 1993;95:509–16.
16. Paige GD. Senescence of human visual-vestibular interactions. 1. Vestibulo-ocular reflex and adaptive plasticity with aging. J Vestib Res 1992;2:133–51.
17. Peterka RJ, Black FO, Schoenhoff MB. Age-related changes in human vestibule-occular reflexes: sinusoidal rotation and caloric test. J Vestib Res 1990; 1:49–59.
18. Teasdale N, Stelmach GE, Breunig A. Postural sway characteristics of the elderly under normal and altered visual and support surface conditions. J Gerontol 1991;46:B238–44.
19. Swinkels A, Newman JH, Allain TJ. A prospective observational study of falling before and after knee replacement surgery. Age Ageing 2009;38:175–81.
20. Doherty TJ. Invited review: aging and sarcopenia. J Appl Physiol 2003;95:1717–27.
21. Kanekar N, Aruin AS. The effect of aging on anticipatory postural control. Exp Brain Res 2014;232: 1127–36.
22. Donoghue OA, Ryan H, Duggan E, et al. Relationship between fear of falling and mobility varies with visual function among older adults. Geriatr Gerontol Int 2014;14:827–36.
23. Toebes MJ, Hoozemans MJ, Furrer R, et al. Associations between measures of gait stability, leg length and fear of falling. Gait Posture 2015;41:76–80.
24. Warren PJ, Olanlokun TK, Cobb AG, et al. Proprioception after knee arthroplasty – the influence of prosthetic design. Clin Orthop Relat Res 1993;297: 182–7.
25. Barrett DS, Cobb AG, Bentley G. Joint proprioception in normal, osteoarthritic and replaced knees. J Bone Joint Surg Br 1991;73:53–6.
26. Fuchs S, Thorwesten L, Niewerth S. Proprioceptive function in knees with and without total knee arthroplasty. Am J Phys Med Rehabil 1999;78:39–45.
27. Gage WH, Frank JS, Prentice SD, et al. Postural responses following a rotational support surface pertuburbation, following knee joint replacement: frontal plane rotations. Gait Posture 2008;27: 286–93.

28. Pap G, Meyer M, Weiler HT, et al. Proprioception after total knee arthroplasty: a comparison with clinical outcome. Acta Orthop Scand 2000;71:153–9.

29. Viton JM, Atlani L, Mesure S, et al. Reorganization of equilibrium and movement control strategies after total knee arthroplasty. J Rehabil Med 2001;34:12–9.

30. Corrigan JP, Cashman WF, Brady MP. Proprioception in the cruciate deficient knee. J Bone Joint Surg Br 1992;74:247–50.

31. Fisher NM, White SC, Yack HJ, et al. Muscle function and gait in patients with knee osteoarthritis before and after muscle rehabilitation. Disabil Rehabil 1997;19:47–55.

32. Horak FB, Nashner LM. Central programming of postural movements: adaption to altered support-surface configurations. J Neurophysiol 1986;55: 1369–81.

33. Bloem BR, Allum JH, Carpenter MG, et al. Triggering of balance corrections and compensatory strategies in a patient with total leg proprioceptive loss. Exp Brain Res 2002;142:91–107.

34. Gauchard GC, Vancon G, Meyer P, et al. On the role of knee joint in balance control and postural strategies: effects of total knee replacement in elderly subjects with knee arthritis. Gait Posture 2010;32: 155–60.

35. Gstoettner M, Raschner C, Dirnberger E, et al. Pre-operative proprioceptive training in patients with total knee arthroplasty. Knee 2011;18:165–270.

36. Thewlis D, Hillier S, Hobbs SJ, et al. Preoperative asymmetry in load distribution during quiet stance persists following total knee arthroplasty. Knee Surg Sports Traumatol Arthrosc 2014;22:609–14.

37. Issac SM, Barker KL, Danial IN, et al. Does arthroplasty type influence knee joint proprioception? A longitudinal prospective study comparing total and unicompartmental arthroplasty. Knee 2007;14: 212–7.

38. Barrack RL, Skinner HB, Cook SD, et al. Effect of articular disease and total knee arthroplasty on knee joint position sense. J Neurophysiol 1983;50: 684–7.

39. Skinner HB, Barrack RL, Cook SD, et al. Joint position sense in total knee arthroplasty. J Orthop Res 1984;1:276–83.

40. Pua YH, Liang Z, Ong PH, et al. Associations of knee extensor strength and standing balance with physical function in knee osteoarthritis. Arthritis Care Res (Hoboken) 2011;63:1706–14.

41. Lewek MD, Ramsey DK, Snyder-Mackler L, et al. Knee stabilization in patients with medial compartment knee osteoarthritis. Arthritis Rheum 2004;52: 2845–53.

42. Heiden TL, Lloyd DG, Ackland TR. Knee joint kinematics, kinetics and muscle co-contraction in knee osteoarthritis patient gait. Clin Biomech 2009;24: 833–41.

43. Cho SD, Hwang CH. Improved single-limb balance after total knee arthroplasty. Knee Surg Sports Traumatol Arthrosc 2013;21:2744–50.

44. Ishii Y, Noguchi H, Takeda M, et al. Changes of body balance before and after total knee arthroplasty in patients who suffered from bilateral knee osteoarthritis. J Orthop Sci 2013;18:727–32.

45. Berth A, Urbach D, Awiszus F. Improvement of voluntary quadriceps muscle activation after total knee arthroplasty. Arch Phys Med Rehabil 2002;83: 1432–6.

46. Venema DM, Karst GM. Individuals with total knee arthroplasty demonstrate altered anticipatory postural adjustments compared with healthy control subjects. J Geriatr Phys Ther 2012;35:62–71.

47. Oehlert K, Hassenpflug J. Coordinative abilities of arthroplasty patients. Z Orthop Ihre Grenzgeb 2004;142:679–84 [in German].

48. Piva SR, Gil AB, Almeida GJ, et al. A balance exercise program appears to improve function for patients with total knee arthroplasty: a randomized clinical trial. Phys Ther 2010;90:880–94.

49. Ritter MA, Davis KE, Meding JB, et al. The role of the posterior cruciate ligament in total knee replacement. Bone Joint Res 2012;1:64–70.

50. Vandekerckhove PJ, Parys R, Tampere T, et al. Does cruciate retention primary total knee arthroplasty affect proprioception, strength and clinical outcome? Knee Surg Sports Traumatol Arthrosc 2015;34:1644–52.

51. Yagishita K, Muneta T, Ju YJ, et al. High-flex posterior cruciate-retaining vs posterior cruciate-substituting designs in simultaneous bilateral total knee arthroplasty: a prospective, randomized study. J Arthroplasty 2012;27:368–74.

52. Viggiano D, Corona K, Cerciello S, et al. The kinematic control during the backward gait and knee proprioception: insights from lesions of the anterior cruciate ligament. J Hum Kinet 2014;41:51–7.

53. Relph N, Herrington L, Tyson S. The effects of ACL injury on knee proprioception: a meta-analysis. Physiotherapy 2014;100:187–95.

54. Dhillon MS, Bali K, Prabhakar S. Proprioception in anterior cruciate ligament deficient knees and its relevance to anterior cruciate ligament reconstruction. Indian J Orthop 2011;45:294–300.

55. Ma Y, Deie M, Iwaki D, et al. Balance ability and proprioception after single-bundle, single-bundle augmentation, and double-bundle ACL reconstruction. ScientificWorldJournal 2014;2014:342012.

56. Douglas MJ, Hutchison JD, Sutherland AG. Anterior cruciate ligament integrity in osteoarthritis of the knee in patients undergoing total knee replacement. J Orthop Traumatol 2010;11:149–54.

57. Hill CL, Seo GS, Gale D, et al. Cruciate ligament integrity in osteoarthritis of the knee. Arthritis Rheum 2005;52:794–9.

58. Pritchett JW. Bicruciate-retaining total knee replacement provides satisfactory function and implant survivorship at 23 years. Clin Orthop Relat Res 2015; 473(7):2327–33.

59. Hurst JM, Berend KR. Mobile-bearing unicondylar knee arthroplasty: the Oxford experience. Clin Sports Med 2014;331:105–21.

60. Suggs JF, Li G, Park SE, et al. Knee biomechanics after UKA and its relation to the ACL—a robotic investigation. J Orthop Res 2006;24:588–94.

61. Matthews DJ, Hossain FS, Patel S, et al. A cohort study predicts better functional outcomes and equivalent patient satisfaction following UKR compared with TKR. HSS J 2013;9:21–4.

62. Labek G, Bohler N. Minimally invasive medial unicompartmental knee replacement. Orthopade 2003;32:454–60.

63. Komistek RD, Allain J, Anderson DT, et al. In vivo kinematics for subjects with and without an anterior cruciate ligament. Clin Orthop Relat Res 2002;404: 315–25 [in German].

64. Stiehl JB, Komistek RD, Cloutier JM, et al. The cruciate ligaments in total knee arthroplasty: a kinematic analysis of 2 total knee arthroplasties. J Arthroplasty 2000;15:545–50.

65. Sabouret P, Lavoie F, Cloutier JM. Total knee replacement with retention of both cruciate ligaments: a 22-year follow-up study. J Bone Joint Surg Br 2013;95:917–22.

66. Christen M, Aghayev E, Christen B. Short-term functional versus patient-reported outcome of the bicruciate stabilized total knee arthroplasty: prospective consecutive case series. BMC Musculoskelet Disord 2014;15:435.

67. Goutallier D, Manicom O, Van Driessche S. Total knee arthroplasty with bicruciate preservation: Comparison versus the same posterostabilized design at eight years follow-up. Rev Chir Orthop Reparatrice Appar Mot 2008;94(6):585–95.

Instability After Total Knee Arthroplasty

Umberto Cottino, MD, Peter K. Sculco, MD, Rafael J. Sierra, MD, Matthew P. Abdel, MD*

KEYWORDS

- Instability • Total knee arthroplasty • Failure • Revision total knee arthroplasty

KEY POINTS

- Instability is not always associated with discomfort, and the diagnosis is largely based on a complete history and physical examination.
- In cruciate-retaining designs, flexion instability may be caused by surgical errors or posterior cruciate ligament failure. In posterior-stabilized designs, the cause is usually unbalanced flexion-extension gaps.
- Genu recurvatum is a rare complication caused by underlying conditions like quadriceps weakness, paralysis, bone deformities, previous high tibial osteotomies, and plantar foot flexion.
- Extension instability can produce rectangular or trapezoidal gaps and thus symmetric or asymmetrical instability, respectively.

INTRODUCTION

Instability is one of the most important causes of failure after total knee arthroplasty (TKA), accounting for 10% to 20% of all knee revision procedures.[1–7] In the United States and Australia, it is one of the most common causes of late revisions.[2–6,8] It has also been reported as one of the most common early complications, found to be as high as 26% in the first 5 years after surgery, and the second most common cause of revision after infection.[9]

Instability is not always associated with discomfort. In addition, the causes are various and include surgical error and poor design selection.[6,10] The treatment of instability is based on an accurate diagnosis, founded on a thorough history and physical examination.[5,11] Onset of signs and symptoms must also be investigated carefully. For instance, a cruciate-retaining (CR) TKA can be unstable in flexion after a period of wellness secondary to a late posterior cruciate ligament (PCL) rupture.

In general, tibiofemoral instability can be classified into 3 different patterns: flexion instability, genu recurvatum, and extension instability.

EVALUATION

The first step is a thorough history and physical examination, focusing on the following aspects[1,12]:

- Original indication for surgery
- Previous deformity or contracture
- Previous knee surgeries
- Wound complications
- Current sense of instability
- Recurrent effusions
- Time of Onset
- Pain localization

The examination should be accurate and focused not only on the knee but also on extra-articular causes of instability. Before addressing the knee, it is useful to search for global or local neuromuscular disorders, hip or ankle deformities,

Department of Orthopedic Surgery, Mayo Clinic, 200 First Street Southwest, Rochester, MN 55905, USA
* Corresponding author.
E-mail address: abdel.matthew@mayo.edu

Orthop Clin N Am 47 (2016) 311–316
http://dx.doi.org/10.1016/j.ocl.2015.09.007

and areas of tenderness (i.e., pes anserine and Gerdy's tubercle).

Varus-valgus testing of the knee should be performed in full extension and at 30° and 90° of flexion to evaluate additional knee stabilizers. Anteroposterior (AP) laxity should be evaluated in both directions with anterior and posterior drawer tests. A useful test is performed with the patient sitting on the examination table, with the knee flexed at 90° and the foot dangling to assess the extent to which the flexion gap increases.[1,10]

When evaluating a painful TKA, the surgeon must first exclude infection as a primary cause of the failure. A contemporary approach has been proposed by the Musculoskeletal Infection Society[13] and is supported by other studies.[14–16] Diagnostic tests include erythrocyte sedimentation rate, C-reactive protein, and an arthrocentesis looking at synovial white blood cell count, differential, and cultures. For this reason, an arthrocentesis is always performed to evaluate the articular fluid and rule out infection. Instability can present with hemarthrosis secondary to intra-articular microtrauma and is another diagnostic clue.[3]

IMAGING ANALYSIS

Radiographic analysis of the knee should investigate implant positioning, limb alignment, and component position. Obligatory radiographs include AP, lateral, full-length weight-bearing, and patellar views. AP radiographs can be completed with varus-valgus stress images to assess the status of the collateral ligaments and if deformities are reducible.[3]

Lateral views can be performed in full extension, 90° of flexion, and full flexion. In the different views, it is possible to measure the tibial translation on the femur, implant positioning, flexion gap, and tibial slope. Full-length radiographs are useful in assessing component positioning compared with anatomic and mechanical axes of the femur and tibia. Radiographs should always be compared with the preoperative and immediate postoperative radiographs to understand the evolution of disease.

Computed tomography scans may be considered when malrotation of the components is suspected.[17] Although rarely indicated, MRI can be used for soft tissue evaluation and component rotation.[18,19] However, this study is technically demanding and difficult to obtain even with metal artifact suppression technology.

FLEXION INSTABILITY

Flexion instability can be seen in patients without radiographic evidence of malalignment or loosening. This problem has been historically underdiagnosed, especially in patients with a CR implant.[1,10] Flexion instability can also occur in patients with posterior-stabilized (PS) prostheses.[20] The signs and symptoms may vary from simple discomfort to a complete knee dislocation.

Factors leading to instability in CR prostheses may include surgical error or late PCL failure. Surgical errors include a loose flexion gap (eg, undersized femoral component or excessive tibial slope) or a misdiagnosed previous PCL rupture. An excessively tight flexion gap has to be avoided as well, because the patient may be more prone to stiffness postoperatively. A subsequent manipulation and PCL overstretching when in flexion may then lead to late PCL rupture and flexion instability. In chronic cases, the PCL can deteriorate, leading to flexion instability. Either way, posterior sag of the tibia is clinically observed against gravity and at 90° of flexion.

In PS implants, frank knee dislocations are prevented by the polyethylene post and the femoral cam mechanism.[21] However, an unbalanced flexion gap can affect stability, leading to anterior tibial translation and instability.[1,22] In 2005, Schwab and colleagues[20] analyzed flexion instability without frank dislocation in 10 patients with a PS design and reported the following classic symptoms:

- Sense of instability without giving away
- Difficulty in ascending and descending stairs
- Recurrent knee swelling
- Anterior knee pain and tenderness

During clinical examination, anterior tibial translation occurs with the knee flexed at 90°. In addition, multiple areas of soft tissue tenderness (i.e., pes anserine, peripatellar region, and hamstrings tendons) and recurrent knee swelling (i.e., hemarthrosis) are appreciated.[20]

In 2014, Abdel and colleagues[22] correlated the radiographic findings of 60 patients revised for isolated flexion instability. These investigators found a strong correlation with decreased condylar offset by 4 mm ($P<.001$), distalization of joint line by 6 mm ($P<.001$), and increased tibial slope up to 5° ($P<.001$) (**Fig. 1**) to be predictive of flexion instability.

Revision procedures must be addressed with a stepwise approach.[22] Usually, the first step is to correct excessive posterior tibial slope and restore axial and rotational alignment.[22] The next step typically involves upsizing the femoral component by a mean of 4 mm. If the flexion gap is still not balanced, a larger distal femoral resection should be performed to match the flexion and extension

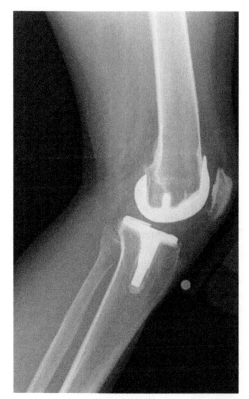

Fig. 1. A lateral radiograph of a 69-year-old male suffering from symptomatic flexion instability with a CR design and greater than 10° of posterior tibial slope.

gaps.[22] A larger polyethylene insert is typically required thereafter.

GENU RECURVATUM

Genu recurvatum, also known as hyperextension instability, is a rare disease identified in only 0.5% to 1% of patients undergoing TKA.[23,24] Commonly, this deformity arises from underlying conditions including quadriceps weakness, paralysis, bone deformities, previous high tibial osteotomies (HTOs), and plantar foot flexion.[24] For these reasons, treatment is usually challenging. Soft tissues are the most important part of correcting a deformity and must be addressed carefully, paying particular attention when selecting the degree of implant constraint. The only exception is made for bony deformities without soft tissue weakness that can be adequately corrected with bone cuts.

Risk factors for genu recurvatum are neuromuscular disorders, rheumatoid arthritis, fixed valgus deformities, and a weak quadriceps muscle.[23,25–27] Poliomyelitis is the most common neuromuscular disorder causing genu recurvatum. This disease typically affects 1 lower limb and causes motor neuron damage, resulting in loss of motor function and consequent flaccid paralysis. The affected knee commonly acquires a valgus deformity, collateral ligament laxity, a recurvatum deformity, and external rotation of the tibia.[25] Total knee arthroplasties in these patients usually produce good pain control but unreliable results with respect to stability and functional outcomes.[25]

Patients with fixed valgus deformities without a neuromuscular disease may have an iliotibial band contracture. With the knee in extension, this structure lies in front of the lateral femoral epicondyle, forcing the knee to hyperextend, causing genu recurvatum.[24] Rheumatoid arthritis can affect stability in hyperextension by damaging the anterior cruciate and collateral ligaments, subsequently leading to laxity and a hyperextension deformity.[23,24,28] Patients with quadriceps weakness have a high recurrence risk of recurvatum after TKA, because they tend to lock the knee during the extension phase of gait to compensate for a weak extensor mechanism and avoid instability.[28] Patients with genu recurvatum who previously received an HTO should be evaluated radiographically, because anterior tibial bone impaction can lead to anterior slope of the tibial plateau.[27]

Over the past few years, many different procedures for the correction of genu recurvatum have been proposed, but only 3 are discussed here. The least technically challenging approach is to tighten the extension gap by underresecting the distal femur, using a thicker polyethylene liner, and placing the femoral component in slight flexion.[28] In this case, a standard implant can be used. Another option is to tighten the collateral ligaments (medial collateral ligament [MCL] and lateral collateral ligament) in extension to obtain a tighter extension gap and prevent a hyperextension deformity.[23] However, the problem with these 2 techniques is that patients typically have poor soft tissue quality, thus increasing the risk of further stretching and recurvatum recurrence. Our preferred technique is to use a rotating-hinge TKA with an extension stop to reduce the risk of hyperextension instability postoperatively (**Fig. 2**).

EXTENSION INSTABILITY

Extension instability can be classified as symmetric or asymmetric according to the shape of the extension gap: rectangular or trapezoidal, respectively.[28]

Symmetric instability can originate from excessive distal femoral or proximal tibial resections. Both events result in inadequate space filling by the implanted components.[29] Excessive bone

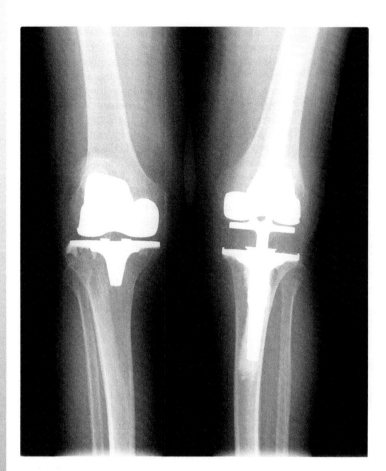

Fig. 2. An AP radiograph showing a rotating-hinge total knee arthroplasty on the left for instability.

removal from the tibia affects both the flexion and extension gaps and is easier to manage. It is typically sufficient to use a thicker polyethylene insert to correct this form of symmetric extension instability.[1] The problem with excessive bone removal from the proximal tibia is long-term fixation of the tibial component, because the bone of the distal tibia is weaker than its proximal counterpart.[29]

In excessive distal femoral resection, the use of a thicker polyethylene is not appropriate because the joint line is elevated even though the extension gap is filled. In addition, the flexion gap is inappropriately tightened.[1] The solution is to restore the joint line height by using distal augments in the femoral component. An exaggerated joint line elevation produces flexion stiffness and patellar overstuffing.

Asymmetric instability is more common and can be a consequence of incomplete correction of a previous angular deformity or surgically induced ligament instability (**Fig. 3**). Preoperative angular deformities of the knee can be undercorrected by the surgeon if too much caution is taken with respect to tissue releases. This problem is usually secondary to the surgeon's fear of excessive laxity in the direction opposite the deformity.[1,5,11] In varus knees, the medial side must be released by subperiosteally elevating the MCL at its insertion. If left too tight, the knee is unstable in extension. In this technique, first described by Insall and colleagues,[30] the foot is externally rotated while the tibial insertion of the MCL is released, avoiding detaching the pes anserine. An excessively tight extension gap on the medial side can lead to medial polyethylene wear from overload[1] and subsequent varus deformity recurrence with TKA failure.

In valgus knees, the risk is underrelease of the lateral aspect of the knee, leaving the medial side loose.[1,11] The medial soft tissues do not recover after surgery and the patient will return with a recurrent deformity.[1] Gap balancing in the setting of this deformity is more challenging because lateral instability is poorly tolerated and the technique needed to perform a lateral release poses more risk to adjacent structures, such as the peroneal nerve.[31]

The technique of release was described by Insall and colleagues[30] and subsequently modified by Laskin.[32] These investigators recommended

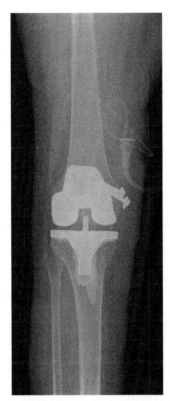

Fig. 3. An AP radiograph of an 87-year-old female who suffered an intraoperative medial femoral condyle fracture treated with open reduction and internal fixation (ORIF). Without ORIF, this patient would be at risk for asymmetric extension instability.

complete release of lateral structures in different orders. However, the results were not reliable and many knees were overcorrected. The solution proposed by Clarke and colleagues[33] in 2005 was pie crusting, a technique that allows more gradual release and thus a more reliable result. The release can be performed with a scalpel or needle while tensioning the lateral space with a lamina spreader. It should include all structures that are tight when palpated.[28] The use of a lamina spreader allows the surgeon to immediately check the effect of the release and to avoid an excessive increase in the width of the lateral compartment. In patients with deformities greater than 20°, the lateral collateral ligament usually has to be released with the pie crusting technique.[33]

Surgically induced ligament instability is usually a consequence of direct damage to the MCL during the tibial bone cut or during overly forceful varus-valgus testing.[33] When a tear in the ligament is complete, a Krackow-type suture can be used to reattach the ligament to its insertion. In complete rupture, augmentation with the use of a hamstring graft is usually required. Typically, the tendons are left intact on the tibial side and secured to the MCL

femoral insertion through a hole in the femoral condyle.[1] After the repair, stability must be tested carefully and constrained implants should be considered.[34,35] Leopold and colleagues[34] reported good results from direct repair and bracing by 6 weeks postoperatively.

SUMMARY

Instability is a common cause of revision TKAs. The diagnosis requires an algorithmic approach to identify the cause and best management option(s). Once identified, and if conservative management has failed, revision surgery is warranted.

REFERENCES

1. Parratte S, Pagnano MW. Instability after total knee arthroplasty. J Bone Joint Surg Am 2008;90(1): 184–94.
2. Callaghan JJ, O'Rourke MR, Saleh KJ. Why knees fail: lessons learned. J Arthroplasty 2004;19(4 Suppl 1):31–4.
3. Fehring TK, Valadie AL. Knee instability after total knee arthroplasty. Clin Orthop Relat Res 1994;(299): 157–62.
4. Vince KG. Why knees fail. J Arthroplasty 2003;18(3 Suppl 1):39–44.
5. Yercan HS, Ait Si Selmi T, Sugun TS, et al. Tibiofemoral instability in primary total knee replacement: a review part 2: diagnosis, patient evaluation, and treatment. Knee 2005;12(5):336–40.
6. Yercan HS, Ait Si Selmi T, Sugun TS, et al. Tibiofemoral instability in primary total knee replacement: a review, part 1: basic principles and classification. Knee 2005;12(4):257–66.
7. Meding JB, Ritter MA, Davis KE, et al. Meeting increased demand for total knee replacement and follow-up: determining optimal follow-up. Bone Joint J 2013;95B(11):1484–9.
8. Graves S, Davidson D, Ingerson L, et al. The Australian Orthopaedic Association national joint replacement registry. Med J Aust 2004;180(5):S31–4.
9. Fehring TK, Odum S, Griffin WL, et al. Early failures in total knee arthroplasty. Clin Orthop Relat Res 2001;392:315–8.
10. Pagnano MW, Hanssen AD, Lewallen DG, et al. Flexion instability after primary posterior cruciate retaining total knee arthroplasty. Clin Orthop Relat Res 1998;356:39–46.
11. Vince KG, Abdeen A, Sugimori T. The unstable total knee arthroplasty: causes and cures. J Arthroplasty 2006;21(4 Suppl 1):44–9.
12. Rossi R, Dettoni F, Bruzzone M, et al. Clinical examination of the knee: know your tools for diagnosis of knee injuries. Sports Med Arthrosc Rehabil Ther Technol 2011;3:25.

13. Parvizi J, Zmistowski B, Berbari EF, et al. New definition for periprosthetic joint infection: from the workgroup of the Musculoskeletal Infection Society. Clin Orthop Relat Res 2011;469(11):2992–4.

14. Qu X, Zhai Z, Liu X, et al. Evaluation of white cell count and differential in synovial fluid for diagnosing infections after total hip or knee arthroplasty. PLoS One 2014;9(1):e84751.

15. Christensen CP, Bedair H, Della Valle CJ, et al. The natural progression of synovial fluid white blood-cell counts and the percentage of polymorphonuclear cells after primary total knee arthroplasty: a multicenter study. J Bone Joint Surg Am 2013; 95(23):2081–7.

16. Alijanipour P, Bakhshi H, Parvizi J. Diagnosis of periprosthetic joint infection: the threshold for serological markers. Clin Orthop Relat Res 2013;471(10): 3186–95.

17. Konigsberg B, Hess R, Hartman C, et al. Inter- and intraobserver reliability of two-dimensional CT scan for total knee arthroplasty component malrotation. Clin Orthop Relat Res 2014;472(1):212–7.

18. Heyse TJ, Figiel J, Hähnlein U, et al. MRI after unicondylar knee arthroplasty: rotational alignment of components. Arch Orthop Trauma Surg 2013; 133(11):1579–86.

19. Heyse TJ, Chong le R, Davis J, et al. MRI analysis for rotation of total knee components. Knee 2012;19(5): 571–5.

20. Schwab JH, Haidukewych GJ, Hanssen AD, et al. Flexion instability without dislocation after posterior stabilized total knees. Clin Orthop Relat Res 2005; 440:96–100.

21. Kocmond JH, Delp SL, Stern SH. Stability and range of motion of Insall-Burstein condylar prostheses. A computer simulation study. J Arthroplasty 1995; 10(3):383–8.

22. Abdel MP, Pulido L, Severson EP, et al. Stepwise surgical correction of instability in flexion after total knee replacement. Bone Joint J 2014;96B(12):1644–8.

23. Krackow KA, Weiss AP. Recurvatum deformity complicating performance of total knee arthroplasty. A brief note. J Bone Joint Surg Am 1990; 72(2):268–71.

24. Meding JB, Keating EM, Ritter MA, et al. Total knee replacement in patients with genu recurvatum. Clin Orthop Relat Res 2001;(393):244–9.

25. Giori NJ, Lewallen DG. Total knee arthroplasty in limbs affected by poliomyelitis. J Bone Joint Surg Am 2002;84A(7):1157–61.

26. Tew M, Forster IW. Effect of knee replacement on flexion deformity. J Bone Joint Surg Br 1987;69(3): 395–9.

27. Insall J. Surgical techniques and instrumentation in total knee arthroplasty. Surgery of the Knee 1993; 1:739–804.

28. Abdel MP, Haas SB. The unstable knee: wobble and buckle. Bone Joint J 2014;96B(11 Supple A):112–4.

29. Brassard MF, Insall JN, Scuderi GR, et al. Complications of total knee arthroplasty. Surgery of the Knee 2001;3:1814–6.

30. Insall JN, Binazzi R, Soudry M, et al. Total knee arthroplasty. Clin Orthop Relat Res 1985;192:13–22.

31. Bruzzone M, Ranawat A, Castoldi F, et al. The risk of direct peroneal nerve injury using the Ranawat "inside-out" lateral release technique in valgus total knee arthroplasty. J Arthroplasty 2010;25(1):161–5.

32. Laskin RS. Total knee replacement. London: Springer-Verlag London Limited; 1991.

33. Clarke HD, Fuchs R, Scuderi GR, et al. Clinical results in valgus total knee arthroplasty with the "pie crust" technique of lateral soft tissue releases. J Arthroplasty 2005;20(8):1010–4.

34. Leopold SS, McStay C, Klafeta K, et al. Primary repair of intraoperative disruption of the medial collateral ligament during total knee arthroplasty. J Bone Joint Surg Am 2001;83A(1):86–91.

35. Easley ME, Insall JN, Scuderi GR, et al. Primary constrained condylar knee arthroplasty for the arthritic valgus knee. Clin Orthop Relat Res 2000;(380):58–64.

The Painful Total Knee Arthroplasty

Mitchell McDowell, DO[a], Andrew Park, MD[b], Tad L. Gerlinger, MD[b,c],*

KEYWORDS

- Total knee arthroplasty • Revision total knee arthroplasty • Painful total knee • Failed total knee

KEY POINTS

- Pain after total knee arthroplasty can be caused by numerous factors, and a systematic evaluation that includes a thorough history, physical, radiographic and laboratory evaluation, and understanding of the differential diagnosis is essential.
- Intra-articular, peri-articular, and extra-articular pathology may cause pain after total knee arthroplasty.
- Revision total knee arthroplasty performed without a firm diagnosis has a high chance of failure.

INTRODUCTION

Total knee arthroplasty (TKA) has been shown to produce good clinical results in approximately 80% of patients at long-term follow-up,[1–6] but the 20% of patients who continue to experience pain following TKA often present a diagnostic challenge to orthopedic surgeons. The evaluation and treatment of these patients relies on a thorough understanding of the differential diagnosis of a painful TKA, and a systematic approach is instrumental to efficiently and effectively resolve their pain.

DEFINITION AND MECHANISM OF PAIN

Pain can serve as a protective mechanism by inducing a reaction to eliminate a harmful stimulus. Excessive pain after a TKA often diminishes one's quality of life.[7–10] Pain has been defined as "what the patient says it is."[11] This simplistic definition emphasizes that pain is a subjective experience with no reliable objective measures. Thus the patient's self-report is the most reliable indicator of pain and should not be discredited.[12] The International Association for the Study of Pain (IASP) defines pain as an "unpleasant sensory and emotional experience associated with actual or potential tissue damage, or described in terms of such damage."[13] This definition emphasizes that pain is a complex, multifactorial experience that involves multiple organ systems. To better understand this complex problem, 2 basic types of pain have been described: nociceptive and neuropathic pain.

Nociceptive Pain

Nociceptive pain is caused by the ongoing activation of sensory neurons in response to a noxious stimulus, such as injury, disease, or inflammation,[14] and it is indicative of real or potential tissue damage. There is generally a close correlation between pain perception and stimulus intensity. Nociceptive pain may be described as visceral or somatic. Somatic pain arises from tissues such as skin, muscle, joint capsules, and bone and is further categorized as superficial and deep somatic pain. Superficial somatic pain presents with a well-localized, sharp, pricking, or burning

Disclosure Statement: The authors have no relevant financial relationships to disclose. Dr T.L. Gerlinger is a paid consultant for Smith & Nephew.
[a] Department of Orthopaedic Surgery, Kaiser Permanente Riverside Medical Center, 10800 Magnolia Avenue, Riverside, CA, USA; [b] Department of Orthopaedic Surgery, Midwest Orthopedics at Rush, 1611 West Harrison Street Suite 300, Chicago, IL, USA; [c] Uniformed Services University of the Health Sciences, Bethesda, MD 20814, USA
* Corresponding author.
E-mail address: tad.gerlinger@rushortho.com

orthopedic.theclinics.com

sensation, whereas deep somatic pain presents as a diffuse, dull, or aching sensation. Deep somatic pain has also been described as a cramping sensation that may be referred to or from other sites (ie, referred pain).

Neuropathic Pain

Neuropathic pain is caused by aberrant signal processing in the peripheral or central nervous system and is broadly categorized as peripheral or central in origin. Animal studies suggest that several changes likely contribute to neuropathic pain:

1. Generation of spontaneous ectopic activity,
2. Loss of normal inhibitory mechanisms in the dorsal horn,
3. Altered primary afferent neuron phenotypes, and
4. Sprouting of nerve fibers leading to altered neural connections.[15]

These changes result in abnormal nerve firing and/or abnormal signal amplification.[16] Common causes of neuropathic pain include nerve transection, inflammation, tumors, toxins, metabolic diseases, infections, and primary neurologic diseases. Neuropathic pain is sometimes called "pathologic" pain because it serves no purpose. A chronic pain state may occur when pathophysiologic changes become independent of the inciting event.[17] Neuropathic pain may be continuous or episodic and is perceived as a variety of different sensations (eg, burning, tingling, prickling, shooting, electric shock–like, jabbing, squeezing, deep aching, spasm, or cold). In contrast to nociceptive pain, neuropathic pain is often unresponsive or poorly responsive to nonsteroidal anti-inflammatory drugs (NSAIDs) and opioids.[18] However, neuropathic pain may respond to antiepileptic drugs, antidepressants, or local anesthetics.[19]

Sensitization has a vital role in the etiology of neuropathic pain. With intense, repeated, or prolonged exposure to inflammatory mediators, nociceptors exhibit a lowered threshold for activation and an increased rate of firing.[20] Peripheral sensitization in turn plays a vital role in central sensitization and clinical pain states such as hyperalgesia and allodynia.[16,21,22] Central sensitization refers to a state of spinal neuron hyperexcitability.[23] Dysregulated activation of certain N-methyl-D-aspartate (NMDA) receptors is responsible for this process.[24] Central sensitization is associated with a reduction in central inhibition, spontaneous dorsal horn neuron activity, the recruitment of responses from neurons that normally only respond to low-intensity stimuli (ie, altered neural

connections), and expansion of dorsal horn neuron receptive fields.[25] Clinically, these changes may manifest as (1) hyperalgesia, (2) allodynia, (3) prolonged pain after a transient stimulus (persistent pain), and (4) the spread of pain to uninjured tissue (ie, referred pain).[25]

Sensitization is likely responsible for most of the continuing pain and hyperalgesia after an injury or surgery.[26] This may be due to noxious stimuli from injured and inflamed tissue or "abnormal" input from injured nerves. Sensitization may serve an adaptive purpose to encourage protection of the injured area during the healing phase; however, these processes may persist long after healing of the injury and lead to chronic pain. Furthermore, sensitization may be why neuropathic pain often exceeds the provoking stimulus, both spatially and temporally.[23] Finally, central sensitization may explain why chronic pain is more difficult to treat than acute pain.[27]

EVALUATION OF PAINFUL TOTAL KNEE ARTHROPLASTY

The management of a painful TKA requires a multidisciplinary team approach that involves orthopedic surgeons, physical therapists, pain management physicians, and primary medical doctors.[10] A full assessment of both the surgical and nonsurgical factors that can cause pain after TKA is often time-consuming, but timely management of the pain is essential and should be approached irrespective of the origin of the pain and whether or not it may be addressed surgically. Depending on the acuity and necessity of surgical intervention, this evaluation may best be done by a pain management specialist, which in itself may help to alleviate anxiety. As a result, the emphasis may be focused on a nonsurgical resolution of the problem.[10]

The use of appropriate analgesics may help to alleviate pain, reduce the sense of urgency for further intervention, and decrease the desperation often felt by patients and their families. Most patients report low pain scores in the first 3 months after TKA, but some report continued pain or even increasing pain as time passes. This often correlates with the cessation of regular pain medications by patients who feel that these medications are not required for such a long period postoperatively. The pain may lead to a reduction in the range of motion, with subsequent stiffness and increased sensitivity around the joint. Patients should be encouraged to take analgesics if warranted, and these should be prescribed according to the World Health Organization (WHO) analgesic ladder (**Fig. 1**).[28] However, medical management

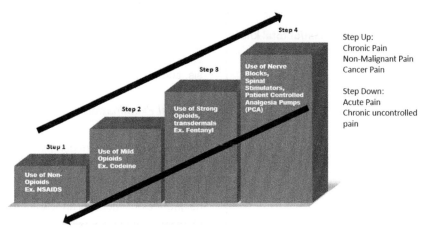

Step 4

Step 3

Step 2

Step 1

Step Up:
Chronic Pain
Non-Malignant Pain
Cancer Pain

Step Down:
Acute Pain
Chronic uncontrolled
pain

Use of Nerve Blocks, Spinal Stimulators, Patient Controlled Analgesia Pumps (PCA)

Use of Strong Opioids, transdermals Ex. Fentanyl

Use of Mild Opioids Ex. Codeine

Use of Non-Opioids Ex. NSAIDS

Fig. 1. WHO new adaption of the analgesic ladder. PCA, patient-controlled analgesia. (*Modified from* World Health Organization. Traitement de la douleur cancéreuse. Geneva (Switzerland): World Health Organization; 1997; with permission.)

of pain should not delay the diagnosis and targeted treatment of the source of the pain by the orthopedic surgeon.

Differential Diagnosis

Laskin[9] categorized etiologies of pain after TKA based on their temporal associations: start-up pain, pain on weight bearing, early postoperative pain, pain associated with full flexion, pain with stair climbing or descent, rest pain, and continuous postoperative pain. For example, start-up pain can indicate loosening of TKA components, whereas pain with stair climbing can be caused by extensor mechanism pathology. Furthermore, the differential diagnosis may be organized according to the anatomic source: intra-articular, peri-articular, and extra-articular (**Box 1**). Pain that was present preoperatively that then persisted without change following TKA suggests an extra-articular etiology. Extra-articular sources of knee pain include lumbar spine and hip conditions, vascular insufficiency, and complex regional pain syndrome (CRPS). With regard to intra-articular pathology, pain that began within the first year after the surgery suggests infection, instability, malpositioned components, or soft tissue impingement. In contrast, pain that began more than 1 year postoperatively suggests wear, osteolysis, aseptic loosening, or infection. A patient's pain trajectory, describing change in magnitude over time, may also be considered when attempting to make the diagnosis within the first 12 months.[29]

Pain that is activity related may indicate a mechanical etiology, whereas pain that is constant and does not abate with rest and activity modifications should raise suspicion of underlying

periprosthetic joint infection. Pain associated with constitutional symptoms such as fevers and chills should also raise suspicion for infection. Activity-related pain associated with recurrent swelling suggests instability. Pain described as burning, tingling, prickling, shooting, electric shock–like, jabbing, squeezing, spasm, or cold may indicate a neuropathic origin. Pain that radiates to the thigh or down to the foot may be referred from the lumbar spine or ipsilateral hip.

History

A comprehensive history is the first step in identifying the etiology of a painful TKA, and it is crucial to use a systematic approach when taking a focused history. The patient's primary symptom should be clearly identified and described in terms of pain, instability, swelling, or stiffness. Information about the initial surgery, including the date, surgeon, approach, implant records, operative reports, and preoperative radiographs and notes regarding physical examination, should be obtained. The nature and extent of the pain is important. *Bates' Guide to Physical Examination and History Taking*[24] suggests 2 mnemonics that can be used to help the physician better clarify pain: OLD CARTS (Onset, Location, Duration, Character, Aggravating/Alleviating Factors, Radiation, and Timing) and OPQRST (Onset, Palliating/Provoking Factors, Quality, Radiation, Site, and Timing).

In addition to clarifying the predominant complaint, details regarding the postoperative course of the index procedure should be obtained. Such examples would include prolonged postoperative wound drainage, delayed wound healing, return trips to the operating room, and treatment

Box 1
Differential diagnosis of the painful total knee arthroplasty

Intra-articular

- Infection
- Aseptic loosening
- Instability
  - ○ Axial
  - ○ Flexion
  - ○ Midflexion
- Malalignment
- Polyethylene wear
- Osteolysis
- Component overhang
- Implant failure
- Arthrofibrosis
- Implant fracture
- Recurrent hemarthrosis
- Loose cement
- Extensor mechanism dysfunction
  - ○ Unsurfaced patella
  - ○ Undersized/oversized patella
  - ○ Patellar baja
  - ○ Lateral facet impingement
  - ○ Patellar clunk
  - ○ Osteonecrosis

Peri-articular

- Periprosthetic fractures
  - ○ Traumatic fracture
  - ○ Tibial stress fracture
  - ○ Patellar stress fracture
- Popliteal tendon impingement
- Biceps tendonitis
- Pes bursitis
- Quadriceps tendonitis/rupture
- Patellar tendonitis/rupture
- Neuroma

Extra-articular

- Hip pathology
- Lumbar spine pathology
- Vascular claudication
- Complex regional pain syndrome

with antibiotics following surgery. Comorbid conditions also should be considered. These conditions include diabetes, renal failure, peripheral vascular disease, lumbar spondylosis and stenosis, and adjacent hip pathology.

Physical Examination

A thorough physical examination must be performed on every patient complaining of continued pain after TKA. The patient should be appropriately disrobed to allow for full evaluation of the limb. Examination should include vital signs, height, weight, general appearance, and gait. A detailed inspection is performed of the skin looking for lesions, erythema, warmth, effusion, vascular changes, and draining sinus tracts. The surgical scar may show evidence of prior wound dehiscence, which may lead one to further consider an infectious etiology. Gait should specifically be analyzed for evidence of antalgia, varus or valgus thrust, and presence of a Trendelenburg sign.

A focused musculoskeletal examination of the knee should include the measurement of active and passive range of motion and the ability to actively maintain full extension without extensor lag. The stability of the knee may be evaluated with varus and valgus forces at 0° and 30°. Stability in the sagittal plane may be assessed with posterior drawer testing at 60° and 90° of flexion to assess for flexion stability. Manual strength testing as well as evaluation for muscle atrophy should be noted. The knee should be palpated to evaluate for swelling, effusion, and focal tenderness. The knee should be assessed for point tenderness along the iliotibial band and pes anserine bursa, which may be indicative of flexion instability or bursitis.[30,31]

Patellar tracking should be assessed closely, as the patellofemoral compartment is a common source of continued pain following TKA. Numerous factors have been associated with painful patellar crepitus, which include previous knee surgery, patellar clunk syndrome, decreased patellar component size, decreased patellar composite thickness, shorter patellar tendon length, increased posterior femoral condylar offset, use of smaller femoral components, thicker tibial polyethylene inserts, and increased flexion of the femoral component.[32] These factors are postulated to increase quadriceps tendon contact forces against the superior aspect of the intercondylar box subsequently increasing the risk of fibrosynovial proliferation.[32]

A neurovascular examination should be performed and the quality and symmetry of the peripheral pulses should be assessed. The strength of the quadriceps and vastus medialis obliquus should be evaluated. Finally, examination of the spine, hip, foot, and ankle should always be undertaken to elucidate extra-articular causes of pain, such as lumbar radiculopathy, referred pain from hip arthritis, and vascular claudication.

Imaging

A comprehensive series of plain radiographs includes standing anteroposterior, lateral, posteroanterior flexed, full-length mechanical axis, and Merchant view radiographs. When possible, serial radiographs may be useful. The anterior-posterior images should be closely evaluated for component size, position, polyethylene gap symmetry, component overhang, bony impingement, osteolysis, progressive radiolucent lines, subsidence, and fracture (**Fig. 2**). The lateral images should be evaluated for femoral component size, posterior femoral offset, patellar height and thickness, and tibial component slope. Osteolysis is typically evident on lateral radiographs along the posterior condyles.[33] High-quality films are important in assessing the prosthesis-bone interface in cementless implants and the bone-cement-implant interface in cemented prostheses. Fluoroscopic examination may be useful in the evaluation of these interfaces as well as assessing varus and valgus stability.[34] The Merchant view should be evaluated for patellar tilt, patellar malalignment, femoral component overhang, component thickness, and patellar facet impingement (**Fig. 3**). Mechanical axis films should be evaluated to assess overall alignment and may provide some additional information on the condition of the hips and spine (**Fig. 4**).

Additional Imaging

Computed tomography (CT) or metal artifact reduction MRI scans are often useful in assessing painful TKAs. These images may be used to accurately assess the rotation of the femoral and tibial components (**Fig. 5**). The femoral component rotation is compared with the transepicondylar axis; the tibial component rotation is compared with the medial one-third of the tibial tubercle. Excessive internal rotation of either component can lead to patellar instability or lateral flexion laxity and result in knee pain and dysfunction. Combined external rotation should be between 0° and 10°.[35] Three-dimensional imaging can aid in accurately determining the extent of osteolytic lesions that may be underestimated or missed entirely on plain radiographs alone.[36] MRI also may be used in detection of a mass or tumor.

Bone scans may be useful in diagnosing aseptic loosening, periprosthetic joint infection, and stress fractures. Nevertheless, these studies are nonspecific and can be falsely positive for up to 2 years postoperatively. Hofman and colleagues[37] demonstrated that technetium bone scans show increased uptake in approximately 90% of tibial components and 65% of femoral components at 1 year following TKA. Technetium scans are unable to distinguish between septic and aseptic loosening. Indium 111–labeled scans have value for the exclusion of infection when they are

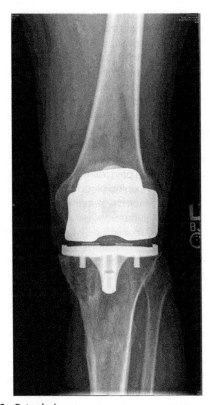

Fig. 2. Osteolysis.

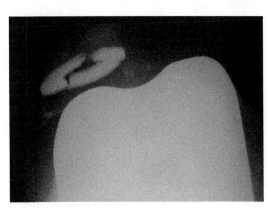

Fig. 3. Patellar maltracking and component failure.

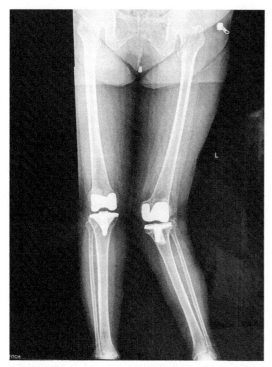

Fig. 4. Alignment films demonstrating tibial component loosening and valgus deformity.

negative, but a high false-positive rate limits their utility.[38,39] PET imaging may also detect periprosthetic infection, and it was recently shown to be superior to combined indium and sulfur colloid bone marrow scans in the detection of infection

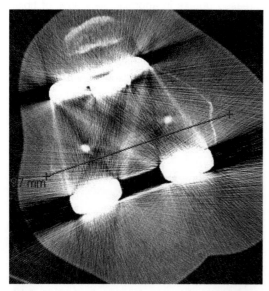

Fig. 5. CT demonstrating appropriate femoral component rotation.

in painful hip and knee prostheses.[40] However, the American Academy of Orthopedic Surgeons (AAOS) clinical practice guidelines for diagnosis of periprosthethic joint infection has a limited recommendation in utilization of these modalities, as evidence of effectiveness is unconvincing.[41] These expensive tests have relatively poor sensitivity and specificity, but they may provide useful information in equivocal cases.

Laboratory Analysis

Periprosthetic joint infection has been reported to be the most common indication for revision TKA and must always be considered in the differential diagnosis of the painful TKA.[42] The AAOS published an algorithm to guide the diagnosis of periprosthetic joint infections of the hip and knee (**Fig. 6**).[41] Serum erythrocyte sedimentation rate (ESR) and C-reactive protein (CRP) as well as synovial fluid cell count and analysis are powerful tools in the diagnosis of periprosthetic joint infection.[41,43–45] The combined use of ESR and CRP is an established "rule-out" test. If the ESR and CRP are both negative, periprosthetic infection is unlikely (negative likelihood ratio 0–0.06). When both tests are positive, periprosthetic infection is likely (positive likelihood ratio 4.3–12.1), and synovial fluid aspiration and analysis are warranted.[41] It is important to note that inflammatory conditions such as rheumatoid arthritis, neoplasms, coronary artery disease, polymyalgia rheumatica, inflammatory bowel disease, and other inflammation-causing diseases may lead to elevation of inflammatory markers as well.

Synovial fluid analysis is of critical importance when considering periprosthetic joint infection. Synovial fluid cultures should be obtained after patients have been off antibiotics for at least 2 weeks.[46] Multiple studies have evaluated the association between periprosthetic joint infection and synovial fluid white blood cell (WBC) count and differential. Reports of synovial WBC counts in the chronically infected knee arthroplasty have ranged from 1100 to 4000 cells/μL, with polymorphonuclear (PMN) percentage ranging from 64% to 69%.[47–49] In patients with acute infections, defined as within 3 months of surgery, a threshold synovial WBC count of 27,800 cells/μL has a positive predicted value of 94% and a negative predictive value of 98%.[50]

Research in the laboratory evaluation of painful TKAs is ongoing, and biomarkers of infection that are currently under investigation include synovial fluid CRP, synovial fluid leukocyte esterase, and molecular markers, such as interleukin-6 and alpha defensin, that may be detected on

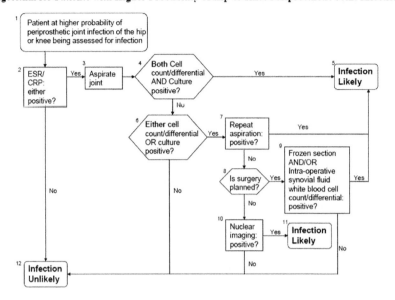

A

Algorithm for Patients with Higher Probability of Hip or Knee Periprosthetic Joint Infection

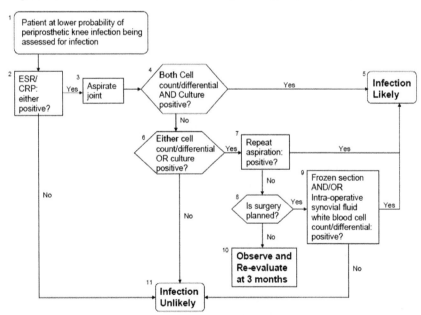

B

Algorithm for Patients with Lower Probability of Periprosthetic Knee Infection

Fig. 6. AAOS algorithms for laboratory diagnosis of periprosthetic joint infections based on high (*A*) and low (*B*) pretest probabilities. (*From* Della Valle C, Parvizi J, Bauer TW, et al. American Academy of Orthopaedic Surgeons clinical practice guideline on: the diagnosis of periprosthetic joint infections of the hip and knee. J Bone Joint Surg Am 2011;93:1355–7; with permission.)

polymerase chain reaction.[51–54] Additionally, metal sensitivity has been hypothesized to be a potential source of pain following TKA, and researchers have evaluated patients with patch testing, lymphocyte transformation testing, and histologic analysis of tissue.[55] Whether these tests prove to be useful in the diagnosis of pain following TKA remains to be seen.

Diagnostic Injections

An intra-articular injection of lidocaine or infiltration of tender points may be a useful adjunct in differentiating intra-articular, extra-articular, or peri-articular diagnoses. This technique may be particularly useful in differentiating between psychosomatic and mechanical sources of reported pain.[33] In cases of suspected CRPS, a sympathetic blockade is often useful.[56]

MANAGEMENT

Because performing a revision TKA without a clear diagnosis is associated with a high rate of failure, a treatment plan should be formulated only after a thorough and systematic evaluation has determined the cause of the pain. Determining the source of the pain and the possible success of revision surgery are often the most difficult aspects of managing a patient with a painful total knee. The most common causes of pain after TKA include infection, aseptic loosening, wear, instability, and extensor mechanism dysfunction,[43] and are amenable to surgical intervention. Whether or not the pain can be relieved with surgical intervention, enlisting the assistance of physical therapists, pain management physicians, and primary medical doctors as a multimodal pain team is often beneficial.

A comprehensive review of surgical management for all causes of the painful TKA is beyond the scope of this article, but a brief discussion of treatment for infection and mechanical causes is highlighted. Treatment of the infected TKA is guided by its acuity as well as by the offending organism. Acute infection may be defined as one that has developed within 4 weeks of the index surgery or within 4 weeks of hematogenous seeding from a distant nidus located elsewhere in the body. An acutely infected TKA generally can be salvaged by treating with surgical irrigation and debridement, exchange of the polyethylene liner, and intravenous culture-specific antibiotics. For chronic (>4 weeks) infections, this treatment modality has a higher rate of failure and is better treated with a staged revision procedure. The process includes explantation of all prosthetic components, placement of an antibiotic-impregnated cement spacer, administration of intravenous antibiotics, and revision TKA once the infection has been eliminated. Infection is felt to have been eradicated once inflammatory markers have normalized and aspiration following an antibiotic holiday is negative.[57] On the other hand, aseptic loosening and instability may be caused by osteolysis and polyethylene wear, suboptimal component positioning and alignment, imbalanced flexion-extension gaps, and a poor cement-bone interface. Patients with pain due to aseptic loosening are typically treated with a 1-stage revision TKA that revises the loose components and addresses the reason for their failure.

Anterior knee pain following TKA may be caused by a number of different factors, including lateral subluxation of the patella, overstuffing of the patellofemoral joint, internal rotation of the femoral or tibial components, and patellar clunk syndrome. The aforementioned issues may all contribute to extensor mechanism dysfunction. Treatment is dependent on the cause of the pain. Component malrotation that is refractory to conservative measures may require revision TKA, whereas patellar clunk syndrome may be treated successfully with arthroscopic debridement of the offending fibrous nodule.[58,59] Another less common condition that has been treated successfully with arthroscopy is popliteus tendon syndrome, in which the popliteus tendon mechanically snaps over the posterior aspect of the prosthetic femoral component.[60] There are numerous reasons that a TKA may be painful, and only with an accurate diagnosis can an appropriate treatment plan be formulated.

SUMMARY

The number of patients who continue to complain of pain following TKA is likely to grow with the increased demand for TKA. Management of a patient with a painful TKA is best done by a multidisciplinary team. Diagnostic workup should not preclude medical treatment of patients' pain. A systematic approach is useful when attempting to identify a cause for pain after TKA. The sources of pain may be broadly defined as intra-articular, peri-articular, and extra-articular. A diagnosis for continued pain must be obtained before consideration for revision TKA, as revision for unexplained pain has a poor prognosis.[33]

REFERENCES

1. Knutson K, Lewold S, Robertsson O, et al. The Swedish knee arthroplasty register: a nation-wide study of 30,003 knees 1976-1992. Acta Orthop Scand 1994;65:375–86.
2. Sharkey PF, Hozack WJ, Rothman RH, et al. Insall Award paper. Why are total knee arthroplasties failing today? Clin Orthop Relat Res 2002;(404): 7–13.
3. Ritter MA. The Anatomical Graduated Component total knee replacement. A long-term evaluation with 20-years survival analysis. J Bone Joint Surg Br 2009;91:45–9.

4. Bourne RB, Chesworth BM, Davis AM, et al. Patient satisfaction after total knee arthroplasty: who is satisfied and who is not? Clin Orthop Relat Res 2010;468(1):57–63.

5. Fehring TK, Christie MJ, Lavernia C, et al. Revision total knee arthroplasty: planning, management and controversies. AAOS Instr Course Lect 2008;57: 341–62.

6. Hawker GA. Who, when, and why total joint replacement surgery? The patient's perspective. Curr Opin Rheumatol 2006;18:526–30.

7. Breugem SJM, Haverkamp D. Anterior knee pain after a total knee arthroplasty: what can cause this pain? World J Orthopedics 2014;5(3):163–70.

8. Dellon AL. Pain solutions 2013. La Vergne (TN): Lightning Source Inc; 2013.

9. Laskin RS. The patient with a painful total knee replacement. In: Lotke PA, Garino JP, editors. Revision total knee arthroplasty. Philadelphia: Lippincott; 1999. p. 91–107.

10. Toms AD, Mandalia V, Haigh R, et al. The management of patients with painful total knee replacement. J Bone Joint Surg Br 2009;91:143–50.

11. Goodwin J, Bajwa ZH. Understanding the patient with chronic pain. In: Warfield CA, Bajwa ZH, editors. Principles and practice of pain medicine. 2nd edition. New York: McGraw-Hill Companies, Inc; 2004. p. 55–60.

12. Jacox AK, Carr DB, Chapman CR, et al. Acute pain management: operative or medical procedures and trauma clinical practice guideline No. 1. Rockville (MD): US Department of Health and Human Services; Agency for Health Care Policy and Research; 1992. AHCPR publication 92–0032.

13. Merskey H, Bugduk N. Classification of chronic pain. Descriptions of chronic pain syndromes and definitions of pain terms. 2nd edition. Seattle (WA): IASP Press; 1994.

14. Coda BA, Bonica JJ. General considerations of acute pain. In: Loeser JD, Butler SH, Chapman CR, et al, editors. Bonica's management of pain. 3rd edition. Baltimore (MD): Lippincott Williams &Wilkins; 2001. p. 222–40.

15. Ru-Rong JI, Woolf CJ. Neuronal plasticity and signal transduction in nociceptive neurons: implications for the initiation and maintenance of pathological pain. Neurobiol Dis 2001;8:1–10.

16. Covington EC. The biological basis of pain. Int Rev Psychiatry 2000;12:128–47.

17. Portenoy RK. Basic mechanisms. In: Portenoy RK, Kanner RM, editors. Pain management: theory and practice. Philadelphia: FD Davis; 1996. p. 19–39.

18. Arner S, Meyerson BA. Lack of analgesic effect of opioids on neuropathic and idiopathic forms of pain. Pain 1988;33:11–23.

19. Covington EC. Anticonvulsants for neuropathic pain and detoxification. Cleve Clin J Med 1998;65(Suppl 1):SI21–9.

20. Neumann S, Doubell TP, Leslie T, et al. Inflammatory pain hypersensitivity mediated by phenotypic switch in myelinated primary sensory neurons. Nature 1996;384:360–4.

21. Alexander J, Black A. Pain mechanisms and the management of neuropathic pain. Curr Opin Neurol Neurosurg 1992;5:228–34.

22. MacDermott AB, Mayer ML, Westbrook GL, et al. NMDA-receptor activation increase cytoplasmic calcium concentration in cultured spinal cord neurons. Nature 1986;321:519–22.

23. Woolf CJ. Evidence for a central component of post-injury pain hypersensitivity. Nature 1983;306:686–8.

24. Bickley LS, Szilagyi PG, Bates B. Bates' guide to physical examination and history taking. Philadelphia: Lippincott Williams & Wilkins; 2007. Print.

25. Cervero F, Laird JM, Pozo MA. Selective changes of receptive field properties of spinal nociceptive neurons induced by noxious visceral stimulation in the cat. Pain 1992;51:335–42.

26. Woolf CJ. Pain. Neurobiol Dis 2000;7:504–10.

27. Wall PD. The prevention of postoperative pain. Pain 1988;33:289–90.

28. World Health Organization. Traitement de la douleur cancéreuse. Geneva (Switzerland): World Health Organization; 1997.

29. Pagé MG, Katz J, Romero Escobar EM, et al. Distinguishing problematic from nonproblematic postsurgical pain: a pain trajectory analysis after total knee arthroplasty. Pain 2015;156(3):460–8.

30. Clarke HD, Scuderi GR. Flexion instability in primary total knee replacement. J Knee Surg 2003;16(2): 123–8.

31. Peralta-Molero JV, Gladnick BP, Lee YY, et al. Patellofemoral crepitation and clunk following modern, fixed-bearing total knee arthroplasty. J Arthroplasty 2014;29(3):535–40.

32. Dennis DA, Kim RH, Johnson DR, et al. The John Insall Award: control-matched evaluation of painful patellar Crepitus after total knee arthroplasty. Clin Orthop Relat Res 2011;469(1):10–1.

33. Meneghini RM. Revision total knee arthroplasty. In: Glassman AH, Lachiewicz PF, Tanzer M, editors. OKU 4: hip and knee reconstruction. Rosemont (IL): AAOS; 2011.

34. Stähelin T, Kessler O, Pfirrmann C, et al. Fluoroscopically assisted stress radiography for varus-valgus stability assessment in flexion after total knee arthroplasty. J Arthroplasty 2003;18(4):513–5.

35. Berger RA, Crossett LS, Jacobs JJ, et al. Malrotation causing patellofemoral complications after total knee arthroplasty. Clin Orthop Relat Res 1998;356: 144–53.

36. Reish TG, Clarke HD, Scuderi GR, et al. Use of multidetector computed tomography for the detection of periprosthetic osteolysis in total knee arthroplasty. J Knee Surg 2006;19(4):259–64.

37. Hofmann AA, Wyatt RW, Daniels AU, et al. Bone scans after total knee arthroplasty in asymptomatic patients. Cemented versus cementless. Clin Orthop Relat Res 1990;251:183–8.

38. Rand JA, Brown ML. The value of indium111 leukocyte scanning in the evaluation of painful or infected total knee arthroplasties. Clin Orthop Relat Res 1990;259:179–82.

39. Scher DM, Pak K, Lonner JH, et al. The predictive value of indium-111 leukocyte scans in the diagnosis of infected total hip, knee, or resection arthroplasties. J Arthroplasty 2000;15(3):295–300.

40. Basu S, Kwee TC, Saboury B, et al. FDG PET for diagnosing infection in hip and knee prostheses: prospective study in 221 prostheses and subgroup comparison with combined (111)In-labeled leukocyte/(99m)Tc-sulfur colloid bone marrow imaging in 88 prostheses. Clin Nucl Med 2014;39(7):609–15.

41. Della Valle C, Parvizi J, Bauer TW, et al. American Academy of Orthopaedic Surgeons clinical practice guideline on: the diagnosis of periprosthetic joint infections of the hip and knee. J Bone Joint Surg Am 2011;93:1355–7.

42. Bozic KJ, Kurtz SM, Lau E, et al. The epidemiology of revision total knee arthroplasty in the United States. Clin Orthop Relat Res 2010;468(1):45–51.

43. Gonzalez MH, Mekhail AO. The failed total knee arthroplasty: evaluation and etiology. J Am Acad Orthop Surg 2004;12(6):436–46.

44. Volin SJ, Hinrichs SH, Garvin KL. Two-stage reimplantation of total joint infections: a comparison of resistant and nonresistant organisms. Clin Orthop Relat Res 2004;427:94–100.

45. Jamsen E, Stogiannidis I, Malmivaara A, et al. Outcome of prosthesis exchange for infected knee arthroplasty: the effect of treatment approach. Acta Orthop 2009;80(1):67–77.

46. Trampuz A, Piper KE, Jacobson MJ, et al. Sonication of removed hip and knee prostheses for diagnosis of infection. N Engl J Med 2007;357(7):654–63.

47. Della Valle CJ, Sporer SM, Jacobs JJ, et al. Preoperative testing for sepsis before revision total knee arthroplasty. J Arthroplasty 2007;22(6 Suppl 2):90–3.

48. Ghanem E, Parvizi J, Burnett RS, et al. Cell count and differential of aspirated fluid in the diagnosis of infection at the site of total knee arthroplasty. J Bone Joint Surg Am 2008;90(8):1637–43.

49. Trampuz A, Hanssen AD, Osmon DR, et al. Synovial fluid leukocyte count and differential for the diagnosis of prosthetic knee infection. Am J Med 2004; 117(8):556–62.

50. Bedair H, Ting N, Jacovides C, et al. The mark coventry award: diagnosis of early postoperative TKA infection using synovial fluid analysis. Clin Orthopaedics Relat Res 2011;469(1):34–40.

51. Parvizi J, Jacovides C, Adeli B, et al. Coventry award: synovial c-reactive protein: a prospective evaluation of a molecular marker for periprosthetic knee joint infection. Clin Orthop Relat Res 2011; 470(1):54–60.

52. Parvizi J, Azzam K, Jacovides C, et al. Diagnosis of periprosthetic joint infection: the role of a simple, yet unrecognized, enzyme. New Orleans (LA): Academy of Orthopaedic Surgeons AAOS; 2010.

53. Deirmengian C, Hallab N, Tarabishy A, et al. Synovial fluid biomarkers for periprosthetic infection. Clin Orthop Relat Res 2010;468(8):2017–23.

54. Deirmengian C, Kardos K, Kilmartin P, et al. The alpha-defensin test for periprosthetic joint infection responds to a wide spectrum of organisms. Clin Orthopaedics Relat Res 2015;473(7):2229–35.

55. Thomas P, Summer B, Krenn V, et al. Allergy diagnostics in suspected metal implant intolerance. Orthopade 2013;42(8):602–6.

56. Schwartz RG. Stem cells for the treatment of complex regional pain syndrome (CRPS)/reflex sympathetic dystrophy (RSD): a case study. Pan Am J Med Thermology 2015;1(2):89–92.

57. Tsukayama DT, Goldberg VM, Kyle R. Diagnosis and management of infection after total knee arthroplasty. J Bone Joint Surg Am 2003;85-A(Suppl 1): S75–80.

58. Sternheim A, Lochab J, Drexler M, et al. The benefit of revision knee arthroplasty for component malrotation after primary total knee replacement. Int Orthop 2012;36(12):2473–8.

59. Costanzo JA, Aynardi MC, Peters JD, et al. Patellar clunk syndrome after total knee arthroplasty; risk factors and functional outcomes of arthroscopic treatment. J Arthroplasty 2014;29(9 Suppl):201–4.

60. Allardyce TJ, Scuderi GR, Insall JN. Arthroscopic treatment of popliteus tendon dysfunction following total knee arthroplasty. J Arthroplasty 1997;12(3): 353–5.

Avoiding Hip Instability and Limb Length Discrepancy After Total Hip Arthroplasty

 CrossMark

Peter K. Sculco, MD*, Umberto Cottino, MD,
Matthew P. Abdel, MD, Rafael J. Sierra, MD

KEYWORDS

- Total hip arthroplasty • Instability • Limb length discrepancy • Preoperative templating
- Component position

KEY POINTS

- Patient risk factors for dislocation include obesity, increasing age, neuromuscular and cognitive disorders, alcoholism, and a previous diagnosis of femoral neck fracture.
- Clinical evaluation includes gait assessment, measurement of true and apparent limb length discrepancies, and identifying a fixed or flexible pelvic obliquity and any periarticular soft tissue contractures.
- Preoperative radiographs help calculate limb length differences and plan intraoperative lengthening, component sizing, and acetabular and femoral component position in relation to radiographic landmarks.
- Larger femoral head sizes ($\geq$32 mm), elevated or lipped liners, high offset stems, and dual mobility devices are implant options that may improve hip stability in higher-risk patients.
- Postoperative hip instability can usually be managed with closed reduction. When this fails, surgical management includes increasing femoral head size, increasing soft tissue tension with higher offset or limb lengthening, and component revision with possible conversion to a dual mobility or constrained liner.

BACKGROUND

Total hip arthroplasty (THA) reduces pain and improves function in patients with end-stage arthritis of the hip[1–3] and is associated with a high satisfaction rate and a low incidence of complications.[4] Two complications after THA are hip instability and limb length discrepancy, and between 2000 and 2007, instability was the most common indication for revision THA.[5] In addition, significant limb length discrepancy after THA is a cause for patient dissatisfaction and possible litigation.[6] The goal of a successful THA is to maximize impingement-free range of motion, recreate appropriate offset, and equalize limb length discrepancies to produce a pain-free and dynamically stable THA. The objective of this article is to review the patient risk factors for dislocation and limb length discrepancy, key elements of the preoperative template, the anatomic landmarks for accurate component placement, the leg positions for soft tissue stability testing, and the management of postoperative instability.

Funding Sources: None.
Conflict of Interest: None (P.K. Sculco, U. Cottino, M.P. Abdel); Zimmer Biomet, consultant and royalties (R.J. Sierra).
Department of Orthopedic Surgery, Mayo Clinic, 200 First Street, Southwest, Rochester, MN 55905, USA
* Corresponding author. 535 East 70th street, New York, NY 10021.
E-mail address: sculcop@hss.edu

Orthop Clin N Am 47 (2016) 327–334
http://dx.doi.org/10.1016/j.ocl.2015.09.006

CLINICAL PATIENT EVALUATION

Patients at risk for postoperative limb length discrepancies include those with previous surgery, trauma, infection, growth plate arrest, and congenital dysplasia. Patients at risk of instability include those with hyperlaxity, connective tissue or neuromuscular disorders, a diagnosis of femoral neck fracture, avascular necrosis, increasing age, alcoholism, obesity, and female sex.[7–9]

PATIENTS AT RISK FOR DISLOCATION

- Female gender
- Obesity
- Diagnosis of femoral neck fracture
- Neuromuscular or cognitive disorders
- Hyperlaxity or connective tissue disorder
- Alcoholism

PATIENTS AT RISK FOR TRUE OR PERCEIVED POSTOPERATIVE LIMB LENGTH DISCREPANCY

- Operative leg longer preoperatively
- Perception of limb length equality when operative leg shorter (block testing)
- Significant (>3 cm) limb length discrepancy
- Fixed pelvic obliquity

Physical examination includes a gait assessment for signs of spasticity or imbalance. The axial skeleton should be assessed for coronal or sagittal plane deformities, such as scoliosis or ankylosing spondylitis. Pelvic obliquity can occur from a spinopelvic deformity or be compensatory and secondary to a limb length discrepancy or soft tissue contracture. If a pelvic obliquity is present, evaluate the patient in both the standing and seated position. A flexible pelvic obliquity corrects in a seated position, whereas a fixed pelvic obliquity does not.

KEY PHYSICAL EXAMINATION FINDINGS

- Gait: spasticity or imbalance
- Fixed or mobile pelvic obliquity
- Soft tissue contractures (flexors, abductors, adductors, external rotators/capsule)
- Abductor strength
- Distal sensation and proprioception
- Actual or perceived limb length discrepancy

Supine range of motion testing should identify any hip or knee contractures that may affect accurate limb length assessment. Abductor strength is tested and should be compared with the contralateral side. A distal sensory examination may identify the presence of a peripheral neuropathy, which may increase the risk of gait imbalance, falls, and subsequent postoperative instability.

LIMB LENGTH ASSESSMENT

True and apparent limb length are the 2 methods used to assess limb length discrepancy. True limb length is measured from the anterior superior iliac spine to the medial malleolus. The apparent limb length is measured from the umbilicus to the medial malleolus. True limb length represents the length of the limb, whereas the apparent limb length takes into account all factors that contribute to differing leg lengths, such as a pelvic obliquity or soft tissue contractures. For this reason, the apparent limb length is a better reflection of the patient's perception because it includes the true limb length difference in addition to any factors that altogether contribute to leg length inequality. Block testing with blocks of different heights placed under the affected extremity helps to quantify the apparent leg length discrepancy (**Fig. 1**).

PREOPERATIVE TEMPLATING AND RADIOGRAPHIC MEASUREMENTS

Standing anteroposterior (AP) pelvic and operative hip radiographs, in addition to a frog-leg or cross-table lateral, are helpful for preoperative planning. A line drawn across 2 fixed reference points on the AP pelvis view and measured from a femoral reference point (lesser trochanter) allows calculation of a radiographic leg length discrepancy. The 3 pelvic reference points include the inferior aspect of the obturator foramen, the ischial tuberosities, and the acetabular teardrop. The teardrop is the most reproducible and accurate when calculating limb length discrepancy[10] but if distorted anatomy makes identification difficult, then another pelvic reference point can be used. **Fig. 2**A shows a pre-operative AP pelvic radiograph and a leg length discrepancy as measured from the teardrop to the midpoint of the lesser trochanter bilaterally.

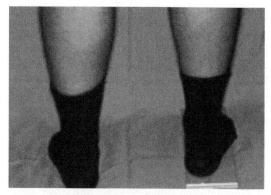

Fig. 1. A block of known thickness is placed under the shorter extremity until the patient perceives leg lengths to be equal.

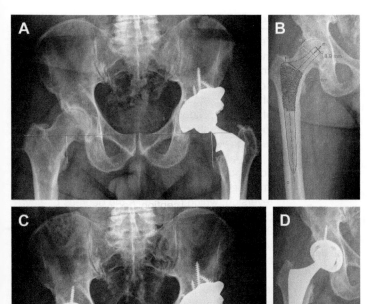

Fig. 2. (*A*) Preoperative AP pelvis radiograph showing a 9-mm limb length discrepancy using the teardrop as the pelvic reference. (*B*) Preoperative template showing planned leg lengthening and planned measured femoral neck resection. Estimated lateral component overhang is recorded for goal acetabular inclination angle. (*C* and *D*) Postoperative radiographs showing restoration of leg length and offset. Acetabular inclination and overhang matches the preoperative template.

PREOPERATIVE TEMPLATING
Tips for Preoperative Templating

- Determine any leg length differences and calculate planned lengthening
- Acetabular component
  - AP radiograph: teardrop, ilioischial line, superolateral acetabulum
  - Measure lateral overhang with cup in desired inclination
- Femoral component
  - Component sizing for canal/metaphyseal fill
  - Standard versus high offset stem
  - Position femoral head center of rotation (COR) above acetabular COR to match planned lengthening
  - Measure neck resection in relation to lesser trochanter
  - Femoral head COR in relation to the tip of the greater trochanter

The most helpful radiographic landmarks for acetabular templating are the teardrop, the ilioischial line, and the superolateral acetabulum. The inferior aspect of the cup should be positioned at the level of the radiographic teardrop and medialized until close to the medial wall (see **Fig. 2**). The acetabular COR affects both leg length and offset, and accurate restoration of the native acetabular

COR optimizes hip biomechanics. The amount of lateral cup overhang from the superolateral aspect of the acetabulum is a helpful intraoperative check for appropriate inclination angle. The femoral component COR should be positioned in the location that best achieves leg length equality and restoration of offset. If the femoral COR is proximal to the acetabular COR, then, the leg is lengthened, and if the femoral COR is medial to the acetabular COR, then, hip offset is increased. High offset or standard femoral stem designs allow for adjustments in offset to match patient anatomy. Once the femoral COR is in a position that best restores leg length and offset, the level of the neck osteotomy is marked and measured in millimeters from the lesser trochanter. Another preoperative method for reproducing the femoral COR is to draw a line perpendicular to the tip of the greater trochanter and mark where it passes through the femoral head. This distance can then be checked intraoperatively once the trial femoral stem is in place. Restoring offset is necessary for overall hip stability and soft tissue tension. If offset is not restored first, then the leg may be inadvertently lengthened to achieve overall hip stability.

Each surgical approach has different advantages and disadvantages in regards to leg length and offset recreation. For the direct anterior approach, the patient is usually supine, which allows for leg length comparison using the medial malleoli as a guide. This comparison is not possible when a fracture table is used, because the feet are secured in traction boots. With fluoroscopy, leg length and offset can be assessed with an AP radiograph of the operative hip and compared with a radiograph of the contralateral side.[11] The direct lateral approach can be performed either supine, with the ability to measure the medial malleoli, or in the lateral decubitus position, in which the tip of the greater trochanter can be easily used as a guide for femoral COR reconstruction. For the posterior approach, the lesser trochanter is the key landmark for making a neck osteotomy of the desired length based on the preoperative template. For patients in the lateral decubitus position, with the knees in the same position, the heels can be assessed clinically and compared with heel position before skin incision.

SURGICAL TECHNIQUE
Acetabular Component

Accurate acetabular and femoral component position is important for producing a dynamically stable THA. The goal of acetabular and femoral component position is to optimize impingement-free range of motion and thus provide stability in a variety of leg positions. The reported safe zone for cup position is 40° of inclination (±10°) and 20° of anteversion (±10°).[12] External reference alignment guides, intraoperative fluoroscopy, and anatomic landmarks can all assist with component positioning. External alignment guides that are fixed angle at 45° and placed on the face of the acetabular component help to assess overall cup position and version but may be altered with patient positioning. Fluoroscopy allows for intraoperative assessment of the inclination and version angles but also depends on accurate patient positioning and magnification. Anatomic landmarks include the transverse acetabular ligament (TAL), the acetabular sulcus on the ischium, the lateral aspect of the acetabulum, and the anterior wall (superior pubic rami). The TAL marks the inferior aspect of the cotyloid fossa and is a helpful intraoperative guide for native hip version.[13] A component that is flush with the acetabular sulcus on the ischium is also a guide for recreation of native acetabular version. Anteriorly, the component should be below the anterior wall to avoid the risk of psoas impingement. For inclination, the amount of lateral cup overhang should be compared with the preoperative radiograph. Because the native acetabulum is 62° on average,[14] there is a few millimeters of lateral component overhang in most cases.

Femoral Component

Femoral neck resection length, which is based on the preoperative template, is an excellent guide for final femoral component position. Most contemporary femoral stem designs come in both high offset and standard offset sizes. High femoral offset may produce direct lateralization or reduce the neck-shaft angle, which increases offset and reduces vertical neck length.

The acetabular and femoral component positions both contribute to overall hip stability and impingement-free range of motion. Combined anteversion, which represents the degrees of elevation of the operative leg with the knee flexed to 90° and the equator of the femoral head parallel to the rim of the acetabular component, should be between 25° and 50°. If the combined anteversion of both the acetabular and femoral component is less than 25°, then the risk for posterior instability increases (particularly in the posterior approach). Likewise, the risk for anterior instability increases if the combined anteversion is greater than 50°.[15]

INTRAOPERATIVE ASSESSMENT OF LIMB LENGTH AND HIP STABILITY
Soft Tissue Trialing

- Full extension, maximum external rotation (posterior impingement?)
- Position of sleep (flexion 45°, adduction) (subluxation?)
- 90° hip flexion, internal rotation (dislocation at <60°?)
- Shuck and drop-kick tests (femoral head clearance? Recoil?)
- Compare medial malleoli (if supine) and heel position (if lateral)

A simple method to assess limb length intraoperatively is to compare the location of the medial malleoli or the heels of both feet. The limb lengths should always be assessed at the beginning of the case and again with the trial components in place. The direct anterior approach or the anterolateral approach are performed supine and allow for direct comparison of the medial malleoli. For the posterior approach, the heels of can be compared before and after trial reduction. In addition, a femoral neck osteotomy in accordance with the preoperative template allows for accurate estimation of planned lengthening. The shuck and drop-kick tests are gross assessments of limb tension.[16] The shuck test refers to manual distraction of the hip prosthesis, and ideally the femoral head should not distract more than 50% of its diameter. The drop-kick test places the hip in neutral extension and then flexes the knee to 90° while assessing for the amount of recoil. A knee that cannot be flexed back to 90° or has excessive recoil with minimal knee flexion may have been lengthened. When performing either of these tests, it is important to recognize that anesthetic medication can increase soft tissue laxity. Alternatively, patients with preoperative soft tissue contractures may have increased recoil without excessive leg lengthening. For this reason, these 2 tests can be unreliable and are based on subjective surgeon experience.

Intraoperative range of motion testing confirms dynamic hip stability. The limb is taken through a series of positions and sites of prosthetic or bony impingement are identified. Leg extension and maximum external rotation identifies any posterior femoral neck-acetabular component impingement. The hip should remain stable in the position of sleep (45° of flexion and adduction). The hip is flexed to 90° with 10° of abduction and then internally rotated. The femoral head should remain reduced until at least 60° to 70° of internal rotation has been achieved. For the anterior or anterolateral approaches, which have intact posterior soft tissue structures, the location of dislocation is often anterior, and external rotation with the leg in full extension is the most important soft tissue test.

An elevated liner or face-changing liner may be used if the femoral head begins to dislocate at less than 60° of internal rotation with well-positioned components. An elevated liner should be placed with the maximum build-up in the location of subluxation, most commonly posterior-superior for the posterior approach. After insertion of an elevated liner, the hip should again be tested in full extension and maximum external rotation to rule out posterior prosthetic impingement.

IMPLANT DESIGN
Implant Options to Improve Hip Stability

- Larger femoral head sizes (32, 36, and 40 mm)
- Elevated or face-changing liners
- High offset stems
- Dual mobility (DM) devices
- Constrained liners

Larger femoral head sizes improve hip stability with better head/neck ratios and a larger jump distance.[9,17,18] With conventional polyethylene, larger head sizes were associated with more volumetric wear, but this problem has not been seen with highly cross-linked polyethylene (XLPE).[18] The downside of larger femoral heads, particularly cobalt-chrome heads on a titanium stem, is the risk of trunnion corrosion and associated adverse local soft tissue reaction, a process that is under investigation.[19] In addition, although XLPE has dramatically reduced wear rates, large femoral heads on thin XLPE should still be used cautiously in young active patients. A DM implant is an alternative bearing option for patients at a high risk for postoperative instability. A DM acetabular component is a tripolar design in which a smaller femoral head (22 or 28 mm) articulates within a larger XLPE bearing that itself articulates with a polished metal acetabular component. The larger outer XLPE bearing has a larger effective head size, which increases jump distance and improves overall stability.[17] The downside of these devices is the unique failure mode of intraprosthetic dislocation, which can occur with long-term wear of the inner articulation.[20]

MANAGEMENT OF INSTABILITY

Dislocation after THA has been classified as early (0–6 months), intermediate (6 months to 5 years), or late (after 5 years), and each time point is associated with a different underlying cause, risk of recurrence, and need for reoperation.[21] An early postoperative hip dislocation can usually be treated with a closed reduction if the components are in an acceptable position. Early dislocation is often secondary to patient risk factors and surgical errors in component position. Late dislocations are often secondary to loss of abductor function, polyethylene wear, osteolysis with trochanteric avulsion, or long-standing component malposition.[22,23] Late dislocations are at a higher risk for recurrence and need for reoperation. The surgical treatments for recurrent instability include revision of 1 or both components, exchange of modular components (femoral head and liner), or acetabular revision with possible conversion to a DM or constrained type device.

CLINICAL WORKUP FOR INSTABILITY
Key Elements of History and Physical Examination

- Duration since surgery
- Number of dislocations, direction, and mechanism
- Radiographs: evidence of osteolysis, trochanteric avulsion, polyethylene wear, component malposition, shortening of operative limb
- Clinical leg length measurements
- Abductor function

The underlying cause for the dislocation should be determined to develop an accurate treatment plan. Important information includes the number of previous dislocations, the time between dislocations, and the duration since surgery. Details of the previous surgical approach with implant information should also be obtained. Physical examination assessment includes evidence of limb length differences, signs of balance or spasticity problems, loss of abductor strength, or decreased peripheral sensation. Standard AP pelvic, lateral hip, and cross-table radiographs provide information regarding component position, leg length, and evidence of polyethylene wear or greater trochanteric fracture. A computed tomography scan is usually not required but may help assess version abnormalities of the acetabular and femoral components. In some cases, the history, physical examination, and radiographs do not elucidate a specific underlying cause for dislocation.

REOPERATION FOR INSTABILITY
Surgical Treatment

- Isolated liner exchange
- Increased head size and liner exchange
- Component revision
- DM device
- Constrained implant
- Abductor repair, reconstruction (allograft, gluteus maximus transfer, mesh)

Revision THA for recurrent instability is challenging problem with a redislocation rates as high as 35% at 15 years.[8] Patients with recurrent instability and acetabular component malposition should undergo component revision, because this intervention has a high likelihood of preventing further instability.[24] A constrained implant cemented into a malpositioned socket is associated with a high rate of failure and should be avoided.[25] Isolated liner exchanges have also been associated with higher rates of failure but an offset, face-changing, or lipped liner can be used effectively in a well-positioned cup when combined with femoral head upsizing.[26] Increasing femoral head size is an effective and simple solution because larger femoral head sizes have been shown to decrease dislocation rates in revision THA.[27] In a review of 539 hips revised for instability, the lowest rate of re-revision and redislocation occurred when a 36 mm or larger femoral head was used along with cup revision.

DM devices have shown excellent results in the treatment of recurrent instability after THA. Wegrzyn and colleagues[28] reviewed 994 revision THAs with a mean follow-up of 7.3 years. Sixty-eight patients were revised for instability with an overall dislocation rate of 1.5%, showing the effectiveness of DM devices in this high-risk group. A second study reported on 180 patients revised for instability to a DM bearing. At 7-year follow-up, there were 7 (4.8%) dislocations for the larger polyethylene articulation, 2 (1.4%) intraprosthetic

dislocations, and 3 re-revisions for instability. These mid-term results seem promising, but longer-term studies are needed to determine if this device can effectively decrease long-term rates of instability and reoperation.

A constrained liner is the final salvage option for recurrent instability. A constrained liner consists of a dual or tripolar articulation with a locking ring that mechanically captures the inner bearing. A constrained liner is best indicated for lower demand patients or those with significant neurologic impairment or abductor deficiency that precludes placement of a less constrained device. Constrained liners reduce range of motion before impingement and transmit greater loads across the bone-implant interface, which can lead to increased wear, osteolysis, and component failure. Guyen and colleagues[24] classified 5 types of failure modes with a tripolar constrained acetabular design and described failures at each interface. The survivorship of constrained liners varies considerably in the literature and is related to length of follow-up, patient cohort, and type of constrained device. A review of 8 studies[29] including 1199 hips with a mean follow-up of 51 months (range, 24–124 months) reported a 10% failure rate.

Soft tissue augmentation is another option in the treatment of recurrent instability but is rarely performed. The indication for these procedures may be deficiency of the hip abductor muscles, resulting in dislocation in the setting of a well-positioned and well-fixed THA. Reconstruction options include gluteus maximus advancement[22] or the use of an Achilles tendon allograft, tensor fascia lata, or even a synthetic mesh.[23] A trochanteric osteotomy and advancement can also be performed to increase soft tissue tensioning and, although rarely performed, it is a reasonable option in a young patient with soft tissue tension deficiency and good bone stock.

MANAGEMENT OF LEG LENGTH INEQUALITY

In most cases, postoperative limb length inequality is functional and is secondary to a flexible pelvic obliquity and resolving periarticular soft tissue contractures.[30] Patients with a true leg length difference are often asymptomatic. When a patient has a symptomatic leg length inequality, a shoe insert for the shorter limb is a simple and effective treatment strategy. For larger limb length inequalities and in patients who do not tolerate a shoe lift, revision surgery can be performed,[31] but the operative extremity should be shortened with caution because of the risk of postoperative instability.

Overview

Prevention of hip instability and limb length inequality after THA requires careful clinical examination and preoperative planning, accurate intraoperative execution, and a systematic approach to soft tissue stability testing. Early identification of patients at risk for postoperative instability and limb length inequality allows the treating surgeon to discuss these risk factors preoperatively and possibly alter surgical approach, implant design, or choice of type of bearing. Larger femoral heads, high offset stems, elevated rim liners, DM, and constrained liners can reduce the risk of postoperative instability when used appropriately. Although closed reduction of an isolated early dislocation is often successful, late or recurrent dislocations often require revision surgery. When possible, identify the underlying cause for dislocation (patient risk factor, component malposition, or soft tissue deficiency). A DM implant can be used with good success, but a constrained liner may be a considered in salvage situations in patients with severe abductor deficiency. Soft tissue reconstructions of the abductor mechanism with muscle transfer, allograft, and trochanteric advancement are rarely performed but could be an option in the young patient with good bone stock.

REFERENCES

1. Lavernia C, Iacobelli D, Brooks L, et al. The costutility of total hip arthroplasty: earlier intervention, improved economics. J Arthroplasty 2015;30(6): 945–9.
2. Chang RW, Pellisier JM, Hazen GB. A cost-effectiveness analysis of total hip arthroplasty for osteoarthritis of the hip. JAMA 1996;275(11):858–65.
3. Khanuja HS, Vakil JJ, Goddard MS, et al. Cementless femoral fixation in total hip arthroplasty. J Bone Joint Surg Am 2011;93(5):500–9.
4. Mahomed NN, Barrett JA, Katz JN, et al. Rates and outcomes of primary and revision total hip replacement in the United States Medicare population. J Bone Joint Surg Am 2003;85A(1):27–32.
5. Bozic KJ, Kurtz SM, Lau E, et al. The epidemiology of revision total hip arthroplasty in the United States. J Bone Joint Surg Am 2009;91(1):128–33.
6. Maloney WJ, Keeney JA. Leg length discrepancy after total hip arthroplasty. J Arthroplasty 2004;19(4 Suppl 1):108–10.
7. Lee BP, Berry DJ, Harmsen WS, et al. Total hip arthroplasty for the treatment of an acute fracture of the femoral neck: long-term results. J Bone Joint Surg Am 1998;80(1):70–5.
8. Jo S, Jimenez Almonte JH, Sierra RJ. The cumulative risk of re-dislocation after revision THA performed for instability increases close to 35% at 15years. J Arthroplasty 2015;30(7):1177–82.
9. Dudda M, Gueleryuez A, Gautier E, et al. Risk factors for early dislocation after total hip arthroplasty: a matched case-control study. J Orthop Surg (Hong Kong) 2010;18(2):179–83.
10. Meermans G, Malik A, Witt J, et al. Preoperative radiographic assessment of limb-length discrepancy in total hip arthroplasty. Clin Orthop Relat Res 2011;469(6):1677–82.
11. Horne PH, Olson SA. Direct anterior approach for total hip arthroplasty using the fracture table. Curr Rev Musculoskelet Med 2011;4(3):139–45.
12. Lewinnek GE, Lewis JL, Tarr R, et al. Dislocations after total hip-replacement arthroplasties. J Bone Joint Surg Am 1978;60(2):217–20.
13. Archbold HA, Mockford B, Molloy D, et al. The transverse acetabular ligament: an aid to orientation of the acetabular component during primary total hip replacement: a preliminary study of 1000 cases investigating postoperative stability. J Bone Joint Surg Br 2006;88(7):883–6.
14. Merle C, Grammatopoulos G, Waldstein W, et al. Comparison of native anatomy with recommended safe component orientation in total hip arthroplasty for primary osteoarthritis. J Bone Joint Surg Am 2013;95(22):e172.
15. Dorr LD, Malik A, Dastane M, et al. Combined anteversion technique for total hip arthroplasty. Clin Orthop Relat Res 2009;467(1):119–27.
16. Longjohn D, Dorr LD. Soft tissue balance of the hip. J Arthroplasty 1998;13(1):97–100.
17. Berry DJ, von Knoch M, Schleck CD, et al. Effect of femoral head diameter and operative approach on risk of dislocation after primary total hip arthroplasty. J Bone Joint Surg Am 2005;87(11):2456–63.
18. Lachiewicz PF, Heckman DS, Soileau ES, et al. Femoral head size and wear of highly cross-linked polyethylene at 5 to 8 years. Clin Orthop Relat Res 2009;467(12):3290–6.
19. Dudda M, Gueleryuez A, Gautier E, et al. Risk factors for early dislocation after total hip arthroplasty: a matched case-control study. J Orthop Surg (Hong Kong) 2010;18(2):179–83.
20. Cooper HJ, Della Valle CJ, Berger RA, et al. Corrosion at the head-neck taper as a cause for adverse local tissue reactions after total hip arthroplasty. J Bone Joint Surg Am 2012;94(18):1655–61.
21. De Martino I, Triantafyllopoulos GK, Sculco PK, et al. Dual mobility cups in total hip arthroplasty. World J Orthop 2014;5(3):180–7.
22. Whiteside LA. Surgical technique: gluteus maximus and tensor fascia lata transfer for primary deficiency of the abductors of the hip. Clin Orthop Relat Res 2014;472(2):645–53.
23. McGann WA, Welch RB. Treatment of the unstable total hip arthroplasty using modularity, soft tissue,

and allograft reconstruction. J Arthroplasty 2001; 16(8 Suppl 1):19–23.

24. Guyen O, Lewallen DG, Cabanela ME. Modes of failure of osteonics constrained tripolar implants: a retrospective analysis of forty-three failed implants. J Bone Joint Surg Am 2008;90(7):1553–60.

25. Callaghan JJ, O'Rourke MR, Goetz DD, et al. Use of a constrained tripolar acetabular liner to treat intraoperative instability and postoperative dislocation after total hip arthroplasty: a review of our experience. Clin Orthop Relat Res 2004;(429):117–23.

26. Pulido L, Restrepo C, Parvizi J. Late instability following total hip arthroplasty. Clin Med Res 2007; 5(2):139–42.

27. Howie DW, Holubowycz OT, Middleton R. Large femoral heads decrease the incidence of dislocation after total hip arthroplasty: a randomized controlled trial. J Bone Joint Surg Am 2012;94(12):1095–102.

28. Wegrzyn J, Tebaa E, Jacquel A, et al. Can dual mobility cups prevent dislocation in all situations after revision total hip arthroplasty? J Arthroplasty 2014;30(4):631–40.

29. Williams JT Jr, Ragland PS, Clarke S. Constrained components for the unstable hip following total hip arthroplasty: a literature review. Int Orthop 2007; 31(3):273–7.

30. Ranawat CS, Rodriguez JA. Functional leg-length inequality following total hip arthroplasty. J Arthroplasty 1997;12(4):359–64.

31. Parvizi J, Sharkey PF, Bissett GA, et al. Surgical treatment of limb-length discrepancy following total hip arthroplasty. J Bone Joint Surg Am 2003; 85A(12):2310–7.

Trauma

Thromboembolic Disease After Orthopedic Trauma

 CrossMark

Paul S. Whiting, MD[a], A. Alex Jahangir, MD, MMHC[b],*

KEYWORDS

- Orthopaedic trauma • Coagulation • Deep venous thrombosis • Pulmonary embolism
- Thromboprophylaxis

KEY POINTS

- Traumatic musculoskeletal injury results in systemic physiologic changes that predispose patients to venous thromboembolism (VTE).
- Combined mechanical and pharmacologic thromboprophylaxis is most efficacious for decreasing VTE incidence.
- Low molecular weight heparin is the preferred agent for pharmacologic thromboprophylaxis.
- Pharmacologic prophylaxis should be initiated as soon as possible, and should be continue for a minimum of 14 days.
- Patients with isolated lower extremity fractures who are ambulatory do not require pharmacologic prophylaxis in the absence of other VTE risk factors.

PHYSIOLOGY AND EPIDEMIOLOGY OF VENOUS THROMBOEMBOLISM IN TRAUMA

Basic Science and Physiology of Trauma and Coagulation

Traumatic injury results in significant physiologic changes. Serum levels of inflammatory cytokines including interleukin-6 (IL-6), IL-8, and tumor necrosis factor-alpha (TNF-α) are increased following traumatic injury and result in a hypercoagulable state.[1] In addition to inflammatory markers, serum levels and activity of procoagulant microparticles are significantly increased following blunt trauma, and peak thrombin levels are correlated to injury severity.[2,3] The systemic inflammatory response triggered by traumatic injury results in a hypercoagulable state that places patients at increased risk of venous thromboembolism (VTE).[4] This hypercoagulability combined with endothelial injury and venous stasis, 2 other conditions often noted

in trauma patients, completes the Virchow Triad. The presence of all 3 elements contributes to venous thrombosis.

Venous Thromboembolism Following Major Trauma

Before the implementation of routine thromboprophylaxis, reported rates of VTE following major trauma were extremely high. Using bilateral lower extremity venography, Geerts and colleagues[5] reported a 58% incidence of lower extremity deep vein thrombosis (DVT) in 349 patients admitted for major traumatic injuries who did not receive thromboprophylaxis. DVT rates varied by anatomic region injured, ranging from 50% in patients with major injuries to the face, chest, or abdomen to 80% in patients with femur fractures. The rate of fatal pulmonary embolism (PE) was 0.9%, and independent risk factors for DVT

Disclosures: Neither author has any potential conflicts of interest.
a Department of Orthopaedics and Rehabilitation, University of Wisconsin, 1685 Highland Avenue, Madison, WI 53705, USA; b Department of Orthopaedics and Rehabilitation, Vanderbilt University Medical Center, 1215 21st Avenue South, MCE South Tower, Suite 4200, Nashville, TN 37232, USA
* Corresponding author.
E-mail address: alex.jahangir@vanderbilt.edu

Orthop Clin N Am 47 (2016) 335–344
http://dx.doi.org/10.1016/j.ocl.2015.09.002
0030-5898/16/$ – see front matter © 2016 Elsevier Inc. All rights reserved.

identified included age, blood transfusion, surgery, fracture of the femur or tibia, and spinal cord injury. Despite its relatively low incidence, PE is still the third most common cause of in-hospital death among trauma patients.[6]

Thromboprophylaxis for Venous Thromboembolism in Trauma Patients

Both chemical and mechanical thromboprophylaxis has been shown to decrease rates of VTE in the setting of trauma.[7,8] Pharmacologic prophylaxis with low molecular weight heparin (LMWH) was shown to significantly decrease the incidence of both DVT and PE in a large cohort of more than 2200 trauma patients.[9] Mechanical prophylaxis with pneumatic sequential compression devices (SCDs) significantly decreased VTE incidence from 11% to 4% ($P = .02$) in a prospective randomized controlled trial of 300 orthopedic trauma patients compared with no VTE prophylaxis.[10] A growing understanding of the importance of thromboprophylaxis in trauma patients has led to the development of institutional protocols for VTE prophylaxis at trauma centers around the world. Additionally, several professional organizations have published clinical guidelines for thromboprophylaxis in trauma patients, which are summarized in **Table 1**.[8,11-13]

More recent literature using larger patient cohorts and routine thromboprophylaxis protocols has better defined the true incidence of clinically relevant VTE following severe trauma. A retrospective review of a multicenter trauma registry containing nearly 8000 major trauma patients identified a VTE incidence of only 1.8% when institutional thromboprophylaxis protocols were used.[14] Despite the relatively low incidence, the presence of VTE (either DVT or PE) nearly doubled the mortality rate (13.7% vs 7.4%), and among patients who developed a PE, the mortality rate was 25.7%. A single-center retrospective review of more than 1300 major trauma patients treated at a level 1 trauma center revealed a 2.3% incidence of PE.[15] All PEs occurred within 15 days of injury, with most being diagnosed within the first week. Age older than 55 years, multisystem injury, cannulation of central veins, and pelvic fractures (but not long-bone fractures) were independent risk factors for developing a PE. Using a statewide trauma database over a 5-year period, Tuttle-Newhall and colleagues[16] reported an overall PE incidence of 0.3% among more than 300,000 trauma patients receiving standard VTE prophylaxis. Age older than 55 was a significant risk factor for development of PE, with an incidence of 0.7% in this demographic. Increasing Injury Severity

Score (ISS) and Abbreviated Injury Scale (AIS) for the extremities, soft tissue, and chest regions were also associated with significantly increased risk of PE.

VENOUS THROMBOEMBOLISM AND ORTHOPEDIC TRAUMA

Compared with the abundance of data relevant to venous thromboembolism in the general trauma population, high-quality evidence specific to VTE prophylaxis and treatment in the orthopedic trauma population is relatively limited. The available literature is summarized as follows and organized by fracture location when possible. In addition, the Orthopedic Trauma Association's Evidence-Based Quality Value and Safety Committee has recently produced a therapeutic algorithm to guide VTE prophylaxis in orthopedic trauma patients. A portion of this algorithm has been presented[13] and publication in its entirety is forthcoming.

Epidemiology and Risk Factors

Using the National Trauma Data Bank (NTDB), Godzik and colleagues[17] investigated the incidence of PE in 200,000 patients with pelvic and lower extremity fractures who received thromboprophylaxis according to the protocols of each institution. The overall incidence of PE was 0.46%, and the in-hospital mortality rate among patients who developed PE was 12%. These investigators also identified independent risk factors for PE in this patient population, including multiple fractures, history of warfarin use, morbid obesity, and emergency department disposition to an intensive care unit or to the operating room. **Table 2** summarizes the literature documenting VTE incidence and risk factors in orthopedic trauma patients.

Thromboprophylaxis

Both mechanical and chemical thromboprophylaxis have been shown to decrease rates of VTE following orthopedic trauma.[7,8,10] Fisher and colleagues[10] conducted a prospective randomized controlled trial comparing pneumatic SCDs with no VTE prophylaxis in 300 orthopedic trauma patients. Mechanical thromboprophylaxis significantly decreased VTE incidence from 11% to 4% ($P = .02$). In another prospective randomized trial, Stannard and colleagues[7] reported equivalent efficacy of mechanical and pharmacologic prophylaxis for DVT prevention following blunt skeletal trauma. The most recent Cochrane database systematic review found that pharmacologic prophylaxis was more effective than mechanical prophylaxis at reducing DVT risk.[8] Thromboprophylaxis in orthopedic trauma patients does not completely eliminate the risk of VTE, however. Using duplex ultrasound and magnetic resonance venography, Stannard and colleagues[18] reported a DVT rate of 11.5% in patients who sustained high-energy skeletal trauma despite pharmacologic prophylaxis.

Anticoagulation Agents

The use of low-dose unfractionated heparin (UH) (5000 units given subcutaneously 2 or 3 times a day) for VTE prophylaxis among orthopedic trauma patients is not supported in the literature.[13] In a prospective randomized trial of trauma patients with an ISS of 9 or greater and no intracranial bleeding, LMWH resulted in a 58% reduction in proximal DVT ($P = .012$) and a 30% reduction in total DVT incidence ($P = .014$) compared with UH and was not associated with increased bleeding complications.[19] All 4 evidence-based guidelines recommend LMWH as the preferred pharmacologic prophylactic agent for VTE prophylaxis following trauma.

Several new oral anticoagulants have been developed that function either as direct thrombin inhibitors or direct factor Xa inhibitors. A recent systematic review of these agents in total joint arthroplasty demonstrated slightly improved efficacy for DVT prevention but slightly increased rates of major bleeding complications.[20] One retrospective cohort study comparing rivaroxaban with LMWH reported a significantly decreased rate of symptomatic VTE in the rivaroxaban group (4.9% vs 8.6%, $P = .008$).[21] A systematic review of semuloparin, an ultra-LMWH, showed improved efficacy of this agent compared with LMWH in VTE prevention following total hip arthroplasty, but there were no differences seen following total knee arthroplasty or hip fractures.[22] Large-scale prospective studies are required to better elucidate the efficacy and safety of these newer anticoagulants.

Complications of Anticoagulation

A recent multicenter study reported outcomes and complications from therapeutic anticoagulation for symptomatic PE following orthopedic trauma.[23] The most common complication of anticoagulation was surgical site bleeding, occurring at a rate of 10%. Other complications reported include gastrointestinal bleeding, anemia, wound complications, compartment syndrome, and death. In light of these serious potential complications, the decision to initiate therapeutic anticoagulation

must involve an assessment of the size and location of the clot as well as the potential risks/benefits of anticoagulant therapy.[24]

Timing of Anticoagulation

Nathens and colleagues[25] reported an 11% incidence of VTE among 315 patients who had hemorrhagic shock after injury and had an intensive care unit stay of at least 7 days. Because anticoagulation was contraindicated in many patients for several days, the impact of timing to prophylaxis on VTE incidence was investigated. A delay in initiation of thromboprophylaxis beyond 4 days was associated with a relative risk of 3.0 for VTE compared with the initiation within 48 hours of injury.

Coordination of care in the polytraumatized patient requires excellent communication between the general surgery trauma service and consulting services, including orthopedic, neurosurgical, urologic, and other surgical specialists. Developing an effective system for regular communication between services can facilitate initiation of VTE prophylaxis as soon as possible while preventing premature anticoagulation in the setting of medical contraindications and avoiding delays in planned surgical interventions.[26] Phelan and colleagues[27] reported no difference in traumatic brain injury progression with enoxaparin versus placebo when started more than 24 hours after injury. The Orthopedic Trauma Association (OTA) evidence-based VTE prophylaxis guidelines include recommendations regarding the safety and timing of initiating anticoagulation in patients with orthopedic trauma with associated solid organ injuries and/or closed head injuries.[13]

Duration of Thromboprophylaxis

The duration of chemical prophylaxis following orthopedic trauma has yet to be elucidated clearly in the literature. A systematic review of standard (7–10 days) versus prolonged (28 days or more) duration of thromboprophylaxis showed a benefit to prolonged therapy in patients with total hip arthroplasty, but data were insufficient to demonstrate the same benefit in patients with hip fracture.[28] However, Rasmussen and colleagues[29] reported that prolonged thromboprophylaxis with LMWH significantly reduced the risk of VTE compared with prophylaxis during hospital admission only. Similarly, Huo and Muntz[30] reported the efficacy and cost-effectiveness of prolonged thromboprophylaxis in surgical patients at high risk for VTE, demonstrating that the increased pharmacy costs associated with prolonged

Table 1
Evidence-based guidelines for venous thromboembolism prophylaxis in orthopedic trauma

Organization	Summary of Findings and Recommendations
Cochrane database systematic review	• Mechanical and pharmacologic prophylaxis independently reduce risk of DVT, RR = 0.43 • Pharmacologic prophylaxis is more effective than mechanical at reducing DVT risk, RR = 0.48 • Combined mechanical and pharmacologic prophylaxis results in the lowest risk of DVT, RR = 0.34 • LMWH reduces DVT risk more effectively than unfractionated heparin, RR = 0.68 • No high-quality evidence that thromboprophylaxis reduces mortality or PE • Recommend the use of any DVT prophylactic method for patients with severe trauma
American College of Chest Physicians (ACCP)	In patients undergoing major orthopedic surgery: • Recommend using a pharmacologic thromboprophylaxis agent (Grade 1B) or IPCDs (Grade 1C) for a minimum of 10–14 d and considering extending pharmacologic thromboprophylaxis for up to 35 d (Grade 2B). • Suggest using LMWH in preference to other pharmacologic agents (Grade 2B/2C) and adding an IPCDs to pharmacologic prophylaxis during the inpatient hospital stay (Grade 2C) • Suggest IPCDs or no prophylaxis for patients at increased bleeding risk (Grade 2C) • Suggest against "prophylactic" IVC filter placement (Grade 2C) and recommend against duplex ultrasound screening for DVT before hospital discharge (Grade 1B) In patients with isolated lower extremity injuries below the knee requiring immobilization without a history of VTE: • Suggest no thromboprophylaxis (Grade 2B)
Eastern Association for the Surgery of Trauma (EAST)	• Risk Factors for VTE: Spinal fractures or SCI (level I), older age, ISS, blood transfusion, long-bone fracture, pelvic fracture, head injury (level II) • Little evidence to support low-dose unfractionated heparin as sole thromboprophylaxis agent (level II) • IPCDs (or foot pumps if the calf is inaccessible) may have some benefit in patients with spine injuries or head trauma (level III) • LMWH may be used in patients with pelvic fractures requiring surgery, complex lower extremity fractures, or complete SCI with motor involvement (level II) • LMWH should be used as primary prophylaxis in trauma patients with ISS >9 and should be considered for several weeks after injury in patients at high risk for VTE (level III) • IVC filters should be inserted for the following indications: ○ Recurrent PE, proximal DVT, or progression of iliofemoral DVT while on full anticoagulation (level I) ○ Large/free-floating IVC/iliac thrombi, following massive PE, during/after surgical embolectomy (level II) • "Prophylactic" IVC filters should be considered in patients with the following high-risk injury patterns: ○ Severe closed head injury (GCS<8), incomplete SCI with motor involvement, complex pelvic fracture with associated long-bone fracture, multiple long-bone fractures (level III) • Duplex ultrasound should be used to assess symptomatic trauma patients with suspected DVT (level I) but should not be used for screening asymptomatic patients (level III) • Ascending venography may be useful for confirming a diagnosis of DVT when ultrasound is equivocal (level III), and there may be a role for MR venography in the diagnosis of DVT in the acute setting, especially in areas in which venography and ultrasound are less reliable (level III)

Orthopedic Trauma Association (OTA)	In hospitalized orthopedic trauma patients:
	• In the absence of contraindications, LMWH is the agent of choice and should be initiated as soon as possible, preferably within 24 h (Strong)
	• Combined LMWH and IPCDs are preferable to either regimen alone (Strong)
	• If anticoagulation is contraindicated, patients at low risk for VTE should be treated with IPCDs (Moderate) and those at high risk should be considered candidates for prophylactic IVC filter placement (Limited)
	• Continuation of VTE prophylaxis for at least 1 mo after discharge may be considered (Limited)
	• Screening for DVT in asymptomatic patients is not recommended (Strong)
	• Anticoagulation can be initiated safely after 24 h in the setting of hemodynamically stable solid organ injuries or closed head injuries in the absence of ongoing bleeding or injury progression. Approval from the treating general or neurosurgeon should be obtained before initiating treatment. (Limited)
	In patients with isolated unilateral lower extremity injury who are ambulatory:
	• Anticoagulation on hospital discharge is not required in the absence of other VTE risk factors (Moderate)

Recommendation Strengths:

• ACCP: 1B = strong recommendation, moderate-quality evidence, benefits clearly outweigh risk and burdens or vice versa; 1C = strong recommendation, low-quality or very low quality evidence, benefits clearly outweigh risks and burdens or vice versa; 2B = weak recommendation, moderate-quality evidence, benefits closely balanced with risks and burdens; 2C = weak recommendation, low-quality or very low quality evidence, uncertainty in the estimates of benefits, risks, and burdens; benefits, risk, and burden may be closely balanced

• EAST: Level I recommendation = convincingly justifiable on the basis of scientific information alone through class I data; level II recommendation = reasonably justifiable on the basis of a preponderance of class II data; level III recommendation = supported only by class III data; Class I data = prospective randomized controlled trial; Class II data = clinical study with prospectively collected data or large retrospective analyses with reliable data; Class III data = retrospective data, expert opinion, or a case report.

• OTA: Strong = >2 high-quality (level I) studies to support the recommendation; Moderate: 1 high-quality (level I) or 2 moderate-quality (level II or III) studies to support the recommendation; Limited = 1 moderate-quality (level II or III) or 2 low-quality (level IV) studies to support the recommendation; Inconclusive = 1 low-quality (level IV) study or lack of evidence to support the recommendation; Consensus = expert work-group opinion (no studies)

Abbreviations: DVT, deep venous thrombosis; GCS, Glasgow Coma Scale; IPCD, intermittent pneumatic compression device; ISS, Injury Severity Score; IVC, inferior vena cava; LMWH, low molecular weight heparin; MR, magnetic resonance; PE, pulmonary embolism; RR, relative risk; SCI, spinal cord injury; VTE, venous thromboembolism.

Data from Refs.[8,11–13]

Table 2
Incidence and risk factors for venous thromboembolism in orthopedic trauma

Study	Study Design, Patient Population	n	Prophylaxis Used?	Incidence of VTE	Risk Factors for VTE Identified
Geerts et al 1994	Single-center prospective cohort, major trauma patients	349	No	58% (1% fatal PE)	Age, blood transfusion, surgery, fracture of the femur or tibia, and spinal cord injury
O'Malley et al 1990	Single-center retrospective cohort, major trauma patients	1316	Yes	2.3% (PE)	Age >55 y, multisystem injury, cannulation of central veins, and pelvic fractures (but not long-bone fractures)
Paffrath et al 2010	Multicenter retrospective cohort, major trauma patients	7937	Yes	1.8% (PE)	ISS score, pelvic AIS score 2 or higher, number of operations, medical comorbidities (diabetes, renal failure, malignancy, coagulation disorders)
Tuttle-Newhall et al 1997	Statewide trauma registry, major trauma patients	318,554	Yes	0.3% (PE)	Age >55 y, increasing ISS and AIS (extremity, soft tissue, chest regions)
Godzik et al 2014	Retrospective database review, orthopedic trauma patients	199,952	Yes	0.46% (PE)	Multiple fractures, history of warfarin use, morbid obesity, ED disposition to ICU or OR
Fisher et al 1995	Prospective RCT (SCDs vs none), orthopedic trauma patients	304	Yes/No	11% vs 4%	11% incidence for control group, 4% incidence in experimental group
Stannard et al 2005	Prospective cohort study, orthopedic trauma patients	312	Yes	11.5%	11.5% incidence of VTE despite prophylaxis

Abbreviations: AIS, Abbreviated Injury Scale; ED, emergency department; ICU, intensive care unit; ISS, Injury Severity Score; OR, operating room; PE, pulmonary embolism; RCT, randomized controlled trial; SCD, sequential compression device; VTE, venous thromboembolism.
Data from Refs.[5,10,14–18]

prophylaxis are offset by the reduction in hospital costs associated with episodes of VTE.

Inferior Vena Cava Filters

The Eastern Association for the Surgery of Trauma (EAST) guidelines, published in 2002, suggested that "prophylactic" IVC filters were warranted in specific trauma patients with risk factors for PE. Subsequent literature has documented a significant reduction in PE rates with IVC filters. However, IVC filters have not shown a clear benefit with respect to mortality and their use may be associated with an increased incidence of symptomatic DVT.[31–33] Two additional studies exploring the cost-effectiveness of prophylactic IVC filters concluded that this practice is not cost-effective.[34] Therefore, as outlined in the OTA evidence-based algorithm, IVC filters should be reserved for PE prophylaxis in high-risk trauma patients with a contraindication to anticoagulation.

SPECIFIC FRACTURE PATTERNS
Pelvic and Acetabular Fractures

As previously mentioned, Fisher and colleagues[10] conducted a prospective randomized controlled trial to assess the effectiveness of pneumatic SCDs in 300 patients with pelvic or hip fractures. VTE incidence was significantly lower in the SCD group compared with the control group (4% vs 11%, $P = .02$). Stannard and colleagues[35] conducted a randomized, controlled trial of 2 methods of mechanical VTE prophylaxis (thigh-calf low-pressure SCDs and calf-foot high pressure pulsatile-compression pumps) in 107 patients with pelvic and acetabular fractures. Compared with patients in the standard SCD group, fewer patients in the pulsatile SCD group developed DVTs (9% vs 19%) and large/occlusive clots (4% vs 13%), although with the number of patients studied, the results did not reach statistical significance. In a prospective cohort of 221 patients who sustained high-energy pelvic trauma, DVT was identified using magnetic resonance venography and duplex ultrasound in 12.2% of patients despite thromboprophylaxis.[18] Forty-eight percent of these clots were in the deep pelvic veins, and duplex ultrasound had a 77% false-negative rate for diagnosing pelvic DVT. Slobogean and colleagues[36] performed a systematic review of the literature with respect to VTE following pelvic and acetabular trauma. Due to significant heterogeneity of the 11 included studies, quantitative pooling was not possible, and the investigators concluded that surgeons have limited high-quality data to guide clinical management of

thromboprophylaxis in this specific patient population.

Fractures Below the Knee

Historically, the literature has recommended routine thromboprophylaxis for lower extremity fractures distal to the knee. The most recent Cochrane database systematic review reported a VTE incidence ranging from 4.3% to 40.0% following lower leg immobilization for nonoperative fracture treatment without thromboprophylaxis.[37] VTE incidence was significantly lower in patients who received LMWH, with an odds ratio of 0.49 compared with no thromboprophylaxis or placebo. Another study identified a 20% incidence of venographic DVT in outpatients immobilized in a plaster cast for a lower leg fracture.[38] The authors recommended routine thromboprophylaxis in this patient population.

However, a growing body of literature suggests that the rate of symptomatic VTE in patients with distal lower extremity fractures is much lower than previously reported, leading several investigators to suggest that routine thromboprophylaxis is not required following fractures distal to the knee.[39–41] In a prospective cohort study of more than 200 patients who underwent foot and ankle surgery and did not receive thromboprophylaxis, Solis and Saxby[39] reported a DVT incidence of only 3.5% using routine bilateral lower extremity duplex ultrasound for diagnosis. On follow-up ultrasound, none of the DVTs identified showed signs of progression or extension proximal to the calf. Using Doppler ultrasound at the time of cast removal, Patil and colleagues[40] reported a 5% incidence of DVT in patients with ankle fractures treated with cast immobilization. None of these patients had clinical signs of DVT, and none of the patients developed PE. Using the NTDB, Shibuya and colleagues[41] reported a 0.28% incidence of DVT and 0.21% incidence of PE in patients with isolated foot and ankle trauma. As routine venography was not performed, only symptomatic DVT and PE were identified in this cohort.

Goel and colleagues[42] conducted a prospective randomized controlled trial of LMWH versus placebo in patients with operatively treated fractures below the knee. Using routine bilateral venography, there was no statistically significant difference in DVT incidence between groups ($P = .22$). Interestingly, due to a cessation in funding, the study was stopped before recruiting the necessary sample size calculated in the power analysis. In the discussion, the investigators acknowledge that the trend toward a decreased incidence of

DVT in the LMWH group (8.7%) compared with the control group (12.6%) might have reached statistical significance with a larger sample size. In a recent multicenter prospective cohort study of 1200 patients with distal lower extremity fractures who did not receive thromboprophylaxis (the knee-to-ankle fracture cohort), Selby and colleagues[43] reported an overall incidence of symptomatic, objectively confirmed VTE of only 0.6%. There were only 5 cases of lower extremity DVT and 2 cases of PE, neither of which was fatal. Based on their findings, the investigators suggested that routine thromboprophylaxis in this patient population is not favorable from a risk-benefit or a cost-effectiveness perspective. Although this study did not compare LMWH with placebo and therefore did not definitively reproduce the findings of Goel and colleagues,[42] the extremely low incidence of symptomatic VTE is compelling evidence that routine thromboprophylaxis is not necessary for fractures below the knee.

Upper Extremity Fractures

The literature exploring VTE following upper extremity trauma is extremely limited. The incidence of VTE in patients with isolated upper extremity injuries is estimated to be between 1% and 5%.[24] Hsu and colleagues[44] identified a cohort of more than 600 patients with isolated upper extremity injuries treated over an 11-year period. Overall VTE incidence was 4.95% (DVT 4.64%, PE 0.31%), a rate equivalent to that in hospitalized patients without upper extremity trauma. The investigators concluded that major upper extremity trauma is not an independent risk factor for VTE, and no additional prophylaxis is required in the absence of other patient risk factors.

HEALTH POLICY AND ECONOMIC CONSIDERATIONS

In the absence of prophylaxis, rates of VTE following orthopedic trauma may be as high as 60%. Institutional protocols for thromboprophylaxis have dramatically reduced the incidence of VTE in this patient population. Nonetheless, quality improvement initiatives often define DVT and PE as preventable events, and health care systems will become increasingly accountable for their occurrence.

With the recent implementation of bundled payment systems for certain orthopedic diagnoses, hospitals will no longer receive additional reimbursement for the costs associated with managing postoperative complications during the 90-day global period following surgery. Consequently, readmissions for DVT or PE following orthopedic trauma admissions will represent a significant burden for health care systems. This reality underscores the importance of developing efficacious protocols for VTE prophylaxis in patients with orthopedic trauma.

In addition, establishing meaningful performance benchmarks for complication rates requires reliable data from which to derive reference standards. Large-scale databases present significant advantages for determining baseline epidemiologic data. However, Kardooni and colleagues[45] have reported on the potential hazards of using the NTDB for this purpose. Due to the significant variability in practices for reporting complications among the institutions that contribute to the NTDB, researchers must be conscientious in carefully selecting the appropriate numerators and denominators when conducting research from large databases that will serve as the benchmarks that define quality care.

SUMMARY

Patients with orthopedic trauma are at significant risk for VTE. Effective mechanical and pharmacologic prophylaxis decreases the risk of developing VTE, most notably symptomatic and fatal PE. High-quality basic science and clinical research are necessary for developing evidence-based protocols, which will in turn serve to decrease the morbidity and mortality associated with VTE following orthopedic trauma.

REFERENCES

1. Riha GM, Kunio NR, Van PY, et al. Uncontrolled hemorrhagic shock results in a hypercoagulable state modulated by initial fluid resuscitation regimens. J Trauma Acute Care Surg 2013;75(1):129–34.
2. Park MS, Owen BA, Ballinger BA, et al. Quantification of hypercoagulable state after blunt trauma: microparticle and thrombin generation are increased relative to injury severity, while standard markers are not. Surgery 2012;151(6):831–6.
3. Owen BA, Xue A, Heit JA, et al. Procoagulant activity, but not number, of microparticles increases with age and in individuals after a single venous thromboembolism. Thromb Res 2011;127(1):39–46.
4. Holley AD, Reade MC. The 'procoagulopathy' of trauma: too much, too late? Curr Opin Crit Care 2013;19(6):578–86.
5. Geerts WH, Code KI, Jay RM, et al. A prospective study of venous thromboembolism after major trauma. N Engl J Med 1994;331(24):1601–6.
6. Shackford SR, Mackersie RC, Holbrook TL, et al. The epidemiology of traumatic death. A

population-based analysis. Arch Surg 1993;128(5): 571–5.

7. Stannard JP, Lopez-Ben RR, Volgas DA, et al. Prophylaxis against deep-vein thrombosis following trauma: a prospective, randomized comparison of mechanical and pharmacologic prophylaxis. J Bone Joint Surg Am 2006;88(2):261–6.

8. Barrera LM, Perel P, Ker K, et al. Thromboprophylaxis for trauma patients. Cochrane Database Syst Hev 2013;(3):CD008303.

9. Gritsiouk Y, Hegsted DA, Schlesinger P, et al. A retrospective analysis of the effectiveness of low molecular weight heparin for venous thromboembolism prophylaxis in trauma patients. Am J Surg 2014; 207(5):648–51 [discussion: 651–2].

10. Fisher CG, Blachut PA, Salvian AJ, et al. Effectiveness of pneumatic leg compression devices for the prevention of thromboembolic disease in orthopaedic trauma patients: a prospective, randomized study of compression alone versus no prophylaxis. J Orthop Trauma 1995;9(1):1–7.

11. Falck-Ytter Y, Francis CW, Johanson NA, et al. American College of Chest Physicians: prevention of VTE in orthopedic surgery patients: antithrombotic therapy and prevention of thrombosis, 9th ed: American College of Chest Physicians evidence-based clinical practice guidelines. Chest 2012;141(2 suppl): e278S–325S.

12. Rogers FB, Cipolle MD, Velmahos G, et al. Practice management guidelines for the prevention of venous thromboembolism in trauma patients: the EAST practice management guidelines work group. J Trauma 2002;53(1):142–64.

13. Sagi HC, Ciesla D, Collinge C, et al. Orthopedic Trauma Association Evidence Based Quality Value and Safety Committee: synopsis of current practice patterns and a suggested evidence-based therapeutic algorithm for venous thromboembolism prophylaxis in orthopaedic trauma patients. Presented at Orthopaedic Trauma Association Annual Meeting. Minneapolis, October 3–6, 2012.

14. Paffrath T, Wafaisade A, Lefering R, et al. Trauma registry of DGU. Venous thromboembolism after severe trauma: incidence, risk factors and outcome. Injury 2010;41(1):97–101.

15. O'Malley KF, Ross SE. Pulmonary embolism in major trauma patients. J Trauma 1990;30(6):748–50.

16. Tuttle-Newhall JE, Rutledge R, Hultman CS, et al. Statewide, population-based, time-series analysis of the frequency and outcome of pulmonary embolus in 318,554 trauma patients. J Trauma 1997;42(1):90–9.

17. Godzik J, McAndrew CM, Morshed S, et al. Multiple lower-extremity and pelvic fractures increase pulmonary embolus risk. Orthopedics 2014;37(6):e517–24.

18. Stannard JP, Singhania AK, Lopez-Ben RR, et al. Deep-vein thrombosis in high-energy skeletal trauma despite thromboprophylaxis. J Bone Joint Surg Br 2005;87(7):965–8.

19. Geerts WH, Jay RM, Code KI, et al. A comparison of low-dose heparin with low-molecular-weight heparin as prophylaxis against venous thromboembolism after major trauma. N Engl J Med 1996; 335(10):701–7.

20. Adam SS, McDuffie JR, Lachiewicz PF, et al. Comparative effectiveness of new oral anticoagulants and standard thromboprophylaxis in patients having total hip or knee replacement: a systematic review. Ann Intern Med 2013;159(4):275–84.

21. Long A, Zhang L, Zhang Y, et al. Efficacy and safety of rivaroxaban versus low-molecular-weight heparin therapy in patients with lower limb fractures. J Thromb Thrombolysis 2014;38(3):299–305.

22. Lassen MR, Fisher W, Mouret P, et al, SAVE Investigators. Semuloparin for prevention of venous thromboembolism after major orthopedic surgery: results from three randomized clinical trials, SAVE-HIP1, SAVE-HIP2 and SAVEKNEE. J Thromb Haemost 2012;10(5):822–32.

23. Bogdan Y, Tornetta P III, Leighton R, et al. Treatment and complications in orthopaedic trauma patients with symptomatic pulmonary embolism. J Orthop Trauma 2014;28(suppl 1):S6–9.

24. Scolaro JA, Taylor RM, Wigner NA. Venous thromboembolism in orthopaedic trauma. J Am Acad Orthop Surg 2015;23(1):1–6.

25. Nathens AB, McMurray MK, Cuschieri J, et al. The practice of venous thromboembolism prophylaxis in the major trauma patient. J Trauma 2007;62(3): 557–62 [discussion: 562–3].

26. Stinner DJ, Brooks SE, Fras AR, et al. Caring for the polytrauma patient: is your system surviving or thriving? Am J Orthop (Belle Mead NJ) 2013;42(5):E33–4.

27. Phelan HA, Wolf SE, Norwood SH, et al. A randomized, double-blinded, placebo controlled pilot trial of anticoagulation in low-risk traumatic brain injury: the Delayed Versus Early Enoxaparin Prophylaxis I (DEEP I) study. J Trauma Acute Care Surg 2012;73(6):1434–41.

28. Sobieraj DM, Coleman CI, Tongbram V, et al. Venous thromboembolism prophylaxis in orthopedic surgery. Rockville (MD): Agency for Healthcare Research and Quality (US); 2012. Report No.: 12-EHC020-EF. Accessed August 14, 2015. http://effectivehealthcare. ahrq.gov/index.cfm/search-for-guides-reviews-and-reports/?productid=999&pageaction=displayproduct.

29. Rasmussen MS, Jørgensen LN, Wille-Jørgensen P. Prolonged thromboprophylaxis with low molecular weight heparin for abdominal or pelvic surgery. Cochrane Database Syst Rev 2009;(1):CD004318.

30. Huo MH, Muntz J. Extended thromboprophylaxis with low-molecular-weight heparins after hospital discharge in high-risk surgical and medical patients: a review. Clin Ther 2009;31(6):1129–41.

31. Young T, Tang H, Hughes R. Vena caval filters for the prevention of pulmonary embolism [review]. Cochrane Database Syst Rev 2010;(2):CD006212.

32. PREPIC Study Group. Eight-year follow-up of patients with permanent vena cava filters in the prevention of pulmonary embolism: the PREPIC (Prevention du Risque d'Embolie Pulmonaire par Interruption Cave) randomized study. Circulation 2005;112(3): 416–22.

33. Rajasekhar A, Lottenberg R, Lottenberg L, et al. Pulmonary embolism prophylaxis with inferior vena cava filters in trauma patients: a systematic review using the meta-analysis of observational studies in epidemiology (MOOSE) guidelines [review]. J Thromb Thrombolysis 2011;32(1):40–6.

34. Chiasson TC, Manns BJ, Stelfox HT. An economic evaluation of venous thromboembolism prophylaxis strategies in critically ill trauma patients at risk of bleeding. PLoS Med 2009;6(6). E1000098.

35. Stannard JP, Riley RS, McClenney MD, et al. Mechanical prophylaxis against deep-vein thrombosis after pelvic and acetabular fractures. J Bone Joint Surg Am 2001;83-A(7):1047–51.

36. Slobogean GP, Lefaivre KA, Nicolaou S, et al. A systematic review of thromboprophylaxis for pelvic and acetabular fractures. J Orthop Trauma 2009;23(5):379–84.

37. Testroote M, Stigter WA, Janssen L, et al. Low molecular weight heparin for prevention of venous thromboembolism in patients with lower-leg immobilization. Cochrane Database Syst Rev 2014;(4): CD006681.

38. Jørgensen PS, Warming T, Hansen K, et al. Low molecular weight heparin (Innohep) as thromboprophylaxis in outpatients with a plaster cast: a venographic controlled study. Thromb Res 2002;105(6):477–80.

39. Solis G, Saxby T. Incidence of DVT following surgery of the foot and ankle. Foot Ankle Int 2002; 23(5):411–4.

40. Patil S, Gandhi J, Curzon I, et al. Incidence of deep-vein thrombosis in patients with fractures of the ankle treated in a plaster cast. J Bone Joint Surg Br 2007;89(10):1340–3.

41. Shibuya N, Frost CH, Campbell JD, et al. Incidence of acute deep vein thrombosis and pulmonary embolism in foot and ankle trauma: analysis of the National Trauma Data Bank. J Foot Ankle Surg 2012; 51(1):63–8.

42. Goel DP, Buckley R, deVries G. Prophylaxis of deep-vein thrombosis in fractures below the knee: a prospective randomised controlled trial. J Bone Joint Surg Br 2009;91(3):388–94.

43. Selby R, Geerts WH, Kreder HJ, et al. Symptomatic venous thromboembolism uncommon without thromboprophylaxis after isolated lower-limb fracture: the knee-to-ankle fracture (KAF) cohort study. J Bone Joint Surg Am 2014;96(10):e83.

44. Hsu JE, Namdari S, Baldwin KD, et al. Is upper extremity trauma an independent risk factor for lower extremity venous thromboembolism? An 11-year experience at a level I trauma center. Arch Orthop Trauma Surg 2011;131(1):27–32.

45. Kardooni S, Haut ER, Chang DC, et al. Hazards of benchmarking complications with the National Trauma Data Bank: numerators in search of denominators. J Trauma 2008;64(2):273–7 [discussion: 277–9].

Arthrofibrosis After Periarticular Fracture Fixation

Ian McAlister, MD, Stephen Andrew Sems, MD*

KEYWORDS

• Arthrofibrosis • Fracture • Periarticular • Shoulder • Elbow • Knee

KEY POINTS

- Arthrofibrosis after periarticular fractures can create clinically significant impairments in both the upper and lower extremities. The shoulder, elbow, and knee are particularly susceptible to the condition.
- Many risk factors for the development of arthrofibrosis cannot be controlled by the patient or surgeon. Early postoperative motion should be promoted whenever possible.
- Manipulations under anesthesia are effective for a period of time in certain fracture patterns, and open or arthroscopic surgical debridements should be reserved for the patient for whom nonoperative modalities fail and who has a clinically significant deficit.

Arthrofibrosis occurs when generalized connective tissue proliferation results in painful joint stiffness.[1] The clinical impact of arthrofibrosis represents a wide spectrum of disease, ranging from minimal to devastating for the patient. Arthrofibrosis may result in a loss of motion of the involved joint, a commonly encountered and challenging problem after fixation of periarticular fractures. Joints across the body tolerate stiffness to a variable degree, with the elbow and knee being less accommodating than the shoulder or ankle. The functional range of motion has been described previously for the shoulder, elbow, and knee, and when arthrofibrosis results in the loss of this functional range, intervention may be indicated.[2–4] Once arthrofibrosis has progressed, activities of daily living (ADLs) can become compromised, with potential resultant limitations in feeding, hygiene, sitting, and ambulation, depending on the degree of motion loss and the joint involved.

Anatomic articular reduction is critical to minimizing posttraumatic arthritis in many periarticular fractures.[5,6] Subsequently, many historic rehabilitation protocols called for prolonged periods of immobilization to minimize the risk of fracture displacement during the period of fracture healing.[7,8] Early motion of the injured joint is now frequently emphasized over a prolonged period of immobilization, as immobilization is a well-established risk factor for the development arthrofibrosis after fixation of periarticular fractures.[1,9]

The clinical appearance of arthrofibrosis is loss of motion in the flexion or extension or both, and develops as the result of diffuse scar tissue and adhesion formation within a joint. Features specific to the patient, the injury, the surgery, and the postoperative rehabilitation seem to play a role in the development of arthrofibrosis.

Regardless of the joint involved, there are a variety of common risk factors for the development of stiffness after intra-articular fracture fixation. Examples include high-energy fracture patterns, the use of an external fixator, prolonged immobilization, and delayed or poor rehabilitation.[1,10,11] The

Disclosures: S.A. Sems receives royalties from Biomet.
Department of Orthopaedic Surgery, Mayo Clinic, 200 First Street Southwest, Rochester, MN 55905, USA
* Corresponding author.
E-mail address: sems.andrew@mayo.edu

Orthop Clin N Am 47 (2016) 345–355
http://dx.doi.org/10.1016/j.ocl.2015.09.003
0030-5898/16/$ – see front matter © 2016 Elsevier Inc. All rights reserved.

orthopedic.theclinics.com

development of an exaggerated pathologic fibrous hyperplasia, however, is not always associated with an overt, identifiable cause. Basic science research has shown that certain cytokines, inflammatory cells, and genetic predisposition play a role in the development of postoperative motion loss.[1]

In this article, we discuss the basic science behind arthrofibrosis, review different anatomic areas while highlighting fractures prone to developing postoperative stiffness, and consider the available treatment options.

BASIC SCIENCE

Scar tissue formation occurs as a normal physiologic response to injury and surgical trauma. Tissue organization after surgery depends on the interplay between local and inflammatory cells, with signaling of growth factors and cytokines playing an integral role. The development of arthrofibrosis is in part the result of excess deposition of matrix proteins such as collagen types I, III, V, and the proliferation of fibroblasts.[1] Specific cytokines that play a key role in the development of excessive fibrous hyperplasia and resultant stiffness have been identified. Transforming growth factor-β (TGF-β) and platelet-derived growth factor (PDGF) are 2 examples of signaling molecules that play a critical role in the process of tissue repair. These factors coordinate cell growth, differentiation, and programmed cell death via paracrine and autocrine signaling pathways. At the site of injury, TGF-β and PDGF initiate a cascade of events resulting in the production of extracellular matrix proteins and protease inhibitors, as well as inhibition of proteolytic enzyme production. Formation of extracellular matrix occurs at the site of injury, consisting of an aggregation of collagen, fibronectin, and proteoglycans. With an increase in local concentration, the autoregulatory mechanism of TGF-β results in feedback inhibition. Overexpression of TGF-β can result in progressive deposition of matrix and tissue fibrosis.[12]

In addition, genetic factors likely also contribute to the development of arthrofibrosis. Studies have shown a possible correlation between specific HLA types and the development of arthrofibrosis after anterior cruciate ligament reconstruction. Further investigation is required to confirm a possible genetic link.[13]

ARTHROFIBROSIS AROUND THE SHOULDER

Functional range of motion of the shoulder requires approximately 120° of forward elevation, 45° of extension, 130° of abduction, 115° of cross-body adduction, 60° of external rotation, and 100° of internal rotation.[1] This motion is significantly less than what has been described as normal shoulder motion (forward elevation 167°, extension 62°, abduction 184°, adduction 140°, external rotation 104°).[2]

Proximal Humerus Fractures

Although some degree of motion loss can be expected after fixation of proximal humerus fractures, with normal motion of the wrist and elbow, the upper limb is typically able to easily accommodate for limited motion without significant functional impairment. Südkamp and colleagues[14] reported the results of open reduction and internal fixation (ORIF) with a locked plate in a prospective, multicenter, observational study. At 1 year follow-up, mean shoulder motion demonstrated 132° forward elevation, 122° abduction, 45° external rotation, and 77° internal rotation. When compared with the uninjured shoulder at 1 year, the shoulder that underwent internal fixation of the proximal humerus had 81% of forward elevation, 79% of abduction, 74% of external rotation, and 93% of internal rotation. These results were consistent with another series that used locked plating of the proximal humerus with the addition of suture fixation, which reported an average forward flexion of 131° in 81 patients at 23 months average follow-up.[15] Duralde and Leddy[16] published their results after plate fixation of proximal humerus fractures also using suture fixation to augment the repair and had an average forward elevation of 156° and 46° of external rotation at an average of 37 months.

A systematic review commented that most of the postoperative rehabilitation protocols of the series of locked plate fixation of proximal humerus fractures were similar, using passive motion initially and active motion 4 weeks later, depending on bone quality and the stability of the fixation.[17]

Postoperative range of motion focusing on daily terminal stretching programs may require several months before maximum benefit is seen. Strengthening of the shoulder should be performed once the clinical and radiographic findings are consistent with fracture healing. Forced manipulation carries the risk of refracture and is rarely required around the shoulder after fixation of proximal humerus fractures. Rarely, postoperative motion loss progresses to adhesive capsulitis that is refractory to conservative treatment.[18] In these instances, shoulder arthroscopy with capsular release is a useful tool that has been shown to improve shoulder motion while allowing the surgeon to evaluate and treat intra-articular conditions.[19] Katthagen and colleagues[19] reported on 37 patients with unsatisfactory results after locked plate fixation of proximal humerus fracture who underwent arthroscopic implant removal with the addition of capsular release (31/37) as necessary. The range of motion improved from 86° to 105° in forward flexion, 77° to 97° in abduction, 30° to 42° in external rotation, and 58° to 81° in internal rotation at 24 months from arthroscopy.

ARTHROFIBROSIS AROUND THE ELBOW

Joint stiffness is a common occurrence after fixation of periarticular fractures involving the elbow. As noted by Morrey, the elbow is a highly sensitive and "unforgiving joint."[20] All patients with traumatic elbow injuries should be counseled about some loss of motion, especially terminal extension.[21] Anatomic restoration of the articular surface will help minimize the risk of posttraumatic arthritis. However, the exposure needed for adequate visualization to achieve this anatomic reduction often results in damage to the surrounding muscle and capsule, leading to scar tissue formation, heterotopic ossification, and a stiff joint.

The cause of posttraumatic motion loss of the elbow is often multifactorial; with causes being classified as either intrinsic or extrinsic. Intrinsic (intra-articular) causes are the result of the articular injury, such as cartilage loss, joint incongruity, or impingement. Extrinsic (extra-articular) causes are related to the periarticular soft tissue and bone, excluding the articular surface. Prolonged pain can produce both voluntary and involuntary guarding of the elbow during motion, eventually leading to contracture of the periarticular soft tissues and resultant stiffness. This pain mechanism is postulated as a possible explanation for stiffness occurring after even relatively minor trauma to the elbow.[22]

Normal range of motion of the elbow joint as defined by the American Academy of Orthopedic Surgeons ranges from 0° (full extension) to 146° of flexion with 71° of pronation and 84° of supination.[23] The goal of treatment when managing stiffness of the elbow is to restore functional range of elbow motion necessary to lead a normal life. Morrey and colleagues[3] defined the functional range of motion of the elbow joint, necessary to carry out most ADLs, to be a 100° arc of motion, from 30° short of full extension to 130° of flexion, along with 50° of pronation and 50° of supination. Deficits in forearm pronation and supination are typically caused by a lesion at the radiocapitellar or proximal radioulnar joints, whereas deficits in flexion and extension are most often caused by ulnohumeral joint lesions.

The goal in the surgical management of periarticular elbow fractures is to anatomically reconstruct the elbow joint with a rigid construct that allows for early mobilization. However, this goal is often difficult to achieve, especially in patients with articular or metaphyseal comminution and associated soft tissue injuries or in elderly patients with osteoporosis. Fracture nonunion frequently results when early motion is attempted in the face of inadequate fixation. Unfortunately, prolonged immobilization to prevent failure of fixation can often lead to loss of elbow motion.

Distal Humerus Fracture

ORIF of distal humerus fractures is typically performed using a posterior approach, which may include an olecranon osteotomy. Loss of elbow motion is the most common sequela after ORIF of these fractures and is often observed even after stable fixation and appropriate rehabilitation. Dual plating, with either biplanar or parallel plating, is the standard fixation construct of intercondylar fractures of the distal humerus.[21] The use of 2 plates on the distal humerus for complete articular fractures greatly assists the reconstruction of the triangle of stability of the distal humerus. Sanchez-Sotelo and colleagues[24] treated 34 complex distal humeral fractures with their parallel plate technique and reported only 41% of elbows obtained at least 30° of extension and 130° of flexion. Other investigators have reported that about one-third of patients failed to regain functional arc of motion after ORIF of intercondylar fractures.[25,26]

Terrible Triad Injury

Posttraumatic stiffness is a common complication after treatment of terrible triad injuries of the elbow. Three studies reporting outcomes after the surgical treatment of terrible triad injuries have documented a mean flexion-extension arc between 112° to 117° and mean rotation of 135° to 137°.[27–29] A delay in treatment and a prolonged period of immobilization has been shown to lead to loss of elbow motion and poor outcomes. Broberg and Morrey[30] similarly noted that immobilization for more than 4 weeks led to consistently poor results in their series of 24 patients. In the setting of a combined bony and ligamentous injury, a surgeon often has to decide between stability and mobilization. A stiff congruent elbow may be more amenable to interventions that result in clinical success than a mobile elbow with residual instability and incongruency.

Olecranon Fractures

Loss of motion is a common problem after fractures about the elbow but is rarely significant in patients with isolated olecranon fractures. A prospective randomized study comparing tension wiring and plate fixation of displaced olecranon fractures reported no difference in elbow range of motion between the 2 groups at final follow-up. The average loss of elbow extension was 10° in the tension band group versus 7° in the plate fixation group, whereas loss of flexion, pronation, and supination each averaged less than 5° in both groups.[31] Patients with isolated injuries typically lose 10° to 15° of extension.[32] However, in patients with associated fractures of the radial head, capitellum, or coronoid, or with a Monteggia fracture dislocation, the range of motion may be more severely compromised. Similarly, comminuted fractures and open injuries are also more likely to result in stiffness.

MANAGEMENT

The management of postoperative elbow stiffness begins with performing internal fixation that results in the elbow being rendered sufficiently stable to allow early rehabilitation and initiation of motion soon after surgery. Frequent follow-up and early identification of patients with elbow stiffness allows the surgeon to intervene before irreversible problems occur. The initial treatment of most patients with elbow stiffness is gentle passive and progressive active assisted stretching exercises under the guidance of a physical therapist. For patients whose motion has plateaued or not improved after a course of therapy, splinting is the next step. Dynamic hinged elbow splints with spring or rubber band tension may be useful to assist with deficits of elbow flexion. However, these devices often lead to spasm and co-contracture of antagonistic muscles, resulting in poor patient compliance. Turnbuckle braces (static progressive splints) are better tolerated and target either flexion or extension deficits. If contracture is present in both directions, the splint can be used in alternating positions.

In a prospective, randomized, controlled trial comparing the use of dynamic versus static progressive splints in the treatment of posttraumatic elbow contractures, Lindenhovius and colleagues[33] showed no difference between the groups in the improvement of the arc of motion. The mean improvement of the flexion-extension arc was 40° versus 39° at 6 months and 47° versus 49° at 12 months, respectively, for the dynamic

and static cohorts. Ten percent of the patients in the dynamic splinting group did not tolerate treatment and requested a change to the static splinting group before 3 months of use. A more recent systematic review of 232 patients with nonoperative management of elbow stiffness also concluded that both dynamic splinting and static progressive splinting were effective as a treatment of elbow stiffness, and that treatment should continue until patients stop making improvement in the elbow range of motion.[34]

Continuous passive motion (CPM) machines may provide some benefit in the immediate postoperative period; however, these devices have a limited role in treating established contractures as they do not possess the mechanical advantage of static progressive splints to affect the end range of motion. If notable elbow stiffness remains despite splinting, further nonsurgical treatment is unlikely to be of benefit. The result of closed manipulation under anesthesia is unpredictable and may even produce loss of motion by producing inflammation and swelling with tearing of soft tissues, causing hemarthrosis and additional fibrosis.

If nonsurgical treatment fails, patients with diminished motion who can cooperate with the required rehabilitation program are candidates for surgical treatment. Assessment of the cause of the stiffness and the degree of functional impairment dictates the surgical approach to be used. For patients with little or no arthritis, soft tissue releases combined with the removal of impinging bone may be helpful. Resection of heterotopic ossification has been recommended after maturation of the bone, theoretically allowing the ossification process to complete and to avoid recurrence.[35] A recent study looked at 2 groups of patients who underwent resection of heterotopic ossification at different time points. The early group had their resection at an average of 6.1 months, and the late group at 23 months. This study showed no difference in the recurrence rate (26% vs 28%) or range of motion or Mayo Elbow Performance score.[36]

For patients without significant bony formation that limits motion, the direction of the greatest limitation of motion dictates the surgical approach and the capsular and tendinous structures to be released. Patients lacking flexion may benefit from ulnar nerve release and transposition, with release of the posterior band of the medial collateral ligament.[37] Using this technique, Park and colleagues[37] were able to improve elbow flexion in patients with posttraumatic stiffness from 89° to 124° on average. These investigators also noted that heterotopic ossification was present in 95% of patients who underwent surgery for elbow stiffness but was only identifiable on preoperative imaging in 54% of patients. The surgeon should have a high index of suspicion for the presence of heterotopic ossification in the patient with posttraumatic elbow stiffness, even if it is not apparent on radiographs. If this technique fails to achieve the desired amount of motion, a posterior capsulotomy can be subsequently performed through the same incision.[38]

In patients lacking elbow extension, release of the anterior capsule is indicated in addition to resection of any bony blocks. Arthroscopic release of the anterior capsule has been shown to improve flexion contractures, with improvements in extension ranging between 17° and 21°.[39,40]

Patients with moderate degenerative changes may be considered for limited bony arthroplasties, which include debridement arthroplasty or the Outerbridge-Kashiwagi ulnohumeral arthroplasty. Younger patients with severe degenerative changes can be treated with fascial interposition arthroplasty, with or without application of a joint distractor during the early healing period. For older or low-demand patients with advanced elbow arthritis, total elbow arthroplasty with a semiconstrained design can restore comfort and mobility.

Elbow arthroscopy has become an increasingly useful tool in the management of elbow stiffness following fracture fixation. Arthroscopic management of elbow stiffness is a viable alternative in certain patients, allowing smaller incisions, decreased soft tissue disruption, and, theoretically, easier rehabilitation. Soft tissue release techniques are being developed and refined. Mild impingement can improve with arthroscopic resection of osteophytes. In addition, elbow arthroscopy may also be beneficial when the status of the articular cartilage is uncertain by providing the surgeon with information needed to make decisions concerning the joint surface. Nguyen and colleagues[41] reported their results of arthroscopic capsular release in 22 patients for the treatment of elbow stiffness. At a mean follow-up of 25 months, average elbow range of motion improved from 38°–122° to 19°–141°, with a 38° improvement in mean arc of motion. The arthroscopic treatment of elbow stiffness is technically demanding and the procedure does carry a significant risk of nerve injury. In a large series of 473 consecutive elbow arthroscopies, a transient nerve palsy occurred at a rate of 2.5%, with most patients regaining complete nerve function within 6 weeks.[42] There were no cases of permanent neurovascular injury.

ARTHROFIBROSIS AROUND THE KNEE

The normal knee allows a range of motion from full extension to 140° of flexion.[43,44] Clinically, full extension allows the patient to stand with the knee locked straight, not requiring chronic quadriceps activation. In order to achieve this goal, the mechanical axis of the leg must pass anterior to the hinge point of the knee. The hinge point on an adult is located at the point where the extension of the posterior femoral cortex intersects the Blumensaat line (**Fig. 1**).

Functional range of motion of the knee requires 63° of flexion while walking, and up to 93° of flexion while standing up from a chair.[45] More motion is required for activities such as getting out of a bathtub (138°), ascending stairs (98.5°), and standing up from a low chair (105°).[4] Although it is the goal to maximize range of motion of the knee after fixation of fractures, these amounts must be considered in order to provide patients with a functional range of motion.

Periarticular fractures around the knee can contribute to loss of motion through varying mechanisms. Malunions may seem to create loss of motion as a result of flexion or extension deformities, and functional deficits that are similar to functional deficits that occur from arthrofibrosis may be encountered. Femoral fractures and fractures that have previously been treated with external

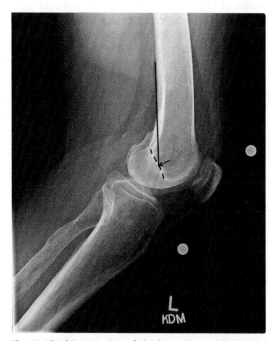

Fig. 1. The hinge point of the knee (*arrow*) is located at the intersection of the Blumensaat line (*dashed line*) and a line extended from the posterior border of the femoral cortex (*solid line*).

fixator with pin sites in the femur may develop adhesions of the quadriceps directly to the femur. Intra-articular fractures may develop arthrofibrosis with adhesions in the parapatellar gutters, patellar tendon, and the patellofemoral joint. Bishop and colleagues[46] performed a case-controlled study to evaluate the factors that predict stiffness after periarticular fractures of the knee. Extensor mechanism disruptions, fasciotomy, need for more than 2 procedures to obtain skeletal stabilization, need for soft tissue coverage, and wounds that precluded early knee range of motion were associated with an increased risk for the development of knee stiffness. Surgical goals include restoring anatomy while providing stable fixation that allows early motion and aggressive postoperative mobilization to minimize the potential for debilitating loss of motion.

Evaluation of Range of Motion

Loss of range of motion after periarticular fracture of the tibia or femur should be assessed clinically and with lateral radiographs of the knee in full extension. A goniometer is placed with 1 axis along the line from the greater trochanter to the lateral femoral condyle, and the other axis is from the lateral malleolus to the fibular head. This method has been shown to be valid with high interobserver reliability (ICC 0.97–0.99).[47] Clinical evaluation of knee motion will identify patients with range of motion deficits, but in patients who have sustained periarticular fractures it does not necessarily diagnose arthrofibrosis. Patients may have perceived loss of motion because of bony deformities, so radiographic evaluation of the sagittal alignment of the limb is also necessary as part of the work up.

Full-length standing lateral radiographs with the knee in full extension are used to assess sagittal alignment. In the normal knee in full extension, a line drawn along the distal one-third of the anterior femoral cortex should be colinear with a line along the anterior tibial cortex. The angle between these lines (**Fig. 2**) represents the amount of flexion or hyperextension present in the knee, depending on the direction of the intersection of the lines.

If the anterior cortices of the tibia and femur are not colinear, the mechanical and anatomic axes of the tibia and femur should be evaluated to determine if the flexion is from bony deformities or caused by soft tissue formation. The posterior distal femoral angle is determined by first establishing the distal femoral joint line. This line is made by connecting the point where the physeal scar intersects the anterior femoral cortex with the point where the physeal scar intersects the

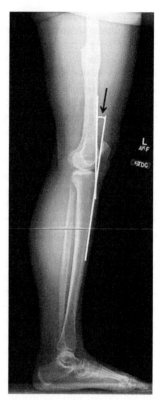

Fig. 2. A standing lateral radiograph to determine contracture of the knee. The patient is instructed to stand with the knee fully extended and the beam is focused on obtaining a perfect lateral radiograph of the knee. The angle between the anterior cortices of the distal third of the femur and tibia is measured (*arrow*).

posterior femoral cortex in a skeletally mature patient. A point along the line that is one-third of the length of the line determined posterior to the anterior femoral cortex is used to connect a line to the center of the femoral head, to determine the modified mechanical axis of the femur. The angle between these lines represents the posterior distal femoral angle (**Fig. 3**). The normal value for this posterior distal femoral angle is 83° ± 4°.[48]

The posterior proximal tibial angle is also evaluated by measuring the slope of the tibia. This is done by connecting the anterior and posterior edges of the tibial articular surface with a line to establish the tibial joint line. A point one-fifth of the length of the line from the anterior edge toward the posterior edge is marked, and this point is connected with a line to the center of the ankle joint on the lateral view (**Fig. 4**). The normal proximal posterior tibial angle is 81° ± 4°.[48]

Evaluation of the radiographic anatomy is critical to determine the contribution that a bony deformity contributes to perceived loss of motion,

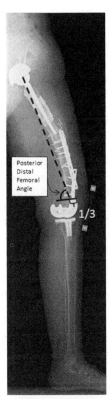

Fig. 3. The distal femoral joint line is determined by connecting the anterior extent of the physeal scar with the posterior extent of the physeal scar (*solid line*). The length of the line is measured and a point is marked one-third of the distance from the anterior end of the line. This point is connected with the center of the femoral head (*dashed line*). The angle between these lines represents the posterior distal femoral angle, which should be 83° (79°–87°). This patient has an abnormal angle of 71° caused by a femoral malunion.

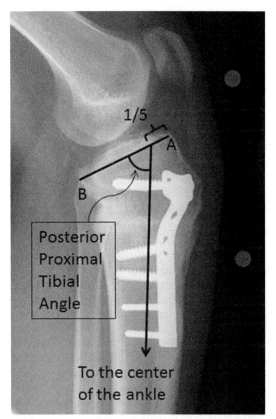

Fig. 4. The posterior proximal tibial angle is measured between the joint line and the mechanical axis of the tibia. The joint line is formed by connecting the anterior margin of the tibial articular surface (A) with the posterior edge of the tibial articular surface (B). A point one-fifth of the distance from anterior to posterior is marked, and a line connecting this point with the center of the ankle is drawn, representing the mechanical axis of the tibia. The posterior proximal tibial angle is measured between these lines.

and to determine what is soft tissue related. Bony deformities that contribute to perceived loss of motion require osteotomy and correction, whereas losses of motion caused by soft tissues are often treated initially with physical therapy modalities.

Supracondylar Femur Fractures

Supracondylar femur fractures that undergo surgical fixation typically lose between 30° to 40° of knee flexion compared with a normal knee.[49] Fixation may be accomplished with multiple techniques, including plating, intramedullary nailing, and external fixation. All 3 techniques are effective at obtaining union and allowing return to function, and all experience similar loss of knee flexion. Kregor and colleagues[50] reported that after submuscular plating of the distal femur, the average range of motion of the knee was from 1° loss of

extension to 109° of flexion. Kolb and colleagues[51] reported that after fixation of supracondylar femoral fractures with the same implant that Kregor had previously reported on, only 13% of patients failed to achieve 90° of knee flexion, with 48% of patients achieving more than 120° of flexion.

Motion after intramedullary nail fixation of distal femur fractures is similar to that reported after plate fixation. Handolin and colleagues[52] reported that 24 of 44 patients treated with retrograde intramedullary nail fixation of distal femoral fractures had no loss of motion compared with the contralateral side, and the other 20 patients only experienced between 5° and 15° of loss of motion. Danzinger and colleagues[53] reported on 16 patients treated with retrograde intramedullary nails for supracondylar femur fractures and found that the average knee range of motion was 109°. However, Demirtaş and colleagues[54] found that 23% of patients who underwent retrograde intramedullary nail fixation had restriction of flexion (100°–124°), and 20% of patients who underwent plate fixation experienced the same loss of flexion.

Loss of extension is less severe after distal femoral fractures. Ehlinger and colleagues[49] reported on 92 cases of plate fixation of distal femur fractures and reported an average extension loss of 8°, with a range from 5° to 20°. Other reports indicate that loss of extension more than 10° is uncommon with either plate or nail fixation.[54]

Tibial Plateau Fractures

Operative fixation of tibial plateau fractures often requires extensive approaches with direct inspection of the articular surface of the tibia. The anterolateral approach involves elevating the anterior compartment from its origin on the proximal tibia, and mobilization of the iliotibial band attachment on the Gerdy tubercle. This exposure allows a submeniscal arthrotomy to gain access to the articular surface and to repair any meniscal injuries. The capsular insertion on the tibia is often traumatized, and the surgical approach further insults this area when the capsule is retracted to visualize the joint when reducing and stabilizing the fracture. Haller and colleagues[11] reviewed 186 patients who underwent surgical fixation of tibial plateau fractures and found that patients who had high-energy injuries, those requiring external fixation, tobacco use, and infection were all associated with the development of arthrofibrosis. The overall need for further interventions to regain motion after tibial plateau fractures was 14.5%, and the use of CPM was associated with less development of arthrofibrosis.

Manipulation Under Anesthesia

Manipulation under anesthesia is an effective technique to regain lost flexion of the knee after surgery. Multiple studies have evaluated the usefulness of manipulation under anesthesia after total knee arthroplasty, but the use of this technique after periarticular fractures is less well studied.[55–58] The largest series reporting on the use of manipulation under anesthesia after tibial plateau fractures showed that manipulations that were successful had less time from injury to manipulation (mean 2.9 months) than unsuccessful manipulations (mean 4.9 months).[11] In a smaller series of 16 patients who sustained tibial plateau fractures fixed through posteromedial approaches, 2 patients (12.5%) required subsequent manipulations

to improve range of motion.[59] The timing of the manipulation is critical, with late manipulations less likely to be successful when compared with manipulations performed within 3 months of injury.

Manipulations of the knee are done under general anesthesia. The patient is placed supine on the operating table and the femur is supported to allow gravity to flex the tibia. A gentle force is then applied to the proximal meta-diaphyseal region of the tibia to increase knee flexion. The amount of force that can be applied must be determined by the surgeon based on the patient's bone quality, presence of hardware, and presence of any stress risers in the bone caused by previous fracture, hardware, or screw holes. The surgeon should avoid applying the force to the ankle or distal tibial area because of the long moment arm that may create significant torque at the knee and cause a fracture. If a manipulation is combined with hardware removal, the manipulation should be completed before the removal of any metal to avoid creating stress risers that may propagate a fracture.

Continuous Passive Motion

CPM machines have been widely used after elective knee arthroplasty in an effort to improve motion.[60] However, studies of this technique in the setting of trauma are less common. Hill and colleagues[61] randomly assigned 40 patients with intra-articular fractures of the knee to CPM or standard physical therapy. They found that, whereas the CPM group had greater knee flexion at 48 hours from surgery, there were no differences at longer outcome points, and 30% of patients in the CPM group were unable to tolerate the device.

In the setting of tibial plateau fractures, Biyani and colleagues[62] looked at 32 elderly patients with tibial plateau fractures and noted better results in the 14 patients who used a CPM for 3 to 7 days after surgery compared with those who did not use a CPM. Haller and colleagues[11] confirmed this finding in tibial plateau fractures, finding that the use of CPM was associated with less development of arthrofibrosis.

CPM is not well tolerated in the immediate postoperative setting, as demonstrated by the 30% of patients who were unable to tolerate CPM immediately after surgery.[11] Addition of regional anesthesia and nerve block catheters may be combined with CPM to improve postoperative pain control and make the use of CPM more tolerable. However, the treating surgeon must weigh the risks and benefits associated with regional anesthesia for pain management as many of the clinical features of compartment syndrome are masked with nerve blocks. Judicious use of regional anesthesia and indwelling nerve block catheters is recommended with injuries at risk of the development of compartment syndrome.

Open Surgical Debridement and Judet Quadricepsplasty

Extension contractures of the knee that persist after 3 months and that affect the patient's clinical function may benefit from open surgical debridement and quadriceps release via a Judet quadricepsplasty. This procedure combines an intra-articular release of adhesions with mobilization of the quadriceps from the femur, performed in a sequential fashion to obtain the desired range of motion.[63] Oliveira and colleagues[64] reported on 45 patients who underwent the procedure for knee stiffness after distal femur fracture (33), femoral shaft fracture (9), and patella fracture (3). They found the increase in knee flexion from 33.6° preoperatively to 105° postoperatively. In the postoperative period, some flexion was lost with a final average flexion of 85°.

This procedure progresses in a stepwise fashion to allow release of the offending structure and minimizes unnecessary releases. The range of motion of the knee should be reassessed after each structure is released, and when the desired amount of motion is achieved, the procedure is concluded.

The procedure starts with a peripatellar release, done through a medial parapatellar approach. The medial retinaculum is released, along with any adhesions in the medial gutter and in the patellofemoral joint. This dissection should proceed to the patellar tendon to release any retro-tendinous adhesions to the tibial eminence. The next step is to release the lateral parapatellar and lateral gutter of the knee, and this incision is extended as far as necessary in the proximal direction to release the vastus lateralis and then the vastus intermedius.

Wang and colleagues[65] described a modification of the open procedure that combines percutaneous release of the lateral patellar retinaculum with arthroscopic releases of intra-articular adhesions in the suprapatellar pouch, patellofemoral compartment, and medial retinaculum. If the desired amount of flexion is not achieved, the vastus intermedius is released, and if still more flexion is desired, a quadriceps tendon lengthening is performed. With this modified technique, the average maximum flexion improved from 27° preoperatively to 141° intraoperatively and 115° at the time of most recent follow-up. All patients who underwent quadriceps lengthening were left with an extension lag.

Open or arthroscopic surgical release combined with quadricep release is an effective method of improving knee flexion after periarticular fracture. after quadricepsplasty, a loss of 20° of motion should be expected between the immediate postoperative range of motion and the motion at final follow-up.

SUMMARY

Arthrofibrosis after periarticular fractures can create clinically significant impairments in both the upper and lower extremities. The shoulder, elbow, and knee are particularly susceptible to the condition. Many risk factors for the development of arthrofibrosis cannot be controlled by the patient or surgeon. Early postoperative motion should be promoted whenever possible. Manipulations under anesthesia are effective for a period of time in certain fracture patterns, and open or arthroscopic surgical debridements should be reserved for the patient for whom nonoperative modalities fail and who has a clinically significant deficit.

REFERENCES

1. Magit D, Wolff A, Sutton K, et al. Arthrofibrosis of the knee. J Am Acad Orthop Surg 2007;15(11):682–94.
2. Namdari S, Yagnik G, Ebaugh DD, et al. Defining functional shoulder range of motion for activities of daily living. J Shoulder Elbow Surg 2012;21: 1177–83.
3. Morrey BF, Askew LJ, Chao EY. A biomechanical study of normal functional elbow motion. J Bone Joint Surg Am 1981;63:872–7.
4. Rowe PJ, Myles CM, Walker C, et al. Knee joint kinematics in gait and other functional activities measured using flexible electrogoniometry: how much knee motion is sufficient for normal daily life? Gait Posture 2000;12:143–55.
5. Knirk JL, Jupiter JB. Intra-articular fractures of the distal end of the radius in young adults. J Bone Joint Surg Am 1986;68:647–59.
6. Matta JM. Fractures of the acetabulum: accuracy of reduction and clinical results in patients managed operatively within three weeks after the injury. J Bone Joint Surg Am 1996;78:1632–45.
7. Slee GC. Fractures of the tibial condyles. J Bone Joint Surg Br 1955;37:427–37.
8. Palmer I. Compression fractures of the lateral tibial condyle and their treatment. J Bone Joint Surg Am 1939;21:674–80.
9. Rasmussen PS. Tibial condylar fractures-impairment of knee joint stability as an indication for surgical treatment. J Bone Joint Surg Am 1973;55:1331–50.

10. Pajarinen J, Björkenheim JM. Operative treatment of type C intercondylar fractures of the distal humerus: results after a mean follow-up of 2 years in a series of 18 patients. J Shoulder Elbow Surg 2002;11:48–52.

11. Haller JM, Holt DC, McFadden ML, et al. Arthrofibrosis of the knee following a fracture of the tibial plateau. Bone Joint J 2015;97-B(1):109–14.

12. Border WA, Noble NA. Transforming growth factor β in tissue fibrosis. N Engl J Med 1994;331:1286–92.

13. Skutek M, Elsner HA, Slateva K, et al. Screening for arthrofibrosis after anterior cruciate ligament reconstruction: analysis of association with human leukocyte antigen. Arthroscopy 2004;20:469–73.

14. Südkamp N, Bayer J, Hepp P, et al. Open reduction and internal fixation of proximal humeral fractures with use of the locking proximal humerus plate. Results of a prospective, multicenter, observational study. J Bone Joint Surg Am 2009;91:1320–8.

15. Badman B, Frankle M, Keating C, et al. Results of proximal humeral locked plating with supplemental suture fixation of rotator cuff. J Shoulder Elbow Surg 2011;20:616–24.

16. Duralde XA, Leddy LR. The results of ORIF of displaced unstable proximal humeral fractures using a locking plate. J Shoulder Elbow Surg 2010;19(4):480–8.

17. Thanasas C, Kontakis G, Angoules A, et al. Treatment of proximal humerus fractures with locking plates: a systematic review. J Shoulder Elbow Surg 2009;18(6):837–44.

18. Clavert P, Adam P, Bevort A, et al. Pitfalls and complications with locking plate for proximal humerus fracture. J Shoulder Elbow Surg 2010;19:489–94.

19. Katthagen JC, Hennecke D, Jensen G, et al. Arthroscopy after locked plating of proximal humeral fractures: implant removal, capsular release, and intra-articular findings. Arthroscopy 2014;30:1061–7.

20. Morrey BF. The elbow and its disorders. 4th edition. Philadelphia: Saunders; 2008.

21. Galano GJ, Ahmad CS, Levine WN. Current treatment strategies for bicolumnar distal humerus fractures. J Am Acad Orthop Surg 2010;18:20–30.

22. Bruno RJ, Lee ML, Strauch RJ, et al. Posttraumatic elbow stiffness: evaluation and management. J Am Acad Orthop Surg 2002;10(2):106–16.

23. American Academy of Orthopaedic Surgeons. Joint motion: method of measuring and recording. Chicago: The American Academy of Orthopaedic Surgeons; 1965.

24. Sanchez-Sotelo J, Torchia ME, O'Driscoll SW. Complex distal humeral fractures: internal fixation with a principle-based parallel-plate technique. J Bone Joint Surg Am 2007;89:961–9.

25. Ek ET, Goldwasser M, Bonomo AL. Functional outcome of complex intercondylar fractures of the distal humerus treated through a triceps sparing approach. J Shoulder Elbow Surg 2008;17:441–6.

26. McKee MD, Wilson TL, Winston L, et al. Functional outcome following surgical treatment of intra-articular distal humeral fractures through a posterior approach. J Bone Joint Surg Am 2000;82:1701–7.

27. Pugh DM, McKee MD. The "terrible triad" of the elbow. Tech Hand Up Extrem Surg 2002;6:21–9.

28. Pugh DM, Wild LM, Schemitsch EH, et al. Standard surgical protocol to treat elbow dislocations with radial head and coronoid fractures. J Bone Joint Surg Am 2004;86:1122–30.

29. Forthman C, Henket M, Ring DC. Elbow dislocation with intra-articular fracture: the results of operative treatment without repair of the medial collateral ligament. J Hand Surg Am 2007;32:1200–9.

30. Broberg MA, Morrey BF. Results of treatment of fracture-dislocations of the elbow. Clin Orthop Relat Res 1987;216:109–19.

31. Hume MC, Wiss DA. Olecranon fractures. A clinical and radiographic comparison of tension band wiring and plate fixation. Clin Orthop Relat Res 1992;(285):229–35.

32. Veillette CJ, Steinmann SP. Olecranon fractures. Orthop Clin North Am 2008;39:229–36.

33. Lindenhovius AL, Doornberg JN, Brouwer KM, et al. A prospective randomized controlled trial of dynamic versus static progressive elbow splinting for posttraumatic elbow stiffness. J Bone Joint Surg Am 2012;94:694–700.

34. Veltman ES, Doornberg JN, Eygendaal D, et al. Static progressive versus dynamic splinting for posttraumatic elbow stiffness: a systematic review of 232 patients. Arch Orthop Trauma Surg 2015;135(5):613–7.

35. Peterson SL, Mani MM, Crawford CM, et al. Postburn heterotopic ossification: insights for management decision making. J Trauma 1989;29:365–9.

36. Chen S, Yu SY, Yan H, et al. The time point in surgical excision of heterotopic ossification of post-traumatic stiff elbow: recommendation for early excision followed by early exercise. J Shoulder Elbow Surg 2015;24(8):1165–71.

37. Park MJ, Chang MJ, Lee YB, et al. Surgical release for posttraumatic loss of elbow flexion. J Bone Joint Surg Am 2010;92(16):2692–9.

38. Everding NG, Maschke SD, Hoyen HA, et al. Prevention and treatment of elbow stiffness: a 5-year update. J Hand Surg Am 2013;38:2496–507.

39. Degreef I, De Smet L. Elbow arthrolysis for traumatic arthrofibrosis: a shift towards minimally invasive surgery. Acta Orthop Belg 2011;77(6):758–64.

40. Cefo I, Eygendaal D. Arthroscopic arthrolysis for posttraumatic elbow stiffness. J Shoulder Elbow Surg 2011;20(3):434–9.

41. Nguyen D, Proper SI, MacDermid JC, et al. Functional outcomes of arthroscopic capsular release of the elbow. Arthroscopy 2006;22(8):842–9.

42. Kelly EW, Morrey BF, O'Driscoll SW. Complications of elbow arthroscopy. J Bone Joint Surg Am 2001; 83(1):25–34.

43. American Academy of Orthopaedic Surgeons. Joint motion: methods of measuring and recording. 6th edition. Edinburgh (United Kingdom): Churchill Livingstone; 1972.

44. Hallaçeli H, Uruç V, Uysal HH, et al. Normal hip, knee and ankle range of motion in the Turkish population. Acta Orthop Traumatol Turc 2014;48(1):37–42.

45. Laubenthal KN, Smidt GL, Kettelkamp DB. A quantitative analysis of knee motion during activities of daily living. Phys Ther 1972;52:34–43.

46. Bishop J, Agel J, Dunbar R. Predictive factors for knee stiffness after periarticular fracture: a case-control study. J Bone Joint Surg Am 2012;94(20): 1833–8.

47. Gogia PP, Braatz JH, Rose SJ, et al. Reliability and validity of goniometric measurements at the knee. Phys Ther 1987;67(2):192–5.

48. Paley D. Principles of deformity correction. Berlin: Springer; 2002.

49. Ehlinger M, Dujardin F, Pidhorz L, et al. SoFCOT. Locked plating for internal fixation of the adult distal femur: influence of the type of construct and hardware on the clinical and radiological outcomes. Orthop Traumatol Surg Res 2014;100(5):549–54.

50. Kregor PJ, Stannard JA, Zlowodzki M, et al. Treatment of distal femur fractures using the less invasive stabilization system: surgical experience and early clinical results in 103 fractures. J Orthop Trauma 2004;18(8):509–20.

51. Kolb W, Guhlmann H, Windisch C, et al. Fixation of distal femoral fractures with the less invasive stabilization system: a minimally invasive treatment with locked fixed-angle screws. J Trauma 2008;65(6): 1425–34.

52. Handolin L, Pajarinen J, Lindahl J, et al. Retrograde intramedullary nailing in distal femoral fractures–results in a series of 46 consecutive operations. Injury 2004;35(5):517–22.

53. Danziger MB, Caucci D, Zecher SB, et al. Treatment of intercondylar and supracondylar distal femur fractures using the GSH supracondylar nail. Am J Orthop (Belle Mead NJ) 1995;24(9):684–90.

54. Demirtaş A, Azboy I, Özkul E, et al. Comparison of retrograde intramedullary nailing and bridge plating in the treatment of extra-articular fractures of the distal femur. Acta Orthop Traumatol Turc 2014; 48(5):521–6.

55. Issa K, Banerjee S, Kester MA, et al. The effect of timing of manipulation under anesthesia to improve range of motion and functional outcomes following total knee arthroplasty. J Bone Joint Surg Am 2014;96(16):1349–57.

56. Ferrel JR, Davis Ii RL, Agha OA, et al. Repeat manipulation under anesthesia for persistent stiffness after total knee arthroplasty achieves functional range of motion. Surg Technol Int 2015;26:256–60.

57. Keating EM, Ritter MA, Harty LD, et al. Manipulation after total knee arthroplasty. J Bone Joint Surg Am 2007;89:282–6.

58. Fox JL, Poss R. The role of manipulation following total knee replacement. J Bone Joint Surg Am 1981; 63:3.

59. Berber R, Lewis CP, Copas D, et al. Postero-medial approach for complex tibial plateau injuries with a postero-medial or postero-lateral shear fragment. Injury 2014;45(4):757–65.

60. Harvey LA, Brosseau L, Herbert RD. Continuous passive motion following total knee arthroplasty in people with arthritis. Cochrane Database Syst Rev 2010;(3):CD004260.

61. Hill AD, Palmer MJ, Tanner SL, et al. Use of continuous passive motion in the postoperative treatment of intra-articular knee fractures. J Bone Joint Surg Am 2014;96(14):e118.

62. Biyani A, Reddy NS, Chaudhury J, et al. The results of surgical management of displaced tibial plateau fractures in the elderly. Injury 1995;26(5):291–7.

63. Moore TJ, Harwin C, Green SA, et al. The results of quadricepsplasty on knee motion following femoral fractures. J Trauma 1987;27:49–51.

64. Oliveira VG, D'Elia LF, Tirico LE, et al. Judet quadricepsplasty in the treatment of posttraumatic knee rigidity: long-term outcomes of 45 cases. J Trauma Acute Care Surg 2012;72(2):E77–80.

65. Wang JH, Zhao JZ, He YH. A new treatment strategy for severe arthrofibrosis of the knee. A review of twenty-two cases. J Bone Joint Surg Am 2006; 88(6):1245–50.

Impact of Infection on Fracture Fixation

Michael Willey, MD*, Matthew Karam, MD

KEYWORDS

- Musculoskeletal trauma • Fracture fixation • Surgical site infection
- Surgical management of infection • Clinical outcomes

KEY POINTS

- Rates of infection are higher in patients undergoing operative fixation of fractures compared with other orthopedic procedures.
- Patients with open fractures are at the highest risk of infection, especially in cases with severe soft tissue injury.
- Re-evaluation of current antibiotic infection prophylaxis in patients with open fracture is warranted.
- A diagnosis of surgical site infection after fracture fixation requires a comprehensive evaluation of clinical examination, serum laboratory values, and imaging studies.
- Surgical site infection can have devastating consequences for patients in orthopedic trauma surgery and innovative methods to prevent these complications must continue to be sought.

INTRODUCTION

The human body is composed of 10^{13} native cells and a surprising 10^{14} symbiotic microbes that coexist to allow a functional, healthy lifestyle.[1] Despite being outnumbered 10 to 1 by microbes, the body is protected by physical barriers, including skin, mucous membranes, and the immune system. Trauma and surgery disrupt these barriers and can disturb the balance, leading to surgical site infection and significant disability. This article discusses the prevention of surgical site infection in patients who undergo operative fixation of fractures and the management of this well-described complication.

Throughout history, surgical site infection has consistently been a barrier to performing operations to treat pathology. Effective anesthesia and antisepsis are justly given credit for allowing advances in surgical treatments. Anesthesia made surgery physically tolerable but especially important to surgical site infection is antisepsis. Well-known individuals in the history of medicine, including Semmelweis, Pasteur, and Lister, are credited with the development of modern asepsis. Ignaz Semmelweis in 1847, before understanding of the germ theory, deduced that unwashed hands of physicians were contaminating women during childbirth. After implementing a policy requiring physicians and medical students to wash their hands in chlorinated lime after leaving the autopsy suite to examine patients on the ward, the mortality mostly due to puerperal fever dropped from 18.3% to 2.2%.[2]

Lister, 20 years later, applied theories developed by Pasteur identifying that microbes causing fermentation could be killed by heat and chemical solutions.[3] He theorized that chemicals could kill microbes on the skin and surgical instruments, preventing inoculation of surgical wounds. Prior to his work, purulence was thought a normal component of the wound

Disclosure Statement: The authors have nothing to disclose related to this article.
Department of Orthopaedic Surgery and Rehabilitation, University of Iowa Hospitals and Clinics, 200 Hawkins Drive, Iowa City, IA 52242, USA
* Corresponding author.
E-mail address: michael-willey@uiowa.edu

Orthop Clin N Am 47 (2016) 357–364
http://dx.doi.org/10.1016/j.ocl.2015.09.004
0030-5898/16/$ – see front matter Published by Elsevier Inc.

healing process. In the American Civil War (1861–1865), gunshot injuries to the extremities with fracture resulted in a 50% rate of amputation and a 26% mortality rate.[4] Exsanguination and infection were the most common complications after amputation.[5] Erysipelas (streptococcal soft tissues infection) was associated with an 87% mortality.[4] During this time, Lister noted that more than half of patients with open fractures developed septicemia and died at the University of Glasgow.[3] Applying theories developed by Pasteur, he treated the wounds of 11 patients who suffered open fractures with carbolic acid, intending to kill infecting microbes. Nine patients healed without infection, which was a drastic improvement from previously reported results.[3] He published his work in 1867, 2 years after the Civil War, and although acceptance of his methods was slow, it led to significant progress in the field of surgery.

By the 1960s, advances in antiseptic technique drove down the rates of surgical site infections enough to allow for development of relatively safe operations. Stevens[6] published a series from this time that reports rates of deep infection as low as 4.35% for all orthopedic operations. Recent published rates of return to the operating room for surgical site infection are 1.18% after primary total hip arthroplasty and 0.90% after primary total knee arthroplasty.[7] These impressive numbers might suggest that this is a minor issue, but rates of surgical site infection have consistently been higher in patients who undergo operative fixation of acute fractures. The procedures with the highest rates of deep surgical site infection in the series published by Stevens in 1964 were "Open reduction with a plate" (13.0%) and "Débridement of open fractures" (12.1%), much higher than the overall average of 4.35%.[6] Recent published series of operative fixation of bicondylar tibial plateau fractures with dual approaches report rates of deep infection requiring operative débridement from 17.6% to 23.6%.[8,9] In patients with compartment syndrome, the rate was 36.4%[8] and with open fracture the rate of deep infection was 43.8%.[9] Two patients with infection in 1 series ultimately required an above-the-knee amputation.[8] Despite advances since the 1960s in minimally invasive techniques for fracture reduction and fixation, surgical site infection rates remain a common complication in the operative treatment of fractures. The rates continue to be significant, and innovative interventions to reduce surgical site infection in this patient population would have significant impact on the field of orthopedic fracture surgery.

TYPE AND TIMING OF PROPHYLACTIC ANTIBIOTICS IN FRACTURE SURGERY

Published series reporting outcomes and antibiotic recommendations for infection prophylaxis in patients with open and closed fractures were developed in the 1970s and early 1980s with little recent change. Since that time, there has been significant increase in the incidence of infection with resistant organisms. In a study that established cephalosporins as the preferred antibiotic to use for prophylaxis in patients with open fracture, Patzakis and colleagues[10] reported that 50% (11/22) patients with infection were culture positive for *Staphylococcus aureus*. In the entire series, infection was seen in 7.1% of all open fractures. They randomized patients with open fractures to no antibiotic prophylaxis, penicillin/streptomycin, and cephalothin. The rate of deep infection was 13.9% in the no antibiotic group, 9.7% in the penicillin and streptomycin group, and 2.3% in the cephalothin group. This study established cephalosporins as the antibiotic of choice for the next 40 years.

Around the same time, Gustilo and Anderson[11] reported results of implementing a débridement, fixation, and intravenous antibiotic protocol for open tibia fractures. They reported that 68.4% of organisms cultured from wound infections were *S aureus*. None of the isolated bacteria in either series was identified as methicillin-resistant *S aureus* (MRSA). *S aureus* first became resistant to penicillins in the 1950s, and, after widespread use of methicillin, MRSA was first isolated in the United Kingdom in 1961.[12] By the mid-1980s, MRSA became a frequently encountered hospital-acquired infecting organism. A recent published series reported a 2.5% rate of MRSA infection in patients with open fractures and 25% of patients with infections were culture positive for MRSA.[13] Another article reporting outcomes of adding intravenous vancomycin as a prophylactic antibiotic identified MRSA as the infecting organism in 18% of cases of open fracture. This trend of increasing rates of MRSA infection over the past 20 years is mirrored in cardiothoracic surgery and hospital-acquired infections.[14,15]

Re-evaluation of the current standard for appropriate prophylactic antibiotics in open and closed injuries is an interesting topic in orthopedic trauma surgery. The previously discussed study by Morris and colleagues[8] reported that 46.5% of wound infections after fixation of bicondylar tibial plateau fractures had cultures positive for MRSA. They discussed the possibility of giving vancomycin as procedural prophylaxis as a standard protocol. Torbert and colleagues[16] published the most comprehensive series of patients who developed infection after fixation of open and closed fractures. They found that bacteria with clinically relevant antibiotic resistance were seen in 36% of patients with deep infection. The standard established antibiotic prophylaxis (cephalosporin) established in the 1970s would not cover more than one-third of the organisms causing infection in this series. Torbert and colleagues[16] also found that gram-negative organisms were isolated in a high number of infections in the pelvis and proximal femur, indicating that physicians should consider prophylactic coverage for these organisms in this area.

There is mounting evidence that S aureus screening and decolonization programs are effective in reducing rates of infection in cardiothoracic, orthopedic, and hospital-acquired infections.[1,14,15,17] High-impact medical journals have published expert opinions recommending S aureus screening and decolonization programs in "all patients receiving an implant."[1] This is a broad reaching statement, but certain operations in orthopedic trauma carry a high risk of surgical site infection[8,9,18] and any potential innovative interventions to prevent the surgical site infection would have an important impact on care delivered. Large randomized studies of medical and surgical patients have demonstrated reduced rates of hospital-acquired and deep surgical site infections with the use of screening and decolonization programs.[17] Specifically in orthopedics, most of the literature has focused on hip and knee arthroplasty.[19,20]

Appropriate timing of antibiotic administration has also been shown important in preventing infection in patients with open fractures. Most literature has suggested that appropriate antibiotics be given as soon as possible after open fractures. Patzakis and Wilkins[21] in a later study found that infection rate was higher in patients who received prophylactic antibiotics longer than 3 hours after injury. In combat soft tissue wounds to a limb, an association with timing and rates of infection has been shown.[22] Lack and colleagues[18] recently examined a series of patients with Gustilo and Anderson type 3 open tibia fractures to look at timing of administration of antibiotics. In a series of 137 patients, 24 developed deep infection (17.5%). Using univariate analysis they found that receiving antibiotics less than 66 minutes after the injury resulted in lower rates of infection. Ultimately they had no infections in patients who received antibiotics within this time frame. The only other factor associated with infection was delay to soft tissue coverage, which has also been shown in other studies of open tibia fractures requiring flap coverage.[23] This study concluded that time to operative débridement did not correlate with infection. There are smaller series that demonstrated delays greater than 8 hours are related to infection in the lower extremity.[24] The upper extremity was not affected in this series by the time to operative débridement. The benefit of early operative débridement of open fractures to prevent infection is debatable. Large systematic reviews have not demonstrated higher rates of deep infection in patients with delayed débridement.[25]

The length of time to administer intravenous antibiotics after definitive closure of an open fracture ranges in clinical practice recommendations from 1 to 3 days. In 1988, Dellinger and colleagues[26] published a randomized study of patients with open fractures who received 1 day of cefonicid, 5 days of cefonicid, or 5 days of cefamandole nafate (both cephalosporins). The findings indicated that infection rates were similar between groups (12%–13%). There was no benefit to giving antibiotics longer than 24 hours after definitive closure.

The recommendations for type of prophylactic antibiotic used in patients with open and closed fractures are currently evolving and clinicians must make decisions based on the best available literature. If rates of MRSA infection are known to be high in a specific region, prophylaxis with vancomycin and a cephalosporin may be indicated for high-risk patients. Screening programs for nasal S aureus colonization may be a more focused methodology to treat high-risk patients with vancomycin, a cephalosporin, and S aureus decolonization programs. Patients with open fractures should be given antibiotics at the earliest possible time because administration less than 1 hour has shown lower infection rates, and trauma systems should consider administration in the field or in transport if this early administration cannot otherwise be accomplished. There is no proved benefit to giving antibiotic longer than 24 hours after definitive closure.

RATES OF INFECTION IN COMMON FRACTURE FIXATION PROCEDURES

The risk of surgical site infection after operative fixation of fractures is variable depending on the location and severity of the injury. The Gustilo and Anderson classification categorizes open fractures based on the severity of the soft tissue injury.[11] Multiple studies have demonstrated that increasing severity of injury in this classification correlates with higher rates of surgical site infection. In their original series, there were 8 deep infections that developed after implementation of the antibiotic and débridement protocol.[11] Six were classified as type 3 and 2 as type 2. In a later series of open fractures by Patzakis and Wilkins,[21] 1.4% of type 1 injuries, 3.6% of type 2 injuries, and 22.7% of type 3 injuries developed deep infections. Another recent series of patients with 106 open tibia fractures reported rates of 0% in type 1 injury, 8.7% of type 2 injuries, and 20.5% of type 3 injuries, highlighting this association.[27]

The infection rate in closed injuries varies depending on type of injury. Rates of infection after intramedullary nailing femoral shaft fractures ranges from 0% to 2.7%.[28,29] Rotational ankle fractures undergoing operative fixation also have described low rates of deep infection at 1.1%.[30] Acetabular fractures treated with the Kocher-Langenbeck approach have an infection rate of 5.2% in large series of experienced surgeons.[31]

The soft tissue envelope around the distal tibia is not robust in a normal state and is notorious for wound healing complications after early fixation of high-energy distal tibia fractures. Ruedi and Allgower[32] reported their results of internal fixation for distal tibia fractures in 1969. They had a lower energy mechanism of injury in most patients and a 5% rate of deep infection in 84 patients. In high-energy fracture of the distal tibia, rates of infection were later reported from 17%[33] to 37%[34] after internal fixation. These alarming rates led to a trend to treat these injuries definitely with external fixation.[35] Sirkin and colleagues[36] reported a series of patients with intra-articular distal tibia fractures who were treated with fixation of the fibula and spanning external fixation within 24 hours of injury. They returned to the operating room an average of 12.7 days after the injury for definitive open reduction internal fixation. In closed injuries, there was 1 deep infection requiring hardware removal (3.4%), indicating that a period of soft tissue healing and reduction of swelling after the injury with the limb stabilized was a moderately safe alternative to early fixation through compromised tissues.

PERIOPERATIVE CONTRIBUTIONS TO SURGICAL SITE INFECTION

Intraoperatively there are unmeasurable techniques that can help prevent infection. Using minimally invasive approaches, limiting periosteal stripping, and preventing muscle and tissue damage during the operation are thought to prevent surgical site infections and wound necrosis. This mostly reflects the skill, training, and experience of the surgeon. Surgical time has been shown to correlate with the incidence of surgical site infection in patients with tibial plateau fractures[37] and acetabular fractures.[31,38] This likely reflects the

complexity of the injury and invasiveness of the approach required to reduce and stabilize the fracture but is also likely linked to the experience of the surgeon. Poorly planned incisions and extensive soft tissue stripping can lead to wound necrosis and subsequent infection (**Fig. 1**).

Other perioperative adjuvants to prevent surgical site infection include placement of antibiotic eluding cement spacers in open fracture wounds/areas of bone loss and other more controversial treatments, such as use of hyperbaric oxygen or placement of vancomycin powder directly in the wound at the time of closure. The latter 2 treatments need further investigations to prove efficacy before general use in orthopedic trauma surgery. Currently, large, randomized clinical trials are investigating the benefits of supplemental oxygen and vancomycin powder to prevent wound complications.

HOST CHARACTERISTICS THAT AFFECT INFECTION RISK

Host factors are important when considering risk of surgical site infection in patients undergoing operative fracture fixation. Cierny-Mader is the most commonly discussed classification when

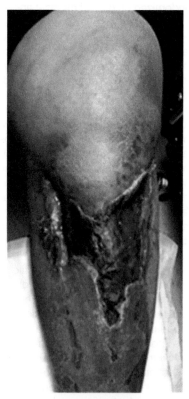

Fig. 1. Anterior knee of a patient who underwent dual approaches to the proximal tibia resulting in necrosis of the soft tissue bridge.

considering characteristics of the bone infection and state of the host. The types of bone infection are described as 4 categories. Type 1 is an intramedullary infection, type 2 infection remains superficial to the bone, type 3 infection penetrates the cortex but the bone remains axially stable, and type 4 is an infection that completely penetrates the bone and renders it axially unstable.[39] The Cierny-Mader classification is unique in that it also considers the physiologic state of the host. It uses 3 categories. A type A host is healthy with no systemic or local compromise, a type B host has systemic or local compromised physiology, and a type C host has multiple severe, irreversible conditions that make the morbidity of the treatment worse than the morbidity of the infection.[39] Examples of systemic physiologic compromise are diabetes, advanced age, vascular disease, malignancy, smoking, chronic hypoxia, and multiple organ failure. Examples of local compromise include previous surgery, scar, and radiation to the infected field. These classifications can be used to help make broad decisions about treatment of infection/osteomyelitis.

Diabetes, smoking, and obesity are commonly encountered in orthopedic trauma patients. These comorbidities need to be considered preoperatively. Diabetic patients with related comorbidities have higher rates of major complications when treated surgically for rotational ankle fractures.[40] Diabetes and smoking are strongly correlated with wound complications in patients who undergo open reduction internal fixation of calcaneus fractures.[41] Patients with these comorbidities should be treated with percutaneous techniques that have lower risk of soft tissue complications[42] or nonsurgically.

DIAGNOSIS OF SURGICAL SITE INFECTION

Often patients with acute surgical site infection after operative fixation of fractures are not difficult to diagnose clinically. They have a draining wound with erythema and either increasing or nonresolving pain after the injury. Systemically they report lethargy and fever. These patients need acute operative débridement of infection. Other times the diagnosis of infection can be difficult and a careful clinical evaluation needs to be combined with diagnostic studies.

Infection should to be suspected in patients with high-risk injuries, including open fracture with severe soft tissue injury; in patients with previous history of infection; or in a type B host with comorbidities, including smoking, substance abuse, malnutrition, and diabetes. Patients often complain of continued pain and nonspecific

symptoms, including fever, weight loss, and difficulty eating. If evaluating a patient for the first time, determine if the wound drained for a prolonged period of time postoperatively.

Radiographs are important because patients with infection often have abnormal healing. Broken hardware or progressive deformity can be signs of nonunion that can be present in infection. Acute infection is often not detected on radiographs unless it is advanced. Soft tissue swelling, periosteal reaction, cortical erosions, and involucrum can be seen on radiographs. Previous imaging studies are useful at follow-up to assess the initial injury and treatment.

Erythrocyte sedimentation rate and C-reactive protein evaluate systematic inflammatory response. These laboratory tests are normally elevated after surgery. C-reactive protein decreases faster than erythrocyte sedimentation rate after surgery, making it more useful for diagnosing infection acutely and evaluating effectiveness of treatment.[43] These laboratory tests are drawn at the initial evaluation so trends can be followed postoperatively. White blood cell count with differential and neutrophil count are often drawn but are less useful for diagnosing infection. In patients with chronic infection, the body has time to compensate and these levels may be low even in the face of infection. Bacteria with low virulence can also have falsely low inflammatory laboratory tests. Blood cultures are useful only in a septic, acutely ill patient.

Advanced imaging is rarely useful for diagnosing a postoperative infection but may be useful in forming a treatment plan. MRI is only useful in patients who have had hardware removed and can diagnose fluid collections/abscesses. CT is less useful for visualizing soft tissue but is better than MRI to evaluate details of bone architecture. CT can be used to identify an involucrum and plan débridement and is also helpful to diagnose nonunion and to plan reconstructive procedures.

Nuclear medicine studies are better able detect infection in patients with hardware. The most common study used is a 2-phase bone scan with technetium tc 99m phosphate. The first phase is a series of dynamic images taken soon after the injection to measure blood flow. The second phase is called the bone pooling phase. The third phase is taken 3 hours later when there is decreased uptake. Infection/osteomyelitis appears hot, or bright, on all phases with focal uptake in the third phase. More recent reports have found that nuclear medicine studies did not contribute to the diagnosis of infection in patients with nonunion.[44]

Intraoperatively, multiple tissue cultures (3–6) must be taken during the débridement to confirm the diagnosis of infection and to determine the speciation and sensitivity to guide postoperative antibiotics. Infection can be confirmed when more than one-third to one-half of the cultures are positive. With better understanding of bacterial biofilms, methods, such as sonication, may greatly improve diagnosis.

In patients with concern for infection/osteomyelitis, a comprehensive evaluation of the patient with clinical examination, serum laboratory values, and imaging is required for diagnosis. A diagnosis of infection is important to know before proceeding with treatment of a patient.

SURGICAL TECHNIQUE IN MANAGEMENT OF INFECTION

Priorities when treating patients with surgical site infection after fracture fixation are

1. Eliminate or suppress the infection
2. Heal the fracture
3. Maintain function of the patient

Most infections after surgical fixation of fractures occur early in the postoperative period before the fracture has healed. If the fixation device is removed, the fracture is unstable. Movement at the fracture site causes irritation of the wound and local soft tissues. Patients also have difficult mobilization with unstable injuries. If fixation hardware is removed, often external fixation can be used to provisionally stabilize the fracture until the infection is cleared and definitive stabilization can be performed. External fixation can also be used for definitive treatment in specific situations.

Infections with orthopedic implants that are colonized with bacterial biofilms make treatment difficult. Bacteria biofilms are adhesive complex networks of bacteria that are resistant to antibiotics and the human immune system. Despite biofilms, retaining hardware in acute infection has shown moderate success. Two series report results of retaining hardware after irrigation and débridement of acute surgical site infections after operative fracture fixation. Berkes and colleagues[45] published a series of patients who developed acute surgical site within 6 weeks of fracture fixation that did not have removal of the hardware. Patients had intraoperative cultures that guided antibiotic therapy. In the entire series, 71% of patients achieved osseous union. This technique was most effective in patients who had fixation with a plate and screws (77%). Surgical site infections in patients with intramedullary nail fixation achieved osseous union in only 46% of cases.[45] This is likely because the device is intramedullary and cannot be directly irrigated intraoperatively. Using a similarly described technique, Rightmire and colleagues[46] reported success in 68% of patients. An average of 2.1 procedures was required to achieve osseous union in patients who were successfully treated.

IMPLICATION OF SURGICAL SITE INFECTION FOR PATIENT OUTCOMES

Surgical site infections after fracture surgery can be devastating for patients who have already suffered a life-altering trauma. Several studies described in this article report the implications of surgical site infection. Patients return to the operating room multiple times,[46] are treated with long courses of intravenous antibiotic therapy,[45] and can suffer amputations if the infection cannot be cleared or bone does not heal.[8]

Duckworth and colleagues[47] reported a large series of patients who developed a deep surgical site infection after fixation of a proximal femur fracture having increased 30-day and 1-year mortality rates. Diabetes and dementia were predictors of mortality in patients with infection. Partanen and colleagues[48] similarly found that patients with deep infection after fixation of a proximal femur fractures had a higher mortality than controls (34.5% vs 24.1%). They also found that patients with infection had impaired walking ability and higher need for assistive devices for ambulation.

Quality of life is significantly diminished in patients with fracture nonunion that is often seen in chronic infection. Brinker and colleagues[49] published a comprehensive series of patients with tibial nonunion to report the effect on clinical health-related outcome scores. In this series, 19% of patients were classified as having infected nonunion. Physical and mental component scores of the Short Form 12 were significantly lower than the population mean. Physical component scores were significantly lower than common debilitating conditions, like myocardial infarction and congestive heart failure.[49] The cost to the health care system as a whole is substantially higher in patients who suffer nonunion of tibia fractures. These patients have higher opioid use, more surgical procedures, and other outpatient services.[50] All these factors contribute to the financial burden for society and to patient suffering.

SUMMARY

Patients who suffer surgical site infection after operative fixation of fractures have significant disability and increased mortality. A significant amount of investigation in orthopedic trauma surgery is dedicated to the prevention of surgical site infection and treatment. Despite these efforts, the rate of this complication is largely unchanged over the past 40 years. This article discusses the history of antisepsis and the care of open fractures, prevention strategies in high-risk patients, important steps to diagnosis of osteomyelitis/infection, and management strategies for osteomyelitis.

REFERENCES

1. Wenzel RP. Minimizing surgical-site infections. N Engl J Med 2010;362:75–7.
2. Lerner BH. Searching for Semmelweis. Lancet 2014; 383:210–1.
3. Jessney B. Joseph Lister (1827-1912): a pioneer of antiseptic surgery remembered a century after his death. J Med Biogr 2012;20:107–10.
4. Blaisdell FW. Medical advances during the Civil War. Arch Surg 1988;123:1045–50.
5. Trombold JM. Gangrene therapy and antisepsis before lister: the civil war contributions of Middleton Goldsmith of Louisville. Am Surg 2011;77:1138–43.
6. Stevens DB. Postoperative orthopaedic infections. A study of etiological mechanisms. J Bone Joint Surg Am 1964;46:96–102.
7. Rasouli MR, Restrepo C, Maltenfort MG, et al. Risk factors for surgical site infection following total joint arthroplasty. J Bone Joint Surg Am 2014;96:e158.
8. Morris BJ, Unger RZ, Archer KR, et al. Risk factors of infection after ORIF of bicondylar tibial plateau fractures. J Orthop Trauma 2013;27:e196–200.
9. Ruffolo MR, Gettys FK, Montijo HE, et al. Complications of high-energy bicondylar tibial plateau fractures treated with dual plating through 2 incisions. J Orthop Trauma 2015;29:85–90.
10. Patzakis MJ, Harvey JP Jr, Ivler D. The role of antibiotics in the management of open fractures. J Bone Joint Surg Am 1974;56:532–41.
11. Gustilo RB, Anderson JT. Prevention of infection in the treatment of one thousand and twenty-five open fractures of long bones: retrospective and prospective analyses. J Bone Joint Surg Am 1976;58: 453–8.
12. Boucher HW, Corey GR. Epidemiology of methicillin-resistant Staphylococcus aureus. Clin Infect Dis 2008;46(Suppl 5):S344–9.
13. Chen AF, Schreiber VM, Washington W, et al. What is the rate of methicillin-resistant Staphylococcus aureus and Gram-negative infections in open fractures? Clin Orthop Relat Res 2013;471:3135–40.
14. Kluytmans JA, Mouton JW, VandenBergh MF, et al. Reduction of surgical-site infections in cardiothoracic surgery by elimination of nasal carriage of Staphylococcus aureus. Infect Control Hosp Epidemiol 1996;17:780–5.
15. Kluytmans JA, Manders MJ, van Bommel E, et al. Elimination of nasal carriage of Staphylococcus aureus in hemodialysis patients. Infect Control Hosp Epidemiol 1996;17:793–7.
16. Torbert JT, Joshi M, Moraff A, et al. Current bacterial speciation and antibiotic resistance in deep infections after operative fixation of fractures. J Orthop Trauma 2015;29:7–17.
17. Bode LG, Kluytmans JA, Wertheim HF, et al. Preventing surgical-site infections in nasal carriers of Staphylococcus aureus. N Engl J Med 2010; 362:9–17.
18. Lack WD, Karunakar MA, Angerame MR, et al. Type III open tibia fractures: immediate antibiotic prophylaxis minimizes infection. J Orthop Trauma 2015;29: 1–6.
19. Chen AF, Heyl AE, Xu PZ, et al. Preoperative decolonization effective at reducing staphylococcal colonization in total joint arthroplasty patients. J Arthroplasty 2013;28:18–20.
20. Rao N, Cannella BA, Crossett LS, et al. Preoperative screening/decolonization for Staphylococcus aureus to prevent orthopedic surgical site infection: prospective cohort study with 2-year follow-up. J Arthroplasty 2011;26:1501–7.
21. Patzakis MJ, Wilkins J. Factors influencing infection rate in open fracture wounds. Clin Orthop Relat Res 1989;(243):36–40.
22. Jackson DS. Sepsis in soft tissue limbs wounds in soldiers injured during the Falklands Campaign 1982. J R Army Med Corps 1984;130:97–9.
23. Gopal S, Majumder S, Batchelor AG, et al. Fix and flap: the radical orthopaedic and plastic treatment of severe open fractures of the tibia. J Bone Joint Surg Br 2000;82:959–66.
24. Malhotra AK, Goldberg S, Graham J, et al. Open extremity fractures: impact of delay in operative debridement and irrigation. J Trauma Acute Care Surg 2014;76:1201–7.
25. Schenker ML, Yannascoli S, Baldwin KD, et al. Does timing to operative debridement affect infectious complications in open long-bone fractures? A systematic review. J Bone Joint Surg Am 2012;94: 1057–64.
26. Dellinger EP, Caplan ES, Weaver LD, et al. Duration of preventive antibiotic administration for open extremity fractures. Arch Surg 1988;123:333–9.
27. Willey MC, Haleem A, Karam M, et al. Antibiotics given for infection prophylaxis in open tibia fractures do not cover common infecting organisms. Las Vegas (NV): American Academy of Orthopaedic Surgery; 2015.
28. Ricci WM, Bellabarba C, Evanoff B, et al. Retrograde versus antegrade nailing of femoral shaft fractures. J Orthop Trauma 2001;15:161–9.
29. Halvorson JJ, Barnett M, Jackson B, et al. Risk of septic knee following retrograde intramedullary

nailing of open and closed femur fractures. J Orthop Surg Res 2012;7:7.

30. Korim MT, Payne R, Bhatia M. A case-control study of surgical site infection following operative fixation of fractures of the ankle in a large U.K. trauma unit. Bone Joint J 2014;96B:636–40.

31. Suzuki T, Morgan SJ, Smith WR, et al. Postoperative surgical site infection following acetabular fracture fixation. Injury 2010;41:396–9.

32. Ruedi T. Fractures of the lower end of the tibia into the ankle joint: results 9 years after open reduction and internal fixation. Injury 1973;5(2):130–4.

33. McFerran MA, Smith SW, Boulas HJ, et al. Complications encountered in the treatment of pilon fractures. J Orthop Trauma 1992;6:195–200.

34. Teeny SM, Wiss DA. Open reduction and internal fixation of tibial plafond fractures. Variables contributing to poor results and complications. Clin Orthop Relat Res 1993;(292):108–17.

35. Marsh JL, Bonar S, Nepola JV, et al. Use of an articulated external fixator for fractures of the tibial plafond. J Bone Joint Surg Am 1995;77:1498–509.

36. Sirkin M, Sanders R, DiPasquale T, et al. A staged protocol for soft tissue management in the treatment of complex pilon fractures. J Orthop Trauma 1999; 13:78–84.

37. Colman M, Wright A, Gruen G, et al. Prolonged operative time increases infection rate in tibial plateau fractures. Injury 2013;44:249–52.

38. Li Q, Liu P, Wang G, et al. Risk factors of surgical site infection after acetabular fracture surgery. Surg Infect (Larchmt) 2015;16:577–82.

39. Cierny G 3rd, Mader JT, Penninck JJ. A clinical staging system for adult osteomyelitis. Clin Orthop Relat Res 2003;(414):7–24.

40. Jones KB, Maiers-Yelden KA, Marsh JL, et al. Ankle fractures in patients with diabetes mellitus. J Bone Joint Surg Br 2005;87:489–95.

41. Folk JW, Starr AJ, Early JS. Early wound complications of operative treatment of calcaneus fractures: analysis of 190 fractures. J Orthop Trauma 1999; 13:369–72.

42. DeWall M, Henderson CE, McKinley TO, et al. Percutaneous reduction and fixation of displaced intra-articular calcaneus fractures. J Orthop Trauma 2010;24:466–72.

43. Greidanus NV, Masri BA, Garbuz DS, et al. Use of erythrocyte sedimentation rate and C-reactive protein level to diagnose infection before revision total knee arthroplasty. A prospective evaluation. J Bone Joint Surg Am 2007;89:1409–16.

44. Stucken C, Olszewski DC, Creevy WR, et al. Preoperative diagnosis of infection in patients with nonunions. J Bone Joint Surg Am 2013;95:1409–12.

45. Berkes M, Obremskey WT, Scannell B, et al. Maintenance of hardware after early postoperative infection following fracture internal fixation. J Bone Joint Surg Am 2010;92:823–8.

46. Rightmire E, Zurakowski D, Vrahas M. Acute infections after fracture repair: management with hardware in place. Clin Orthop Relat Res 2008;466: 466–72.

47. Duckworth AD, Phillips SA, Stone O, et al. Deep infection after hip fracture surgery: predictors of early mortality. Injury 2012;43:1182–6.

48. Partanen J, Syrjala H, Vahanikkila H, et al. Impact of deep infection after hip fracture surgery on function and mortality. J Hosp Infect 2006;62:44–9.

49. Brinker MR, Hanus BD, Sen M, et al. The devastating effects of tibial nonunion on health-related quality of life. J Bone Joint Surg Am 2013;95:2170–6.

50. Antonova E, Le TK, Burge R, et al. Tibia shaft fractures: costly burden of nonunions. BMC Musculoskelet Disord 2013;14:42.

Nonunion of the Femur and Tibia: An Update

Anthony Bell, MD[a], David Templeman, MD[b],*, John C. Weinlein, MD[c]

KEYWORDS

- Nonunion • Tibial nonunion • Femoral nonunion • Dynamization • Exchange nailing • Bone grafting
- Atypical femur fractures • Bisphosphonates

KEY POINTS

- Lower extremity nonunions, particularly of the tibia, have significant impact on both the patient and society.
- Radiographic union score for tibia fractures (RUST) is a method for more objectively describing fracture healing based on plain films.
- Fracture-specific and treatment-related risk factors have been associated with nonunion.
- Patient-related risk factors, both modifiable and nonmodifiable, have been associated with nonunion.
- Evaluating for the presence of infection is extremely important in the treatment of nonunion.

DEMOGRAPHICS AND ECONOMIC IMPACT

A retrospective review in the United States of 2006 managed care claims at 24 months after injury in 853 patients with tibial shaft fractures noted a 12% incidence of nonunion. This study also documented the increased costs of tibial nonunions for inpatient and outpatient services, as well as increased costs associated with narcotic usage (**Table 1**).[1,2]

According to one retrospective review of a prospective database collected by two level 1 trauma centers, patients with delayed union or nonunion also have significant lost productivity resulting in indirect costs. Records of 489 patients with 260 femur fractures and 282 tibia fractures were reviewed. Of the 423 patients who went on to known healing outcome, 138 (25%) experienced delayed union or nonunion. Seventy-two percent of patients with united fractures returned to work at 1 year, compared with 59% of patients with a delayed union or nonunion.[3]

DEFINITION

Fracture healing is assessed by a combination of clinical and radiographic criteria. Clinical markers of union include resolution of pain with weight bearing and radiographs that show progressive healing and cortical bridging of fracture lines.

The development of the radiographic union score for tibia fractures (RUST) is an attempt to objectively determine the extent of healing by scoring the degree of fracture healing from each of the 4 cortices, as viewed from anteroposterior and lateral radiographs. A recent modification of the initial scoring system differentiates bridging and nonbridging callus in an attempt to improve intraobserver agreement and the accuracy of predicting union (**Table 2**). Use of the scoring system results in a score ranging from 4 (no callus any of 4 cortices) to 16 (complete remodeling of all 4 cortices). A summary of the initial findings comparing the readings of academic orthopedic traumatologists defines that healing corresponds

[a] Department of Orthopaedics and Rehabilitation, Ambulatory Care Center, University of Florida College of Medicine-Jacksonville, 2nd Floor, 655 West 8th Street, C126, Jacksonville, FL 32209, USA; [b] Department of Orthopaedics, Hennepin County Medical Center, University of Minnesota, 701 Park Avenue S, Minneapolis, MN 55404, USA; [c] Regional One Health, University of Tennessee-Campbell Clinic, Memphis, TN, USA
* Corresponding author.
E-mail address: templ015@umn.edu

Orthop Clin N Am 47 (2016) 365–375
http://dx.doi.org/10.1016/j.ocl.2015.09.010
0030-5898/16/$ – see front matter © 2016 Elsevier Inc. All rights reserved.

Table 1
Increased costs associated with nonunion of the tibia

	Tibial Nonunion	Tibial Union
Inpatient	$7263.96	$2868.56
Outpatient	$1300.95	$490.14
Narcotics	$1,0300.95	$605.44

Data from Antonova E, Le TK, Burge R, et al. Tibia shaft fractures: costly burden of nonunions. BMC Musculoskelet Disord 2013;14:42.

to bridging callus on at least 3 cortices. However, these findings remain to be correlated with clinical outcomes.[4,5]

The score for each individual cortex is summed yielding a score between 4 and 16.

In addition to the RUST, computed tomography is helpful for evaluating suspected nonunions.[6]

A nonunion is generally defined as radiographic evidence of nonprogression of healing for at least 3 months, or lack of healing by 9 months since injury. Although the clinical and radiographic criteria discussed above are routinely used by most surgeons, there is a lack of consensus as to the real-time functional definition of nonunion.[7] It can be agreed, however, that nonunion is the cessation of both endosteal and periosteal healing responses without bridging callus.[8]

CLASSIFICATION

The classification of nonunions has not changed, and both the biological and mechanical characteristics must be evaluated for each case. The most important biological factor is the presence or absence of sepsis. Mechanical characteristics are frequently described as

- Hypertrophic-exuberant callous but not united, indicating a lack of stability but good biology;

Table 2
Radiographic union score for tibia fractures, modified

Score	Radiographic Description
1	No evident callus
2	Callus present
3	Bridging callus
4	Remodeling – no fracture visible

Data from Litrenta J, Tornetta P III, Mehta S, et al. Determination of radiographic healing: an assessment of consistency using RUST and modified RUST in metadiaphyseal fractures. J Orthop Trauma 2015;29(11):516–20.

- Atrophic-absent or minimal callous, which indicates a poor biological healing response;
- Oligotrophic-incomplete callous formation, which completes the spectrum between hypertrophic and atrophic.

FRACTURE-SPECIFIC AND TREATMENT-RELATED RISK FACTORS

Opening of the fracture site,[9] severe open injuries,[10] and the presence or development of infection[10] have been associated with nonunion after intramedullary nailing of the long bones.

PATIENT-RELATED RISK FACTORS
Metabolic, Endocrine, and Other Systemic Factors

The importance of bone metabolism is increasingly recognized as a key component of fracture care. Brinker and colleagues[11] examined the results of endocrinology referrals for 37 patients with nonunion. Criteria for referral included an unexplained nonunion without obvious technical error or other cause (26 patients), a history of multiple low-energy fractures with at least 1 progressing to a nonunion (8 patients), or nonunion of a nondisplaced pubic rami or sacral alar fracture (3 patients). They found that 31 of 37 patients (84%) who met screening criteria had a new diagnosis of a metabolic or an endocrine abnormality. Twenty-four patients (65%) had more than 1 metabolic or endocrine abnormality. Eight patients (22%) healed with medical treatment alone. Among the new diagnoses, 87% had a vitamin D deficiency or abnormal calcium regulation, 24% had thyroid dysfunction, 22% had reproductive hormone dysregulation, 13% had pituitary dysfunction, and 11% had parathyroid dysfunction.[11]

25-Hydroxyvitamin D (25[OH]D) deficiency and insufficiency has been well documented in orthopedic trauma patients. Prevalence is high, as a majority (66%–86%) of patients have levels deemed insufficient (<30 ng/mL), whereas approximately half (40%–53%) are deficient (<20 ng/mL).[12–15] Dark-skinned individuals are disproportionately affected,[14,15] as are those between the ages of 18 and 60 years versus older or younger individuals.[12,14]

The ramifications of insufficiency or deficiency on fracture healing and risk of nonunion are still unknown. A recent review notes that fracture may result in higher interosseous vitamin D metabolites and lower serum vitamin D metabolites; however, this finding is not consistent among studies.[16] The prevalence of vitamin D deficiency in nonunion patients is also debated, as at least one small case-control study demonstrates higher prevalence of deficiency in nonunion patients,[17] whereas another study seems to refute this.[18] The effect of vitamin D supplementation on fracture healing is unclear; although animal studies demonstrate promising results, the few small human studies do not consistently demonstrate benefit.[19,20] Thus, the role of vitamin D supplementation in fracture healing and nonunion treatment remains to be elucidated.

The medical comorbidities of the patients are correlated with increased risk of nonunion. Insulin-dependent and insulin-independent diabetes, as well as rheumatoid arthritis, have been linked to nonunion.[21,22] HIV infection seems to correlate with nonunion, but data are limited.[23]

Tobacco

Smoking may be the most well-documented modifiable patient factor correlated with nonunion and longer healing times. Meta-analysis of high-quality studies confirm the increased risk of nonunion for all fractures, but this seems to be particularly evident for open fractures and tibial fractures. Smoking is also associated with a trend toward increasing the time to union and increasing the rates of superficial and deep infections.[24] These findings have been confirmed prospectively.[25]

The potential for smoking cessation programs to improve fracture healing is unknown. The only published, prospective, randomized study demonstrated a trend toward lower superficial wound infections in the acute phase of postoperative fracture care but did not follow patients long enough to document the effect of smoking cessation on union rates.[26] Of the 287 eligible patients who met the inclusion criteria, 182 (63%) declined to participate; thus patient compliance with smoking cessation programs in the setting of fracture care remains unknown. No studies have evaluated the isolated effect of smoking cessation on established nonunions.

Medications (Nonsteroidal Anti-inflammatory Drugs)

A link between nonsteroidal anti-inflammatory drugs (NSAIDs) and nonunion has been demonstrated in animal studies. This has been shown for both selective and nonselective cox inhibitors, although the effects may be reversible after short-term treatment.[27] Human studies have been slow to follow.[28,29] An association between NSAID use and nonunion has now been shown in a small retrospective study of femoral nonunion,[30] a large retrospective level 1 trauma center study of long bone fracture nonunions,[31,32] and a large

retrospective national database review of both long- and small-bone fracture nonunions.[21]

TREATMENT
Nonsurgical Treatment Adjuncts

Ultrasound
Few small randomized controlled trials of low intensity pulsed ultrasound (LIPUS) exist. One study demonstrated shorter healing times for conservatively treated acute tibia fractures,[33–35] whereas another did not find any difference with acute tibias treated with reamed and statically locked intramedullary nailing.[36] Use of LIPUS for established nonunion healing is purported to promote healing in 73% to 86% of cases[37–40]; however, these are retrospective studies without control groups, and no randomized trials exist.

Teriparatide
Teriparatide (rhPTH 1-34) has been demonstrated to result in clinically significant radiographic and functional healing of pelvic fractures in elderly women in a quasi-randomized clinical trial.[41] Promising results for use in nonunion cases have been presented in case reports; however, no randomized trials exist to date.

Lee and colleagues[42,43] presented a series of 3 nonunion cases, 1 femoral shaft fracture treated by previous intramedullary nail, 1 distal femur fracture treated by open reduction and internal fixation, and 1 femoral neck fracture treated by closed reduction and internal fixation with cannulated screws. All 3 cases were without any identifiable risk factors or infection, and all 3 achieved radiographic union with PTH and no further surgery within 3 months after start of treatment.

A similar case of an atrophic humeral shaft fracture nonunion, previously treated by flexible nails, has been presented. The only identifiable risk factor in that case was a 3-week course of NSAIDs during the early treatment. The fracture demonstrated complete healing within 3 to 5 months of PTH treatment without further surgery.[44] This same group reported successful treatment of a previously nonoperatively treated atrophic humeral shaft nonunion in a smoker with multiple psychiatric disorders and polysubstance abuse. PTH treatment alone resulted in union after 4 months.[45]

Preoperative Assessment

Once a nonunion has been identified, thorough assessment of possible causes should be performed. The first step is to assess the initial treatment. Assessment of the reduction, choice of fixation, fracture characteristics, and condition of soft tissues should be assessed in all nonunion cases. If the fracture was open, the adequacy of debridement and loss of soft tissues should be analyzed.

A thorough medical history should be obtained, particularly in diabetics who require blood sugar and A1C laboratory assessment. Their history should be explored for rheumatoid arthritis or other autoimmune disorders, HIV, renal, respiratory, or any other significant chronic disease.

The past medical history should include any previous history of wound problems; a history of bisphosphonate use or NSAIDs administration; and social factors including smoking and alcoholism; and social barriers that imply difficulty in access and follow-up to medical care.

All nonunion patients should have their vitamin D level assessed. Consideration should also be given to obtaining laboratory values of calcium, thyroid, parathyroid, and reproductive hormone, as these are also common abnormalities. Referral to an endocrinologist may be warranted.

The possibility of infection should be assessed, with the patient's history and laboratory values, including white blood cell (WBC) count, erythrocyte sedimentation rate (ESR), and C-reactive protein (CRP) levels. Even with a negative history and laboratory workup, intraoperative cultures from multiple sites should be taken from all nonunion cases to detect occult infections. Limited data demonstrate that polymerase chain reaction (PCR) of intraoperative samples may be warranted when available to the operating surgeon.

The applicability and role of a trial of nonoperative treatment should be assessed and discussed with the patient. This may vary on a case-specific basis, and may include correction of risk factors such as diabetes, smoking, and endocrine abnormalities. The use of nonsurgical adjuncts such as ultrasound or PTH may also be applicable in certain cases either before or in conjunction with surgery.

Infection

Diagnosis of infection

For surgical planning purposes, the possibility of infection requires preoperative evaluation in all nonunion cases.

Inflammatory laboratory values

The use of the WBC count, the ESR, and the CRP levels are accurate predictors of infection in nonunions. Stucken and colleagues[46] demonstrated that the likelihood of infection increases with each additional positive test. Based on their analysis, the predicted probabilities for 0, 1, 2, and 3 risk factors were 20%, 19%, 56%, and

100%, respectively. Their study also documented that expensive nuclear bone scans did not improve the predictive value of the WBC, ESR, and CRP.

Tissue culture

Intraoperative cultures remain the gold standard for diagnosing infections and the isolation of pathogenic organisms at the site of nonunions. Neither superficial swabbing nor needle biopsy is sufficient for the diagnosis or identification of pathogenic organisms. Perry[47] compared intraoperative superficial swabs with intraoperative needle biopsy and found that swabbing of wounds and needle biopsy identified organisms in only 55% to 62% of cases. In 10 cases of tibial nonunion with latent infection, as identified by intraoperative cultures, needle biopsy failed to result in any organism in 9 (90%) cases.

Harvest of tissue from multiple culture sites of suspected or known infections is recommended. Patzakis and colleagues[48] demonstrated the frequent polymicrobial nature of traumatic osteomyelitis in a series of 30 patients. Using aerobic, anaerobic, and fungal cultures of specimens harvested from the sinus track, purulent fluid, soft tissue, bone obtained from curettage, and the bed of the involved bone, multiple organisms were identified in 21 (70%) patients. Eleven patients (37%) had more than 3 organisms present.

Polymerase Chain Reaction

The role of biofilms has come to light in recent years, and this characteristic of pathogenic organisms, and the difficulty in culturing biofilm organisms may make even intraoperative cultures less reliable.[49] In the near future, PCR of intraoperative tissue may become the standard of care. Palmer and colleagues[50–52] compared intraoperative culture and molecular examination of harvested tissues via PCR of 34 nonunions. PCR assessed for the presence of bacterial 16S and 18S rDNA, and this was confirmed by fluorescent in situ hybridization. Eight cases (24%) were both culture positive and PCR positive, whereas 22 cases (65%) were culture negative and PCR positive. Only 4 cases (12%) were negative by both methods. Similar to the findings of Patzakis,[48] 21 of 30 infected cases (70%) were PCR positive for multiple organisms. Although this method is highly sensitive, it is not routinely available to most surgeons.

Treatment of Infected Nonunions

Operative treatment of infected nonunions requires adequate debridement of the nonunion site, appropriate fracture stabilization, and bone grafting when necessary. Both single- and multiple-staged procedures have been proposed.

One case series reviewed the treatment of 42 infected long bone nonunions. The investigators recommended single-stage debridement and bone grafting for nondraining quiescent infections and staged debridement and bone grafting for active infections. They also recommended fixation and bone grafting for gaps up to 4 cm, with distraction osteogenesis for gaps over that threshold.[53]

A review of published nonunion case series was unable to make recommendations for either single- or multiple-staged procedures. They found single-stage procedures to result in union in 70% to 100% of cases, with persistent infection in 0% to 55%. Similarly 2-staged strategies resulted in union in 66% to 100% of cases with persistent infection in 0% to 50%. They did, however, find that the use of an antibiotic-eluting device decreased persistent infection in planned staged debridement with secondary bone grafting. Cases with debridement and secondary bone grafting alone resulted in union in 75% to 100% of cases with 0% to 60% persistent infection, whereas in cases with debridement, antibiotic device placement and secondary bone grafting resulted in union in 93% to 100% of cases with 0% to 18% persistent infection.[54] Thus, although it is unclear if single- versus multiple-staged procedures are superior, if delayed bone grafting is planned, interim placement of an antibiotic-eluting device is beneficial to both healing and persistent infection.

Bone grafting: iliac crest bone graft versus reamer irrigator aspirator

Although iliac crest bone graft (ICBG) is the traditional biological adjuvant, the reamer irrigator aspirator (RIA) has emerged as an alternative for autograft harvest. The device allows a method of bone graft harvest from the intramedullary canal of the femur or tibia that rivals the gold standard ICBG in terms of both volume and osteogenic potential, while potentially decreasing donor site morbidity.[55] The potential for unique complications exist, including the risk of femoral neck fracture and shaft cut out with poor technique because of the sharp reamers.[55–58] The risk of postoperative fracture seems to be increased when RIA is used in patients with thin cortices or with overaggressive harvesting and/or reaming by the surgeon.[59] Significant blood volume loss caused by prolonged aspiration has also been reported.[56]

A recent review of the literature noted that RIA harvest has relatively low complication rates when there is adequate preoperative planning and a good technique is used. Four of 233 patients (1.7%) reported chronic pain. There were 4 fractures (1.7%) and 4 breaches of the anterior cortex (1.7%) that did not lead to other fractures, 1 violation of the knee joint, 1 vascular injury, but no nerve injuries. One episode of bradycardia and hypotension caused by prolonged aspiration led to a volume loss requiring transfusion. These investigators also noted that one case with excessive reaming of the femoral neck could have been avoided by use of a lateral entry point rather than via the piriformis.[60,61] A review of ICBG from the anterior iliac crest (AIC) and posterior iliac crest (PIC) in that same article noted 204 of 3180 (6.4%) and 164 of 1909 (8.6%) of AIC and PIC patients reported chronic pain, respectively. Sensory disturbances surrounding the harvest site were the second most common complication with 5.2% and 7.3% of AIC and PIC patients reporting them, respectively.[60]

Ex-vivo transcriptional and histologic analysis has demonstrated similar expression of osteogenic genes[62] and stem cell populations between RIA and ICBG samples.[62,63] A randomized controlled trial of RIA-harvested graft versus AIC or PIC-harvested ICBG demonstrated similar union rates and statistically, but likely not clinically, significant increased volume of bone graft and reduced harvest time with RIA compared with ICBG. Patients also reported less pain at the donor site with RIA compared with ICBG.[64]

Bone grafting: bone morphogenetic protein

Although recombinant human bone morphogenetic protein-2 (BMP-2) may provide a benefit in terms of reduced need for bone grafting or secondary procedures for acute Gustilo-Anderson type-III open tibial fractures,[65] it may not have a substantial role in nonunion treatment. A retrospective review has demonstrated that ICBG autograft results in a nonstatistically significant trend toward improved healing in established nonunion, compared with BMP-2 combined with allograft cancellous bone chips (85.1% vs 68.4%, respectively).[66,67] According to one retrospective review of a prospective database, there is no apparent advantage for use of BMP-2 with ICBG autograft versus ICBG autograft alone in treatment of established nonunion.[68] Thus, there is likely no role for BMP-2 when a suitable high-quality autograft such as ICBG or RIA graft is available.

In a single randomized controlled trial, recombinant human osteogenic protein-1 (rhOP-1 or BMP-7) demonstrated results equivalent to autograft (type not specified) (81% vs 85%) in terms of radiographic and clinical healing at 9 months, and with a similar need for further surgical treatment (5% vs 10%). The BMP-7 group consisted of a higher proportion of atrophic nonunion than the bone graft group (65% vs 41%).[69] A small prospective nonrandomized comparative study of the direct medical costs associated with BMP-7 versus ICBG noted higher initial costs associated with BMP-7 treatment, in large part because of the cost of BMP-7.[70]

Specific Treatment of Tibial Shaft Fractures

Tibial nail dynamization and exchange nailing

Exchange nailing and nail dynamization are two common methods for treating aseptic nonunion of the tibia. Dynamization is performed by removing the interlocking bolts that are most distant from the fracture site, and it relies on weight bearing to compress the fracture site; theoretically this stimulates union by mechanical compression. Exchange nailing involves reaming the intramedullary canal and using a larger nail. The reaming is believed to biologically stimulate fracture healing by depositing the reamings as a local bone graft and also by generating a revascularization of the fracture site. In addition, insertion of a larger nail improves the stability of the fracture site. Two recent studies have re-addressed these techniques. Litrenta and colleagues[4,5] retrospectively compared a series of 194 tibial nonunions treated with either dynamization (97 patients) or exchange nailing (97 patients). High union rates were achieved in both groups with dynamization and exchange nailing resulting in 83% and 90% union, respectively. The investigators noted that gaps of greater than 5 mm were associated with a 78% union rate compared with a 90% union rate with no gap at the fracture site. Because this was a retrospective study, the indications for dynamization or exchange nailing were based on the preferences of the treating surgeons and do not clearly establish either the indications or the benefits of one procedure over the other.

Swanson and colleagues[71,72] treated 46 tibial nonunions with exchange nailing and achieved a success rate of 98%. This protocol included reaming, increasing the nail diameter by at least 2 mm, static interlocking, and low incidence of fibulectomy. Achieving cortical contact with a minimum of 50% cortical contact was an important inclusion criterion in this series. All cases were statically locked, but other series have recommended dynamic locking at the time of exchange nailing, so no conclusions can be made regarding the benefits of static versus dynamic interlocking at the time of exchange nailing.

Although dynamization and exchange nailing can be effective in the treatment of delayed and nonunion, waiting to intervene is also important. The SPRINT trial (Study to Prospectively Evaluate Reamed Intramedullary Nails in Patients with Tibial Fractures) documents that nonunion rates and secondary events are significantly reduced by allowing a minimum 6-month postoperative period for tibial fractures to heal after intramedullary nailing. With this protocol, the trial observed only a 4.6% rate of exchange nailing or bone grafting for treating nonunions.[54,73] Although the study was initially designed to compare the relative merits of reamed versus nonreamed nailing techniques for closed and open fractures, the greatest benefit seems to be establishing that, by avoiding "fracture site gaps" at the time of intramedullary nailing, most fractures will progress to union, with a slight advantage for reamed nailing in closed tibia fractures.

While waiting to intervene in many tibia fractures may be appropriate, this approach may cause some patients unnecessary and prolonged morbidity. Yang and colleagues[74–76] have shown that experienced orthopedic trauma surgeons can use mechanism of injury and radiographic parameters at 3 months to determine patients who will ultimately proceed to nonunion. It is to be hoped that future investigation will clarify the fracture, treatment, and patient characteristics that predict nonunion and lead to early effective intervention.

Specific Treatment of Femoral Shaft Fractures

Nonunion of femoral shaft fractures treated by intramedullary nailing is uncommon. Union rates as high as 98% to 99% have been reported with reamed intramedullary nailing, which is the standard of care for closed fractures of the femoral shaft.[77–79] Nonunion has been associated with open fractures and delayed weight bearing,[80] as well as Arbeitsgemeinschaft für Osteosynthesefragen/Orthopaedic Trauma Association (AO/OTA) fracture classification.[81]

Femoral Exchange Nailing

Exchange nailing seems to be successful in the treatment of femoral nonunions. Swanson and colleagues[71,72] recently reported 100% union rate with exchange nailing of aseptic nonunions. This technique was used even with atrophic nonunions (7/50) and bone grafting was not used. Treatment was focused on increasing the stability of the construct by placing an intramedullary nail at least 2 mm larger than the original one. The method of intramedullary nail placement (antegrade vs retrograde) was also chosen to optimize stability in meta-diaphyseal fractures with short segments, as 6 exchange nailings were performed in the opposite direction of the original intramedullary nailing.

Plating/Bone Grafting over a Nail

Exchange nailing may not be as successful with meta-diaphyseal nonunions.[74–76] Hakeos and colleagues[82] have recently described, in a very small series, open plating of proximal and distal meta-diaphyseal fractures while leaving the intramedullary nail in place. These investigators report a 100% union rate with this technique. Bone grafting was used with this technique of open plating. A second small series (7/11 nonunions were of the femur) also demonstrated a 100% union rate with plating and bone grafting around an intramedullary nail.[83] Unfortunately, neither of these small studies had a comparison group, so determining the effectiveness of the plating and bone grafting individually is impossible.

Atypical Femoral Fractures and Bisphosphonates

Osteoporosis was believed to be a risk factor for delayed healing and nonunion; however, early studies were not age matched.[84] Osteoporosis and decreased bone density are not risk factors for nonunion when matched for age and sex.[85] These findings are confirmed in a large retrospective national database review of both long- and small-bone fracture nonunions.[21] Thus, it seems that nonunion in advanced age is more significantly related to the healing capacity of bone, which declines with age, rather than trabecular density.

Bisphosphonates are a major treatment of osteoporosis and prevent bone loss by inhibiting osteoclastic mediated bone resorption. However, this effect also inhibits the osteoclastic activity during normal bone healing and seems to increase the risk of nonunion. In one study of 17 femur fractures in 15 patients treated with bisphosphonates for an average of 7.8 years, 7 of 12 (58%) subtrochanteric and midshaft femoral fractures treated with intramedullary nailing required secondary surgery.[86] Revisions varied from dynamization, to exchange nailing, to conversion to blade plate. Another study of 41 atypical femur fractures treated by intramedullary nailing in 33 patients with a history of bisphosphonate treatment for an average of 8.8 years demonstrated that, although 98% of patients appeared to have radiographically united, only 66% of patients were pain free at the fracture site at 1 year.[87] A third retrospective study of 33 consecutive female patients presenting with atypical subtrochanteric femur fractures after bisphosphonate therapy demonstrated 6.7 months to full weight bearing, 10.9 months to radiologic union, a revision rate of 38%, and an implant failure rate of 29% in 21 patients treated with extramedullary implants, versus 8.2 months to full weight bearing, 7.7 months to radiologic union, 22% revision rate, and 11% implant failures in 9 patients treated with intramedullary implants (**Table 3**).[88]

Intramedullary implants are recommended for the treatment of bisphosphonate-related fractures[89]; however, as mentioned previously, a significant known failure rate has now been demonstrated.[86–88] Some investigators have recommended treatment with compression plating, which may result in more reliable healing.[90,91] Further research to assess the optimal fixation strategy is necessary. Although bone grafting is frequently considered at the time of nonunion surgery in the presence of prolonged bisphosphonate therapy, the patient's autogenous bone graft will also have been subjected to the effects of bisphosphonates and may not promote union. For recalcitrant bisphosphonate nonunions, segmental resection of sclerotic bone should be considered until there is better evidence to guide treatment.

PTH is known to increase bone turnover. Animal studies have demonstrated that use of PTH may help re-establish bone and bisphosphonate metabolism in animals previously treated with bisphosphonates.[92,93] This is supported by a retrospective review of atypical femur fractures treated with or without PTH after cessation of bisphosphonate treatment. Patients treated with PTH demonstrated faster times to union and decreased frequency of delayed or nonunion.[94]

Table 3
Intramedullary versus extramedullary fixation in atypical femur fractures associated with prolonged bisphosphonate therapy

	Intramedullary	Extramedullary
Time to weight bearing	8.2 mo	6.7 mo
Radiographic union	7.7 mo	10.9 mo
Revision surgery	22%	38%
Implant failures	11%	29%

Data from Teo BJ, Koh JS, Goh SK, et al. Post-operative outcomes of atypical femoral subrochanteric fracture in patients on bisphosphonate therapy. Bone Joint J 2014;96-B(5):660.

SUMMARY

Delayed union and nonunion of tibial and femoral shaft fractures are common problems that an orthopedic surgeon encounters. It is hoped that, through an improved understanding of the current trends and recent literature surrounding tibial and femoral nonunions, the orthopedic surgeon will be more comfortable dealing with these difficult problems.

REFERENCES

1. Antonova E, Le TK, Burge R, et al. Tibia shaft fractures: costly burden of nonunions. BMC Musculoskelet Disord 2013;14:42.
2. Audige L, Griffin D, Bhandari M, et al. Path analysis of factors for delayed healing and nonunion in 416 operatively treated tibial shaft fractures. Clin Orthop Relat Res 2005;438:221–32.
3. Tay WH, de Steiger R, Richardson M, et al. Health outcomes of delayed union and nonunion of femoral and tibial shaft fractures. Injury 2014;45(10):1653–8.
4. Litrenta J, Tornetta P III, Mehta S, et al. Determination of radiographic healing: an assessment of consistency using RUST and modified RUST in metadiaphyseal fractures. J Orthop Trauma 2015;29(11):516–20.
5. Litrenta J, Tornetta P III, Vallier H, et al. Dynamization and exchanges; success rates and indications. J Orthop Trauma 2015;29(12):569–73.
6. Kuhlman JE, Fishman EK, Magid D, et al. Fracture nonunion: CT assessment with multiplanar reconstruction. Radiology 1988;167(2):483–8.
7. Bhandari M, Fong K, Sprague S, et al. Variability in the definition and perceived causes of delayed unions and nonunions: a cross-sectional, multinational survey of orthopaedic surgeons. J Bone Joint Surg Am 2012;94(15):e1091–6.
8. Marsh D. Concepts of fracture union, delayed union, and nonunion. Clin Orthop Relat Res 1998;(355 Suppl):S22–30.
9. Malik MH, Harwood P, Diggle P, et al. Factors affecting rates of infection and nonunion in intramedullary nailing. J Bone Joint Surg Br 2004;86(4):556–60.
10. Harley BJ, Beaupre LA, Jones CA, et al. The effect of time to definitive treatment on the rate of nonunion and infection in open fractures. J Orthop Trauma 2002;16(7):484–90.
11. Brinker MR, O'Connor DP, Monla YT, et al. Metabolic and endocrine abnormalities in patients with nonunions. J Orthop Trauma 2007;21(8):557–70.
12. Bee CR, Sheerin DV, Wuest TK, et al. Serum vitamin D levels in orthopaedic trauma patients living in the northwestern United States. J Orthop Trauma 2013; 27(5):e103–6.
13. Bhandari M, Tornetta P 3rd, Hanson B, et al. Optimal internal fixation for femoral neck fractures: multiple screws or sliding hip screws? J Orthop Trauma 2009;23(6):403–7.
14. Bogunovic L, Kim AD, Beamer BS, et al. Hypovitaminosis D in patients scheduled to undergo orthopaedic surgery: a single-center analysis. J Bone Joint Surg Am 2010;92(13):2300–4.
15. Zellner BS, Dawson JR, Reichel LM, et al. Prospective nutritional analysis of a diverse trauma population demonstrates substantial hypovitaminosis D. J Orthop Trauma 2014;28(9):e210–5.
16. Gorter EA, Hamdy NA, Appelman-Dijkstra NM, et al. The role of vitamin D in human fracture healing: a systematic review of the literature. Bone 2014;64:288–97.
17. Tauber C, Noff D, Noff M, et al. Blood levels of active metabolites of vitamin D3 in fracture repair in humans. A preliminary report. Arch Orthop Trauma Surg 1990;109(5):265–7.
18. Haining SA, Atkins RM, Guilland-Cumming DF, et al. Vitamin D metabolites in patients with established non-union of fracture. Bone Miner 1986;1(3):205–9.
19. Eschle D, Aeschlimann AG. Is supplementation of vitamin d beneficial for fracture healing? A short review of the literature. Geriatr Orthop Surg Rehabil 2011;2(3):90–3.
20. Fong K, Truong V, Foote CJ, et al. Predictors of nonunion and reoperation in patients with fractures of the tibia: an observational study. BMC Musculoskelet Disord 2013;14:103.
21. Hernandez RK. Patient-related risk factors for fracture-healing complications in the United Kingdom general practice research database. Acta Orthop 2012;83(6):653–60.
22. Hoffman MF, Jones CB, Sietsema DL, et al. Clinical outcomes of locked plating of distal femoral fractures in a retrospective cohort. J Orthop Surg Res 2013;8:43.
23. Hao J. An observational case series of HIV-positive patients treated with open reduction internal fixation for a closed lower extremity fracture. Eur J Orthop Surg Traumatol 2015;25(5):815–9.
24. Scolaro JA, Schenker ML, Yannascoli S, et al. Cigarette smoking increases complications following fracture: a systematic review. J Bone Joint Surg Am 2014;96(8):674–81.
25. Moghaddam A, Zimmermann G, Hammer K, et al. Cigarette smoking influences the clinical and occupational outcome of patients with tibial shaft fractures. Injury 2011;42(12):1435–42.
26. Nåsell H, Adami J, Samnegård E, et al. Effect of smoking cessation intervention on results of acute fracture surgery: a randomized controlled trial. J Bone Joint Surg Am 2010;92(6):1335–42.
27. Gerstenfeld LC, Al-Ghawas M, Alkhiary YM, et al. Selective and nonselective cyclooxygenase-2 inhibitors and experimental fracture-healing. Reversibility of effects after short-term treatment. J Bone Joint Surg Am 2007;89(1):114–25.

28. Kurmis AP, Kurmis TP, O'Brien JX, et al. The effect of nonsteroidal anti-inflammatory drug administration on acute phase fracture-healing: a review. J Bone Joint Surg Am 2012;94(9):815–23.

29. Kuzyk PR, Bhandari M, McKee MD, et al. Intramedullary versus extramedullary fixation for subtrochanteric femur fracture. J Orthop Trauma 2009;23(6):465–70.

30. Giannoudis PV, MacDonald DA, Matthews SJ, et al. Nonunion of the femoral diaphysis. The influence of reaming and non-steroidal anti-inflammatory drugs. J Bone Joint Surg Br 2000;82(5):655–8.

31. Jeffcoach DR, Sams VG, Lawson CM, et al. Nonsteroidal anti-inflammatory drugs' impact on nonunion and infection rates in long-bone fractures. J Trauma Acute Care Surg 2014;76(3):779–83.

32. Kayal RA, Tsatsas D, Bauer MA, et al. Diminished bone formation during diabetic fracture healing is related to the premature resorption of cartilage associated with increased osteoclast activity. J Bone Miner Res 2007;22(4):560–8.

33. Heckman JD, Ryaby JP, McCabe J, et al. Acceleration of tibial fracture-healing by non-invasive, low-intensity pulsed ultrasound. J Bone Joint Surg Am 1994;76(1):26–34.

34. Hedström M. Are patients with a nonunion after a femoral neck fracture more osteoporotic than others? BMD measurement before the choice of treatment?: a pilot study of hip BMD and biochemical bone markers in patients with femoral neck fractures. Acta Orthop Scand 2004;75(1):50–2.

35. Heetveld MJ, Raaymakers EL, van Eck-Smit BL, et al. Internal fixation for displaced fractures of the femoral neck. Does bone density affect clinical outcome? J Bone Joint Surg Br 2005;87(3):367–73.

36. Emami A, Petrén-Mallmin M, Larsson S. No effect of low-intensity ultrasound on healing time of intramedullary fixed tibial fractures. J Orthop Trauma 1999;13(4):252–7.

37. Rutten S, Nolte PA, Guit GL, et al. Use of low-intensity pulsed ultrasound for posttraumatic nonunions of the tibia: a review of patients treated in the Netherlands. J Trauma 2007;62(4):902–8.

38. Watanabe Y, Arai Y, Takenaka N, et al. Three key factors affecting treatment results of low-intensity pulsed ultrasound for delayed unions and nonunions: instability, gap size, and atrophic nonunion. J Orthop Sci 2013;18(5):803–10.

39. Wang SH, Yang JJ, Shen HC, et al. Using a modified Pauwels method to predict the outcome of femoral neck fracture in relatively young patients. Injury 2015;46(10):1969–74.

40. Zura R, Della Rocca GJ, Mehta S, et al. Treatment of chronic (>1 year) fracture nonunion: heal rate in a cohort of 767 patients treated with low-intensity pulsed ultrasound (LIPUS). Injury 2015;46(10):2036–41.

41. Peichl P, Holzer LA, Maier R, et al. Parathyroid hormone 1-84 accelerates fracture-healing in pubic bones of elderly osteoporotic women. J Bone Joint Surg Am 2011;93(17):1583–7.

42. Lee YK, Ha YC, Koo KH. Teriparatide, a nonsurgical solution for femoral nonunion? A report of three cases. Osteoporos Int 2012;23(12):2897–900.

43. Liporace F, Gaines R, Collinge C, et al. Results of internal fixation of Pauwels type-3 vertical femoral neck fractures. J Bone Joint Surg Am 2008;90(8):1654–9.

44. Oteo-Alvaro A, Moreno E. Atrophic humeral shaft nonunion treated with teriparatide (rh PTH 1-34): a case report. J Shoulder Elbow Surg 2010;19(7):e22–8.

45. Oteo-Alvaro A, et al. Nonunion of the humeral shaft successfully treated with teriparatide [rh (1-34) PTH]. Case Rep Clin Med 2013;2(1):11–5.

46. Stucken C, Olszewski DC, Creevy WR, et al. Preoperative diagnosis of infection in patients with nonunions. J Bone Joint Surg Am 2013;95(15):1409–12.

47. Perry CR, Pearson RL, Miller GA. Accuracy of cultures of material from swabbing of the superficial aspect of the wound and needle biopsy in the preoperative assessment of osteomyelitis. J Bone Joint Surg Am 1991;73(5):745–9.

48. Patzakis MJ, Wilkins J, Kumar J, et al. Comparison of the results of bacterial cultures from multiple sites in chronic osteomyelitis of long bones. A prospective study. J Bone Joint Surg Am 1994;76(5):664–6.

49. Costerton JW. Biofilm theory can guide the treatment of device-related orthopaedic infections. Clin Orthop Relat Res 2005;437:7–11.

50. Palmer MP, Altman DT, Altman GT, et al. Can we trust intraoperative culture results in nonunions? J Orthop Trauma 2014;28(7):384–90.

51. Parker MJ, Raghavan R, Gurusamy K, et al. Incidence of fracture-healing complications after femoral neck fractures. Clin Orthop Relat Res 2007;458:175–9.

52. Parker MJ. Prediction of fracture union after internal fixation of intracapsular femoral neck fractures. Injury 1994;25(Suppl 2):B3–6.

53. Jain AK, Sinha S. Infected nonunion of the long bones. Clin Orthop Relat Res 2005;(431):57–65.

54. Struijs PA, Poolman RW, Bhandari M, et al. Infected nonunion of the long bones. J Orthop Trauma 2007;21(7):507–11.

55. Belthur MV, Conway JD, Jindal G, et al. Bone graft harvest using a new intramedullary system. Clin Orthop Relat Res 2008;466:2973–80.

56. Quintero AJ, Tarkin IS, Pape HC. Technical tricks when using the reamer irrigator aspirator technique for autologous bone graft harvesting. J Orthop Trauma 2010;24(1):42–5.

57. Ricci WM, Streubel PN, Morshed S, et al. Risk factors for failure of locked plate fixation of distal femur fractures: an analysis of 335 cases. J Orthop Trauma 2014;28(2):83–9.

58. Rodriguez EK, Boulton C, Weaver MJ, et al. Predictive factors of distal femoral fracture nonunion after lateral locked plating: a retrospective multicenter case-control study of 283 fractures. Injury 2014; 45(3):554–9.

59. Pratt DJ, Papagiannopoulos G, Rees PH, et al. The effects of medullary reaming on the torsional strength of the femur. Injury 1987;18(3):177–9.

60. Dimitriou R, Mataliotakis GI, Angoules AG, et al. Complications following autologous bone graft harvesting from the iliac crest and using the RIA: a systematic review. Injury 2011;42(Suppl 2):S3–15.

61. Drosos GI, Bishay M, Karnezis IA, et al. Factors affecting fracture healing after intramedullary nailing of the tibial diaphysis for closed and grade I open fractures. J Bone Joint Surg Br 2006;88(2):227–31.

62. Sagi HC, Young ML, Gerstenfeld L, et al. Qualitative and quantitative differences between bone graft obtained from the medullary canal (with a Reamer/Irrigator/Aspirator) and the iliac crest of the same patient. J Bone Joint Surg Am 2012; 94(23):2128–35.

63. Henrich D, Seebach C, Sterlepper E, et al. RIA reamings and hip aspirate: a comparative evaluation of osteoprogenitor and endothelial progenitor cells. Injury 2010;41(S2):S62–8.

64. Dawson J, Kiner D, Gardner W 2nd, et al. The reamer-irrigator-aspirator as a device for harvesting bone graft compared with iliac crest bone graft: union rates and complications. J Orthop Trauma 2014;28(10):584–90.

65. Swiontkowski MF, Aro HT, Donell S, et al. Recombinant human bone morphogenetic protein-2 in open tibial fractures. A subgroup analysis of data combined from 2 prospective randomized studies. J Bone Joint Surg Am 2006;88(6):1258–65.

66. Tressler MA, Richards JE, Sofianos D, et al. Bone morphogenetic protein-2 compared to autologous iliac crest bone graft in the treatment of long bone nonunion. Orthopedics 2011;34(12):e877–84.

67. Upadhyay A, Jain P, Mishra P, et al. Delayed internal fixation of fractures of the neck of the femur in young adults. A prospective, randomised study comparing closed and open reduction. J Bone Joint Surg Br 2004;86(7):1035–40.

68. Takemoto R, Forman J, Taormina DP, et al. No advantage to rhBMP-2 in addition to autogenous graft for fracture nonunion. Orthopedics 2014; 37(6):e525–30.

69. Friedlaender GE, Perry CR, Cole JD, et al. Osteogenic protein-1 (bone morphogenetic protein-7) in the treatment of tibial nonunions. J Bone Joint Surg Am 2001;83-A(Suppl 1(Pt 2)):S151–8.

70. Dahabreh Z, Calori GM, Kanakaris NK, et al. A cost analysis of treatment of tibial fracture nonunion by bone grafting or bone morphogenetic protein-7. Int Orthop 2009;33(5):1407–14.

71. Swanson EA, Garrard EC, O'Connor DP, et al. Results of a systematic approach to exchange nailing for the treatment of aseptic tibial nonunions. J Orthop Trauma 2015;29(1):28–35.

72. Swanson EA, Garrard EC, Bernstein DT, et al. Results of a systematic approach to exchange nailing for the treatment of aseptic femoral nonunions. J Orthop Trauma 2015;29(1):21–7.

73. SPRINT Investigators. A randomized trial of reamed and unreamed intramedullary nailing of tibial shaft fractures. J Bone Joint Surg Am 2008;90:2567–78.

74. Yang JJ, Lin LC, Chao KH, et al. Risk factors for nonunion in patients with intracapsular femoral neck fractures treated with three cannulated screws placed in either a triangle or an inverted triangle configuration. J Bone Joint Surg Am 2013;95(1):61–9.

75. Yang KS. Can tibial nonunion be predicted at 3 months after intramedullary nailing? J Orthop Trauma 2013;27(11):599–603.

76. Yang KH, Kim JR, Park J. Nonisthmal femoral shaft nonunion as a risk factor for exchange nailing failure. J Trauma Acute Care Surg 2012;72(2):E60–4.

77. Brumback RJ, Uwagie-Ero S, Lakatos RP, et al. Intramedullary nailing of femoral shaft fractures. Part II: fracture-healing with static interlocking fixation. J Bone Joint Surg Am 1988;70(10):1453–62.

78. Winquist RA, Hansen ST Jr, Clawson DK, et al. Closed intramedullary nailing of femoral fractures. A report of five hundred and twenty cases. J Bone Joint Surg Am 1984;66(4):529–39.

79. Xia L, Zhou J, Zhang Y, et al. A meta-analysis of reamed versus unreamed intramedullary nailing for the treatment of closed tibial fractures. Orthopedics 2014;37(4):e332–8.

80. Taitsman LA, Lynch JR, Agel J, et al. Risk factors for femoral nonunion after femoral shaft fracture. J Trauma 2009;67(6):1389–92.

81. Metsemakers W, Roels N, Belmans A, et al. Risk factors for nonunion after intramedullary nailing of femoral shaft fractures - remaining controversies. Injury 2015;46(8):1601–7.

82. Hakeos WM, Richards JE, Obremskey WT. Plate fixation of femoral nonunions over intramedullary nail with autogenous bone grafting. J Orthop Trauma 2011;25(2):84–9.

83. Nadkarni B, Srivastav S, Mittal V, et al. Use of a locking compression plate for long bone nonunions without removing existing intramedullary nail: review of literature and our experience. J Trauma 2008; 65(2):482–6.

84. Nikolaou VS, Efstathopoulos N, Kontakis G, et al. The influence of osteoporosis in femoral fracture healing time. Injury 2009;40(6):663–8.

85. van Wunnik BP, Weijers PH, van Helden SH, et al. Osteoporosis is not a risk factor for the development of nonunion: a cohort nested case-control study. Injury 2011;42(12):1491–4.

86. Weil YA, Rivkin G, Safran O, et al. The outcome of surgically treated femur fractures associated with long-term bisphosphonate use. J Trauma 2011; 71(1):186–90.

87. Egol KA, Park JH, Rosenberg ZS, et al. Healing delayed but generally reliable after bisphosphonate-associated complete femur fractures treated with IM nails. Clin Orthop Relat Res 2014;472(9): 2728–34.

88. Teo BJ, Koh JS, Goh SK, et al. Post-operative outcomes of atypical femoral subtrochanteric fracture in patients on bisphosphonate therapy. Bone Joint J 2014;96-B(5):658–64.

89. Das DS, Setiobudi T, Shen L, et al. A rational approach to management of alendronate-related subtrochanteric fractures. J Bone Joint Surg Br 2010;92(5):679–86.

90. Grady MK, Watson JT, Cannada LK. Treatment of femoral fracture nonunion after long-term bisphosphonate use. Orthopedics 2012;35(6): e991–5.

91. Haidukewych GJ, Rothwell WS, Jacofsky DJ, et al. Operative treatment of femoral neck fractures in patients between the ages of fifteen and fifty years. J Bone Joint Surg Am 2004;86-A(8):1711–6.

92. Murphy CM, Schindeler A, Cantrill LC, et al. PTH(1-34) treatment increases bisphosphonate turnover in fracture repair in rats. J Bone Miner Res 2015;30(6):1022–9.

93. Murphy DK, Randell T, Brennan KL, et al. Treatment and displacement affect the reoperation rate for femoral neck fracture. Clin Orthop Relat Res 2013; 471(8):2691–702.

94. Miyakoshi N, Aizawa T, Sasaki S, et al. Healing of bisphosphonate-associated atypical femoral fractures in patients with osteoporosis: a comparison between treatment with and without teriparatide. J Bone Miner Metab 2015;33(5):553–9.

Pediatrics

Complications of Pediatric Elbow Fractures

Brad T. Hyatt, MD, Matthew R. Schmitz, MD, Jeremy K. Rush, MD*

KEYWORDS

- Pediatric elbow fractures • Malunion • Nonunion • Tardy ulnar nerve palsy

KEY POINTS

- Cubitus varus can lead to increased risk of subsequent fracture, elbow instability, and tardy ulnar nerve palsy, and can typically be treated with a correctional osteotomy.
- Displaced lateral condyle fractures found acutely are best treated with open reduction and internal fixation (ORIF); fractures found late can be corrected with various osteotomies. The treatment of subacute fractures (3–12 weeks) is controversial, with recent literature advocating ORIF.
- Medial epicondyle nonunion is common but rarely causes functional deficits.
- Elbow stiffness in pediatric patients is a rare but challenging complication.
- Missed osteochondral lesions and missed Monteggia fractures have poor outcomes and providers evaluating patients with elbow injuries and normal plain films should have a low threshold for obtaining advanced imaging.

INTRODUCTION

Fractures about the elbow are common in children and adolescents and comprise 5% to 10% of fractures in this age group.[1–4] They also account for most operatively treated injuries, up to 85% in some series.[2,3] Supracondylar humerus fractures are the most common injury in this region, followed by lateral condyle and medial epicondyle fractures. The unique developmental anatomy of the elbow makes radiographs sometimes difficult to interpret. Combined with the potential for complications in the growing child, this often provokes anxiety in referring primary care providers, emergency medicine physicians, or even treating orthopedic surgeons. This article discusses the diagnosis and management of the most common complications encountered by treating orthopedic surgeons.

SUPRACONDYLAR HUMERUS FRACTURES
Malunion

Cubitus varus is defined as a loss of carrying angle of more than 5° compared with the contralateral elbow. It is the most common angular deformity following supracondylar humerus fractures.[5,6] Historically, it has been reported in up to 58% of nonoperatively treated patients.[7] Pirone and colleagues[8] observed a 3% incidence after operative management of supracondylar humerus fractures. In current practice, an estimated 5% to 10% of supracondylar humerus fractures develop cubitus varus[8]; although rates are lower with operative treatment, varus deformity can occur, typically caused by suboptimal Kirschner wire (K-wire) placement.[7] The typical deformity includes varus malalignment, internal malrotation, and hyperextension or recurvatum (**Fig. 1**).[9]

Department of Orthopaedics and Rehabilitation, San Antonio Military Medical Center, 3551 Roger Brooke Drive, Fort Sam Houston, TX 78234, USA
* Corresponding author.
E-mail address: jeremy.k.rush.mil@mail.mil

Orthop Clin N Am 47 (2016) 377–385
http://dx.doi.org/10.1016/j.ocl.2015.09.011
0030-5898/16/$ – see front matter Published by Elsevier Inc.

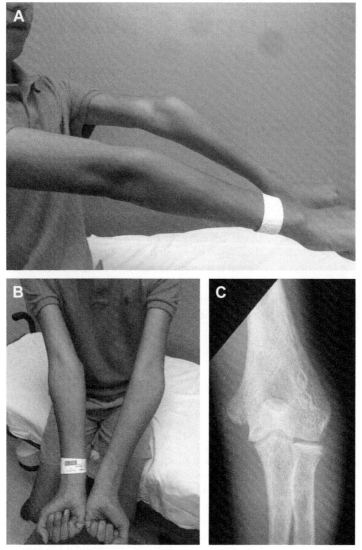

Fig. 1. (*A, B*) Clinical photographs and (*C*) anterior-posterior (AP) radiograph showing left cubitus varus malunion following supracondylar humerus fracture.

Cubitus varus has traditionally been regarded as a cosmetic concern but recent studies have shown the potential for functional complications. Two recent studies have identified cubitus varus as a risk factor for subsequent fracture.[10,11] Davids and colleagues[10] reported on 6 children who sustained lateral condyle fractures at an average of 32 months after their initial elbow fracture. These patients had cubitus varus as a sequela of their initial injury (supracondylar fracture in 5 and lateral condyle in 1), and the investigators suggest that varus deformity increases both the shear force and torsional moment generated by a fall. In a similar study, Takahara and colleagues[11] described 9 patients with previous supracondylar fractures

who sustained epiphyseal injuries (8 lateral condyle fractures and 1 physeal separation). These patients all had cubitus varus deformity following their initial fracture, and sustained the second fracture at an average of 18 months after the first.

Cubitus varus from remote fracture was also identified as a contributing factor in 18 patients with posterolateral rotatory instability (PLRI).[12] The average varus was 15° and the tardy PLRI presented more than 20 years following the fracture. The investigators illustrate the mechanism whereby cubitus varus leads to chronic attenuation of the lateral collateral ligament complex.

Multiple studies have also identified cubitus varus as a precursor to tardy ulnar nerve palsy, despite being more commonly associated with cubitus valgus. Various mechanisms by which varus deformity leads to ulnar nerve symptoms have been described. In 14 of their 15 patients, Abe and colleagues[13] found the ulnar nerve to be constricted by a fibrous band between the 2 heads of the flexor carpi ulnaris; 9 of these patients also had an ulnar nerve that ran anterior to the deformity. Spinner and colleagues[14] reported on 5 patients with snapping (dislocation) of the medial portion of the triceps with the ulnar nerve, leading to either friction neuritis or compression of the ulnar nerve by the snapping triceps muscle. In contrast, Mitsunari and colleagues[15] showed a significant association between tardy ulnar palsy and the internal rotation deformity that occurred as a sequela of supracondylar humerus fracture, rather than the varus deformity. They proposed that the internal rotation involves posterior displacement of the distal medial fragment, which causes stretching of the ulnar nerve with elbow flexion.

Various osteotomies have been advocated, all of which attempt to correct varus angulation; complex and dome osteotomies may also improve rotation or hyperextension, or minimize lateral prominence. Proponents of complex osteotomies cite better correction and cosmesis,[9,16] whereas advocates for simple closing wedge osteotomies cite functional improvement and lower complication rates.[17,18]

In most cases, a simple closing wedge osteotomy fixed with percutaneously placed K-wires suffices.[19,20] In a systematic review of 40 studies involving nearly 900 patients, Sofelt and colleagues[20] found a mean angular correction of 27.6° across all osteotomy types. No technique showed statistically significant superiority to another, and there were no differences in

complication rates. The overall complication rate was 14.5%, with transient nerve palsy being the most common. In a recent retrospective study of 90 patients treated with a French osteotomy (a lateral closing wedge osteotomy that relies on an intact medial hinge and lateral screw and wire tension-band construct), North and colleagues[18] reported a complication rate of 3.3% and no nerve injuries.

The timing of corrective osteotomy is controversial. At a minimum, surgery should be delayed until the fracture has healed, remodeling is mature, and range of motion has reached maximum improvement. Ippolito and colleagues[21] recommended waiting until close to skeletal maturity because several of their patients showed loss of correction with continued growth. However, Voss and colleagues[22] found that 11% of the patients in their series showed disruption of medial-sided growth. They thought that this could lead to progressive worsening of deformity and recommended corrective osteotomy at least 1 year after injury, but not necessarily waiting until skeletal maturity.

LATERAL CONDYLE FRACTURES
Nonunion and Malunion

Nonunion is more common in lateral condyle fractures than supracondylar humerus fractures (**Fig. 2**). The reason for this is likely multifactorial and may involve the intra-articular nature of the fracture, poor blood supply of the epiphyseal fragment, and the pull of the common forearm extensor tendon.[23,24] Risk factors for nonunion include delayed diagnosis and nonoperative treatment.[7,23] Symptomatic patients may complain of ulnar nerve dysfunction, pain, instability, or deformity.[25] Treatment depends on the timing of

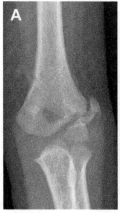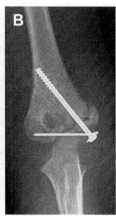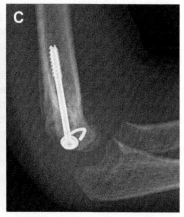

Fig. 2. Lateral condyle nonunion in a 5-year-old boy. (*A*) At 7 weeks postinjury, the lateral condyle shows evidence of nonunion on this AP radiograph. (*B*) AP and (*C*) lateral radiographs following open reduction and internal fixation.

diagnosis and the distinction between delayed union and nonunion.[26] Most investigators agree that acute fractures (<3 weeks from injury) with more than 2 mm of displacement should be reduced and stabilized surgically.[27,28] In addition, there is agreement that symptomatic nonunions (>12 weeks from injury) also benefit from surgery.[26,29]

Delayed presentation (3–12 weeks from injury) of a displaced fracture continues to be a controversial problem. Cited reasons for nonoperative treatment include the possibility of asymptomatic malunion with immobilization alone, difficulty with reduction given soft tissue swelling and callus formation, tenuous blood supply to the distal fragment, and the risk of physeal arrest.[26,30] Although older studies found no benefit with surgery in patients treated greater than 3 to 6 weeks after injury,[30–32] newer studies advocate open reduction and fixation.[33,34] Wattenberger and colleagues[33] reported on 9 patients who underwent open reduction and pin fixation greater than 3 weeks postinjury. Union was universal and there was no avascular necrosis. Similarly, Agarwal and colleagues[34] treated 22 patients greater than 4 weeks from injury with open reduction and pinning or screw fixation in older children. They reported overall favorable results, with 2 cases each of nonunion and physeal arrest, and 1 case of avascular necrosis. Both studies emphasized the importance of maintaining the posterior soft tissue attachments in order to avoid avascular necrosis.

Treatment of an established nonunion should be guided by the severity of symptoms, patient age, and functional goals, as well as the patient's and family's expectations and commitment to participate in therapy.[26,29] Risks of surgery include osteonecrosis, loss of range of motion, physeal arrest, and persistent nonunion.[30,35,36] Long-standing nonunions from fractures extending lateral to the capitellotrochlear groove (Milch type I) are more likely to be symptomatic, and may benefit from surgical correction more than fractures with an intact radiocapitellar joint.[37]

Given the complexity of lateral condyle nonunion, multiple surgical strategies have been suggested.[26,28,35,37–41] Papandrea and Waters[26] describe the surgeon's dilemma as choosing between fixation in situ with the potential for angular deformity, or reduction with the potential for avascular necrosis. Either choice may also require a supracondylar osteotomy, bone grafting, and nerve decompression/transposition, which can be performed at the time of fracture fixation or in a staged fashion.[26,37]

High union rates with good functional outcomes have been reported with fibrous take-down,

reduction, and fixation with K-wires, as long as soft tissue stripping is minimized.[35,36] These investigators recommend ranging the joint after provisional anatomic fixation; if range of motion is decreased compared with baseline, the fragment is replaced in its displaced location and stabilized. They also recommend fixation adjuncts, as needed, including cancellous screws for large fragments, a tension-band technique, or a narrow plate. If the pull of the common extensor tendon makes reduction difficult, a lengthening of the common extensor aponeurosis can be performed.[41]

An alternative is in situ stabilization with supracondylar osteotomy to treat the resulting valgus angulation.[28,38] Knight and colleagues[40] showed good results with fragment compression alone using a percutaneously placed cancellous screw, as long as the interval between injury and nonunion diagnosis was less than 16 weeks.

The timing of corrective osteotomy is subject to the same considerations cited earlier for varus deformity. Correction is generally delayed until the child has neared skeletal maturity and most investigators recommend waiting at least 1 year from initial injury before pursuing late angular correction.

In the rare case of lateral condyle malunion, an intra-articular osteotomy can improve elbow range of motion by more than 35°; there was a trend toward better results in Milch type I fractures.[39] For all treatment strategies of nonunions and malunions, the authors emphasize the importance of maintaining the posterior soft tissue attachments to the lateral fragment in order to avoid osteonecrosis.

Lateral spurring or overgrowth following lateral condyle fracture is common. In a study of 212 fractures, spurring was seen in 73%, and the size of the spur correlated with the degree of displacement.[42,43] Range of motion was not significantly affected in this series. Although potentially a cosmetic concern, the lateral spur seems to be of no functional importance.[26,42,43]

MEDIAL EPICONDYLE FRACTURES
Nonunion

Medial epicondyle nonunion or fibrous union is reported in most displaced fractures treated nonoperatively[44,45]; however, only 21% of all nonunions are symptomatic.[46] Symptoms may include pain, weakness, decreased range of motion, and ulnar nerve compression. Treatment should be tailored accordingly.[46] Fragment excision and fixation have both been advocated. Smith and colleagues[46] reported union in 7 out of 8 patients and return to athletics in all patients treated with open reduction and screw fixation. In 5 patients with valgus instability at an average of 10 years from injury, Gilchrist and McKee[47] performed fragment excision and advancement of the ulnar collateral ligament; all patients had good patient-reported outcome scores. In contrast, Farsetti and colleagues[45] reported poor results from fragment excision at 34 years of follow-up. Complications included pain, weakness, paresthesias, and instability. In an effort to decrease hardware-related complications, Shukla and Cohen[48] performed open reduction and internal fixation (ORIF) using a tension-band technique for symptomatic nonunions in 5 patients. They achieved union in all patients and reported high satisfaction and no complaints related to elbow stiffness or prominent hardware.

STIFFNESS

Function-limiting stiffness following elbow fractures is uncommon in the pediatric population. Studies uniformly show a rapid gain in range of motion within the first month following discontinuation of immobilization, then gradual improvements for up to a year.[49-53] Most children have no significant side-to-side difference in elbow range of motion. Factors associated with longer recovery time include increasing patient age, length of immobilization, severity of injury, intra-articular fracture, and need for surgical intervention.[49-53] In order to optimize treatment, stiffness should be classified based on cause. Intrinsic causes include intra-articular malunion, callus formation, and degenerative changes. Extrinsic causes include heterotopic ossification and soft tissue contracture.[54] Given the potential for improvement in motion over a long time period and data from a large study showing that surgery for elbow stiffness in children is less effective than in adults,[55] splinting and physical therapy should be the first-line treatment. Experienced investigators emphasize unrestricted play (especially swimming) over formal physical therapy.[26,54] Indications for surgery are a functional deficit caused by stiffness in a child at least 6 months after injury who has undergone an appropriate trial of nonoperative treatment.

Three studies in the past 20 years have specifically reported outcomes of open surgical release in children with stiff elbows.[55-57] Common themes include the need to address both intrinsic and extrinsic blocks to motion, release and/or transposition of the ulnar nerve (especially in cases in which flexion is improved), and the use of a continuous passive motion machine with adequate pain control (with either a peripheral nerve block or patient-

controlled analgesia) postoperatively. Lateral,[57] medial,[56] and combined[55-57] approaches have proved successful, and no comparisons have been studied to suggest superiority of a given approach. Each patient was treated individually, and the most common procedures were anterior and posterior capsulotomies; olecranon tip excision; and removal of hardware, osteophytes, and loose bodies.

Mih and Wolf[57] studied 9 patients and showed an increase in arc of motion of 53°; Bae and Waters[56] reported a similar gain of 54°. This finding is consistent with the adult literature, with gains in arc of motion reported around 45° to 50° in large cohorts.[58-60] However, in their study of 37 patients, Stans and Morrey[55] reported less favorable results, with an average gain in arc of motion of 28°, including 2 patients who lost motion and 1 who gained none. Unlike the previous 2 studies, Stans and colleagues[55] did not perform muscle or tendon lengthening as part of their treatment, which may account for the discrepancy in results.

Only 1 study has reported the results of arthroscopic treatment of elbow stiffness in children, the indications being stiffness recalcitrant to nonoperative treatment in athletic patients.[61] All procedures included joint debridement and release of flexion contracture. Six patients were available for follow-up, with an average improvement of 63° in the arc of motion.

MISSED INJURIES AND DELAYED DIAGNOSIS

The complication of delayed diagnosis or missed injury merits special attention. At birth, only the distal humeral metaphysis is ossified with the secondary ossification centers appearing in a well-described manner.[62-64] This unique and complex developmental anatomy makes interpretation of radiographs difficult at times. An understanding of normal anatomy is a prerequisite for interpreting the radiographs of injured children. The number of missed injuries and delayed diagnoses is minimized by obtaining a thorough history and physical examination followed by high-quality appropriate radiographic views. A low threshold for advanced imaging, including MRI and ultrasonography, must be held.

Waters and colleagues[65] described several of these potentially missed injuries as TRASH (the radiographic appearance seemed harmless) lesions. These injuries include (1) transphyseal distal humerus fractures, (2) displaced medial condyle fracture before ossification of the trochlea, (3) capitellar shear fractures, (4) radial head fracture with subsequent progressive radiocapitellar subluxation, and (5) intra-articular osteochondral fractures.

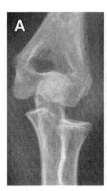
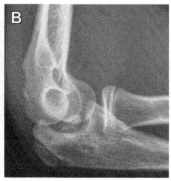
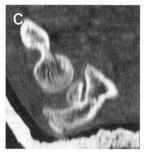

Fig. 3. Medial epicondyle fracture. (*A*) AP and (*B*) lateral radiographs showing a medial epicondyle incarcerated in the ulnohumeral joint following closed reduction of an elbow dislocation. (*C*) Computed tomography showing the incarcerated fragment. (*From* Martin JR, Mazzini JP. Posterolateral elbow dislocation with entrapment of the medial epicondyle in children: a case report. Cases J 2009;2:6603.)

Recognizing common features of TRASH lesions minimizes missed injuries. TRASH lesions are usually caused by a high-energy mechanism (eg, a fall from a significant height in a small child). These predominantly osteochondral lesions are commonly the result of a spontaneously reduced elbow dislocation. Swelling is usually more than would be expected for the misinterpreted benign radiographs, and restrictions to range of motion are greater than would be expected for a sprain or contusion. Along with careful scrutiny of quality plain films, providers should have a low threshold for obtaining advanced imaging (MRI or ultrasonography) in suspected cases.

Medial epicondyle fracture with the fracture fragment entrapped in the joint has also been recognized as a potentially missed injury (**Fig. 3**).[66–68] This pattern typically occurs following an elbow dislocation, with or without spontaneous reduction, and is associated with up to 18% of medial epicondyle fractures[68] and up to 25% of elbow dislocations.[66] Clinical findings include a block to motion (especially full extension) and radiographs showing the fracture fragment at the level of the joint. In this scenario, the fragment must be considered to be in the joint until proven otherwise.[66] When promptly treated with ORIF, 13 out of 13 patients achieved excellent range of motion and functional outcome scores.[68]

In addition, although often grouped with forearm injuries, Monteggia injuries (proximal ulna fractures associated with a radial head dislocation)

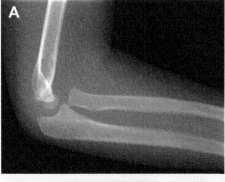
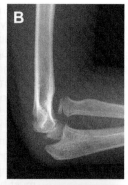
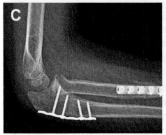
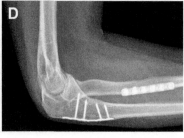

Fig. 4. Missed Monteggia fracture. (*A*) This 5-year-old girl presented with elbow pain after falling from a tree. This radiograph was read as normal; note that the radial head does not align with the capitellum and the subtle bow of the ulna, representing plastic deformation. (*B*) At 33 months postinjury, the dislocated radial head shows chronic changes, including erosion of the distal humerus. (*C*) At 39 months postinjury, the patient is 8 years old and has undergone osteotomies of the radius and ulna and annular ligament reconstruction. (*D*) At 9 years postinjury, the elbow shows advanced arthrosis.

merit special attention because missed injuries can lead to poor outcomes (**Fig. 4**).[69] A complete discussion of reconstruction strategies is beyond the scope of this article. What is clear is that clinicians should always assess the radiocapitellar joint in any patient with a forearm fracture. Likewise, clinicians should be wary of a diagnosis of isolated radial head dislocation and ensure there is not a subtle fracture of the ulna, including plastic deformation. Although the radial head may be reducible, the reduction is often lost if the concomitant ulna fracture is not simultaneously reduced. Orthogonal radiographs should show a concentric radiocapitellar joint in all views and the ulna should have no bow in the sagittal plane.[70]

REFERENCES

1. Herring JA, Ho C. Upper extremity injuries. In: Tachdjian's pediatric orthopaedics. 5th edition. Philadelphia: Elsevier/Saunders; 2014. p. 1264.
2. Landin LA. Fracture patterns in children. Analysis of 8,682 fractures with special reference to incidence, etiology and secular changes in a Swedish urban population 1950-1979. Acta Orthop Scand Suppl 1983;202:1–109.
3. Landin LA. Epidemiology of children's fractures. J Pediatr Orthop B 1997;6:79–83.
4. Landin LA, Danielsson L. Elbow fractures in children: an epidemiological analysis of 589 cases. Acta Orthop Scand 1986;57:309–12.
5. Abzug JM, Herman MJ. Management of supracondylar humerus fractures in children: current concepts. J Am Acad Orthop Surg 2012;20:69–77.
6. Otsuka NY, Kasser JR. Supracondylar fractures of the humerus in children. J Am Acad Orthop Surg 1997;5:19–26.
7. Flynn JM, Sarwark JF, Waters PM, et al. The operative management of pediatric fractures of the upper extremity. J Bone Joint Surg Am 2002;84:2078–89.
8. Pirone AM, Graham HK, Krajbich JI. Management of displaced extension-type supracondylar fractures of the humerus in children. J Bone Joint Surg Am 1988; 70:641–50.
9. Davids JR, Lamoreaux DC, Brooker RC, et al. Translation step-cut osteotomy for the treatment of posttraumatic cubitus varus. J Pediatr Orthop 2011;31: 353–65.
10. Davids JR, Maguire MF, Mubarak SJ, et al. Lateral condylar fracture of the humerus following posttraumatic cubitus varus. J Pediatr Orthop 1994; 14:466–70.
11. Takahara M, Sasaki I, Kimura T, et al. Second fracture of the distal humerus after varus malunion of a supracondylar fracture in children. J Bone Joint Surg Br 1998;80:791–7.
12. O'Driscoll SW, Spinner RJ, McKee MD, et al. Tardy posterolateral rotatory instability of the elbow due to cubitus varus. J Bone Joint Surg Am 2001;83: 1358–69.
13. Abe M, Ischizu T, Shirai H, et al. Tardy ulnar nerve palsy caused by cubitus varus deformity. J Hand Surg Am 1995;20:5–9.
14. Spinner RJ, O'Driscoll SW, Davids JR, et al. Cubitus varus associated with dislocation of both the medial portion of the triceps and the ulnar nerve. J Hand Surg Am 1999;24:718–26.
15. Mitsunari A, Muneshige H, Ikuta Y, et al. Internal rotation deformity and tardy ulnar nerve palsy after supracondylar humeral fracture. J Shoulder Elbow Surg 1995;4:23–9.
16. Banerjee S, Sabui KK, Mondal J, et al. Corrective dome osteotomy using the paratricipital (triceps-sparing) approach for cubitus varus deformity in children. J Pediatr Orthop 2012;32:385–93.
17. Kumar K, Sharma VK, Sharma R, et al. Correction of cubitus varus by French or dome osteotomy: a comparative study. J Trauma 2000;49:717–21.
18. North D, Held M, Dix-Peek S, et al. French osteotomy for cubitus varus in children: a long-term study over 27 years. J Pediatr Orthop 2015. [Epub ahead of print].
19. Oppenheim WL, Clader TJ, Smith C, et al. Supracondylar humeral osteotomy for traumatic childhood cubitus varus deformity. Clin Orthop Relat Res 1984; 188:34–9.
20. Solfelt DA, Hill BW, Anderson CP, et al. Supracondylar osteotomy for the treatment of cubitus varus in children: a systematic review. Bone Joint J 2014; 96:691–700.
21. Ippolito E, Moneta MR, D'Arrigo C. Post-traumatic cubitus varus. Long-term follow-up of corrective supracondylar humeral osteotomy in children. J Bone Joint Surg Am 1990;72:757–65.
22. Voss FR, Kasser JR, Trepman E, et al. Uniplanar supracondylar humeral osteotomy with preset Kirschner wires for posttraumatic cubitus varus. J Pediatr Orthop 1994;14:471–8.
23. Flynn JC, Richards JF Jr, Saltzman RI. Prevention and treatment of non-union of slightly displaced fractures of the lateral humeral condyle in children. An end-result study. J Bone Joint Surg Am 1975; 57:1087–92.
24. Hardacre JA, Nahigian SH, Froimson AI. Fractures of the lateral condyle of the humerus in children. J Bone Joint Surg Am 1971;53:1083–95.
25. Toh S, Tsubo K, Nishikawa S, et al. Long-standing nonunion of fractures of the lateral humeral condyle. J Bone Joint Surg Am 2002;84:593–8.
26. Papandrea R, Waters PM. Posttraumatic reconstruction of the elbow in the pediatric patient. Clin Orthop Relat Res 2000;370:115–26.
27. Weiss JM, Graves S, Yang S, et al. A new classification system predictive of complications in surgically

treated pediatric humeral lateral condyle fractures. J Pediatr Orthop 2009;29:602–5.

28. Song KS, Waters PM. Lateral condylar humerus fractures: which ones should we fix? J Pediatr Orthop 2012;32:5–9.

29. Wilkins KE. Residuals of elbow trauma in children. Orthop Clin North Am 1990;21:291–314.

30. Jakob R, Fowles JV, Rang M, et al. Observations concerning fractures of the lateral humeral condyle in children. J Bone Joint Surg Br 1975;57:430–6.

31. Dhillon KS, Sengupta S, Singh BJ. Delayed management of fracture of the lateral humeral condyle in children. Acta Orthop Scand 1988;59:419–24.

32. Zionts LE, Stolz MR. Late fracture of the lateral condyle of the humerus. Orthopedics 1984;7:541–5.

33. Wattenbarger JM, Gerardi J, Johnston CE. Late open reduction internal fixation of lateral condyle fractures. J Pediatr Orthop 2002;22:394–8.

34. Agarwal A, Qureshi NA, Gupta N, et al. Management of neglected lateral condyle fractures of humerus in children: a retrospective study. Indian J Orthop 2012;46:698–704.

35. Shimada K, Masada K, Tada K, et al. Osteosynthesis for the treatment of non-union of the lateral humeral condyle in children. J Bone Joint Surg Am 1997;79: 234–40.

36. Masada K, Kawai H, Kawabata H, et al. Osteosynthesis for old, established non-union of the lateral condyle of the humerus. J Bone Joint Surg Am 1990;72:32–40.

37. Toh S, Tsubo K, Nishikawa S, et al. Osteosynthesis for nonunion of the lateral humeral condyle. Clin Orthop Relat Res 2002;(405):230–41.

38. Tien YC, Chen JC, Fu YC, et al. Supracondylar dome osteotomy for cubitus valgus deformity associated with a lateral condylar nonunion in children. J Bone Joint Surg Am 2005;87:1456–63.

39. Bauer AS, Bae DS, Brustowicz KA, et al. Intra-articular corrective osteotomy of humeral lateral condyle malunions in children: early clinical and radiographic results. J Pediatr Orthop 2013;33:20–5.

40. Knight DM, Alves C, Alman B, et al. Percutaneous screw fixation promotes healing of lateral condyle nonunion in children. J Pediatr Orthop 2014;34:155–60.

41. Gaur SC, Varma AN, Swarup A. A new surgical technique for old ununited lateral condyle fractures of the humerus in children. J Trauma 1993;34:68–9.

42. Pribaz JR, Bernthal NM, Wong TC, et al. Lateral spurring (overgrowth) after pediatric lateral condyle fractures. J Pediatr Orthop 2012;32:456–60.

43. Koh KH, Seo SW, Kim KM, et al. Clinical and radiographic results of lateral condylar fracture of distal humerus in children. J Pediatr Orthop 2010;30(5): 425–9.

44. Josefsson PO, Danielsson LG. Epicondylar elbow fracture in children. 35-year follow-up of 56 unreduced cases. Acta Orthop Scand 1986;57:313–5.

45. Farsetti P, Potenza V, Caterini R, et al. Long-term results of treatment of fractures of the medial humeral epicondyle in children. J Bone Joint Surg Am 2001; 83:1299–305.

46. Smith JT, McFeely ED, Bae DS, et al. Operative fixation of medial humeral epicondyle fracture nonunion in children. J Pediatr Orthop 2010;30:644–8.

47. Gilchrist AD, McKee MD. Valgus instability of the elbow due to medial epicondyle nonunion: treatment by fragment excision and ligament repair–a report of 5 cases. J Shoulder Elbow Surg 2002;11:493–7.

48. Shukla SK, Cohen MS. Symptomatic medial epicondyle nonunion: treatment by open reduction and fixation with a tension band construct. J Shoulder Elbow Surg 2011;20:455–60.

49. Wang YL, Chang WN, Hsu CJ. The recovery of elbow range of motion after treatment of supracondylar and lateral condylar fractures of the distal humerus in children. J Orthop Trauma 2009;23:120–5.

50. Spencer HT, Wong M, Fong YJ, et al. Prospective longitudinal evaluation of elbow motion following pediatric supracondylar humeral fractures. J Bone Joint Surg Am 2010;92:904–10.

51. Bernthal NM, Hoshino CM, Dichter D, et al. Recovery of elbow motion following pediatric lateral condylar fractures of the humerus. J Bone Joint Surg Am 2011;93:871–7.

52. Schmale GA, Mazor S, Mercer LD, et al. Lack of benefit of physical therapy on function following supracondylar humeral fracture: a randomized controlled trial. J Bone Joint Surg Am 2014;96:944–50.

53. Fletcher ND, Schiller JR, Garg S, et al. Increased severity of type III supracondylar humerus fractures in the preteen population. J Pediatr Orthop 2012;32: 567–72.

54. Stans AA, Morrey BF. Post-traumatic elbow stiffness in children. In: Morrey BF, Sanchez-Sotelo J, editors. The elbow and its disorders. 4th edition. Philadelphia: Saunders Elsevier; 2009. p. 326–33.

55. Stans AA, Maritz NG, O'Driscoll SW, et al. Operative treatment of elbow contracture in patients twenty-one years of age or younger. J Bone Joint Surg Am 2002;84:382–7.

56. Bae DS, Waters PM. Surgical treatment of posttraumatic elbow contracture in adolescents. J Pediatr Orthop 2001;21:580–4.

57. Mih AD, Wolf FG. Surgical release of elbow-capsular contracture in pediatric patients. J Pediatr Orthop 1994;14:458–61.

58. Gates HS, Sullivan FL, Urbaniak JR. Anterior capsulotomy and continuous passive motion in the treatment of post-traumatic flexion contracture of the elbow. A prospective study. J Bone Joint Surg Am 1992;74:1229–34.

59. Mansat P, Morrey BF. The column procedure: a limited lateral approach for extrinsic contracture of the elbow. J Bone Joint Surg Am 1998;80:1603–15.

60. Bręborowicz M, Lubiatowski P, Długosz J, et al. The outcome of open elbow arthrolysis: comparison of four different approaches based on one hundred cases. Int Orthop 2014;38:561–7.

61. Micheli LJ, Luke AC, Mintzer CM, et al. Elbow arthroscopy in the pediatric and adolescent population. Arthroscopy 2001;17:694–9.

62. Silberstein MJ, Brodeur AE, Graviss ER, et al. Some vagaries of the medial epicondyle. J Bone Joint Surg Am 1981;63:524–8

63. Silberstein MJ, Brodeur AE, Graviss ER, et al. Some vagaries of the olecranon. J Bone Joint Surg Am 1981;63:722–5.

64. Haraldsson S. On osteochondrosis deformas juvenilis capituli humeri including investigation of intraosseous vasculature in distal humerus. Acta Orthop Scand Suppl 1959;38:1–232.

65. Waters PM, Beaty J, Kasser J. Elbow "TRASH" (the radiographic appearance seemed harmless). J Pediatr Orthop 2010;30:77–81.

66. Gottschalk HP, Eisner E, Hosalkar HS. Medial epicondyle fractures in the pediatric population. J Am Acad Orthop Surg 2012;20:223–32.

67. Pathy R, Dodwell ER. Medial epicondyle fractures in children. Curr Opin Pediatr 2015;27:58–66.

68. Tarallo L, Mugnai R, Fiacchi F, et al. Pediatric medial epicondyle fractures with intra-articular elbow incarceration. J Orthop Traumatol 2015;16:117–23.

69. Lloyd-Roberts GC, Bucknill TM. Anterior dislocation of the radial head in children: aetiology, natural history and management. J Bone Joint Surg Br 1977;59:402–7.

70. Ring D, Jupiter JB, Waters PM. Monteggia fractures in children and adults. J Am Acad Orthop Surg 1998;6:215–24.

Surgical Site Infections After Pediatric Spine Surgery

Lorena V. Floccari, MD, Todd A. Milbrandt, MD*

KEYWORDS

- Surgical site infection • Pediatric spine • Scoliosis • Infection prevention

KEY POINTS

- There is a higher incidence of surgical site infection (SSI) in neuromuscular patients (5.3% to 14%) than in idiopathic patients (0.5% to 2.7%).
- Risk factors include incontinence, inappropriate perioperative antibiotics, prominent implants, length of fusion, obesity, malnutrition, pelvic fixation, increased operative time, blood loss/transfusion, and length of hospital stay.
- Back acne is a risk factor for delayed infection with *Propionibacterium acne*.
- Best practice guidelines include use of chlorhexidine skin wash, nutritional assessment, urine cultures, limiting operating room traffic, vancomycin powder, minimizing dressing changes, and antibiotic prophylaxis with cefazolin and gram-negative antimicrobial for high-risk patients.
- Treatment of acute infection includes aggressive debridement and antimicrobial therapy, whereas delayed infection requires implant removal.

INTRODUCTION

Surgical site infection (SSI) after pediatric spinal deformity surgery is a complication that results in substantial morbidity and cost. The 2015 updated Centers for Disease Control and Prevention's (CDC) guidelines[1,2] defines a superficial SSI as infection involving skin or subcutaneous tissue of the incision within 30 days of surgery, whereas a deep SSI involves deeper soft tissue structures within 90 days of surgery, in association with clinical signs or symptoms of infection, purulent drainage, positive cultures, or abscess formation.

In a 2009 retrospective case series, Hedequist and colleagues[3] found that the mean number of hospital days related to an SSI was 29 (range 6–171 days) and hospitalization cost $157,537 (range $26,877–$961,722). Prolonged courses of intravenous (IV) antibiotics and multiple surgeries for debridement, implant removal, and revision impose tremendous burden to patients, families, physicians, hospitals, and payers. The in-hospital costs pale in comparison with the personal and societal costs, including missed school, lost parental days of work, and psychological stresses to the involved patients and families.[4]

Given the high morbidity and cost incurred with this complication, SSI after pediatric spinal surgery is a major topic of research. This review focuses on recent advancements in the identification of risk factors, prevention strategies, diagnosis, and treatment of surgical SSIs in pediatric spine patients.

INCIDENCE

Despite modern advances in infection-preventative strategies, the postoperative SSI incidence has remained substantial, with an overall rate of 2.2% to 8.5% in series that combine deep and superficial

Disclosures: The authors have nothing to disclose.
Department of Orthopedic Surgery, Mayo Clinic, 200 1st Street Southwest, Rochester, MN 55905, USA
* Corresponding author.
E-mail address: Milbrandt.Todd@mayo.edu

Orthop Clin N Am 47 (2016) 387–394
http://dx.doi.org/10.1016/j.ocl.2015.09.001
0030-5898/16/$ – see front matter © 2016 Elsevier Inc. All rights reserved.

SSIs from all patients with scoliosis.[4–11] Previous literature demonstrates that patients with neuromuscular scoliosis (NMS) are at higher risk than patients with adolescent idiopathic scoliosis (AIS) for SSI, with a 0.5% to 2.7% rate in patients with AIS[4–6,12] versus 5.3% to 14.0% in the NMS population.[4–6,13–16] A retrospective review of 20,424 pediatric patients with scoliosis in the Scoliosis Research Society database supported these trends; the overall infection rate was 2.6%, with a 5.5% rate in patients with NMS versus 1.4% in idiopathic patients.[7]

RISK FACTORS

In recent years, an important focus of pediatric spinal SSI research has concentrated on defining risk factors for infection in order to clarify targets for preventative strategies. Glotzbecker and colleagues[17] performed a systematic review of risk factors for pediatric spine SSI and rated studies as grade A evidence (good), grade B (fair), or grade C (poor). Although there is a lack of high-quality evidence in the literature, several level II to IV studies revealed the risk factors as listed in **Box 1**.

Subramanyam and colleagues[18] also completed a systematic review of risk factors for SSI in a pooled population of pediatric patients with spinal

deformity and found the following 5 factors statistically predictive of SSI:

- Inappropriate antibiotic use (wrong drug, only clindamycin, incorrect dose or timing, and/or continuation beyond 24 hours after surgery)
- Neuromuscular scoliosis
- Instrumentation
- Increased length of hospitalization
- Residual postoperative curve (considered to be a marker of surgical invasiveness or length of procedure)

Speculation as to the reason for a higher risk in patients with NMS includes a higher rate of urinary and fecal incontinence leading to wound contamination, excessive tension on the wound from body habitus, and poor preoperative nutritional status.

PREVENTATIVE STRATEGIES

Despite increased awareness of risk factors for SSI, there is a void in the literature of high quality evidence for infection prevention strategies. Glotzbecker and colleagues[4] performed a survey in 2013 among Pediatric Orthopedic Society of North America/Scoliosis Research Society (POSNA/SRS) members and found significant variability in the current practices of spinal deformity surgeons.

Box 1
Risk factors for SSI in pediatric spine patients

Grade B

    Urinary or bowel incontinence

    Positive preoperative urine culture

    Inappropriate antibiotic prophylaxis

    Prominent implants

    First-generation stainless steel implants (compared with newer titanium implants)

Grade C

    Malnutrition

    Obesity

    Blood loss

    Blood transfusion

    Increased number of levels fused

    Extension to pelvis/sacrum

    Increased operative time

    No use of drain

Risk factors were graded A (good evidence), B (fair evidence), or C (conflicting or poor-quality evidence).
From Glotzbecker MP, Riedel MD, Vitale MG, et al. What's the evidence? Systematic literature review of risk factors and preventive strategies for surgical site infection following pediatric spine surgery. J Pediatr Orthop 2013;33(5):485; with permission.

It was postulated that this variability results from lack of good evidence and may reflect suboptimal care. Glotzbecker and colleagues's[17] systematic review found insufficient evidence to recommend numerous preventative tactics, highlighting the need for high-quality research.

The best attempt thus far to fill this void is the 2013 seminal article in which Vitale and colleagues[19] developed a best practice guideline (BPG) for SSI prevention in high-risk pediatric spine patients. Given the lack of high-quality literature, the BPG relies heavily on the expert opinion of experienced pediatric spine surgeons and pediatric infectious disease specialists. Agreement of greater than 80% of the panel constituted consensus for 14 prevention strategies. These guidelines are listed in **Box 2**. No consensus (<80% agreement) was reached on preoperative methicillin-resistant *Staphylococcus aureus* (MRSA) screening, chlorhexidine skin prep, titanium versus cobalt chrome implants, saline versus dilute povidone-iodine irrigation, pulse lavage, gentamicin in bone graft, and postoperative subcutaneous drains, thereby highlighting targets for additional research.

The important question is whether combined strategies, when placed into a care plan, will successfully reduce SSI risk. Vitale and colleagues[20] surveyed all sites involved in the creation of the BPG; after 1 year of implementation at their respective institutions, the rates of adherence to the guidelines were high and infection rates for high-risk spine patients remained stable or decreased almost universally.

Ryan and colleagues[8] described a standardized multidisciplinary infection-prevention protocol at a large children's hospital that led to an absolute risk reduction of 3.6% after implementation. Another large academic center's infection-prevention protocol decreased infection rates from 7.8% to 4.5% overall and from 12.9% to 6.5% in high-risk pediatric patients. Although these numbers did not reach statistical significance, the results were clinically meaningful with a relative risk reduction approaching 50%, demonstrating the effectiveness of these multidisciplinary infection-prevention protocols.[21]

Although implementing systemic changes has the laudable end goal to reduce SSIs, careful long-term assessment of these systems needs to occur in order to guarantee that the positive reductions in infections represent true sustainable changes rather than simply an example of the Hawthorne effect. Determining which strategies are

---

Box 2
Vitale and colleagues' consensus guidelines for high risk patients

Preoperative

  Chlorhexidine skin wash the night before surgery

  Urine cultures and treatment

  Nutrition assessment

  Patient education sheet

Perioperative

  Clipping rather than shaving hair

  Prophylactic IV cefazolin

  Gram-negative bacilli prophylaxis

  Monitor adherence to perioperative antimicrobial regimens

  Limit operating room access during surgery

  Ultraviolet lights not needed

  Intraoperative wound irrigation

  Vancomycin powder in bone graft and/or surgical site

Postoperative

  Impervious dressings

  Minimize dressing changes before discharge

From Vitale MG, Riedel MD, Glotzbecker MP, et al. Building consensus: development of a best practice guideline [BPG] for surgical site infection [SSI] prevention in high-risk pediatric spine surgery. J Pediatr Orthop 2013;33(5):475; with permission.

most effective at reducing SSI rate should continue to be a major focus of research in future years.

ANTIBIOTIC PROPHYLAXIS

Despite widespread antibiotic availability and improved knowledge of causative organisms of SSI in pediatric spine patients, there remains considerable variability in hospital protocol for antibiotic prophylaxis.[4,22] Traditional first-line therapy is prophylaxis against gram-positive bacteria with a first-generation cephalosporin, such as cefazolin.[17,22] The recommended prophylactic dosing of cefazolin has recently increased from 20 mg/kg to a higher dose of 30 mg/kg for pediatric patients.[15,23] The use of clindamycin alone is no longer considered adequate, as literature shows it is an independent risk factor associated with SSI.[24]

Although no study has systematically examined the benefits of broad-spectrum antimicrobials (such as aminoglycosides or third/fourth-generation cephalosporins), grade B evidence in Glotzbecker and colleagues's[17] systemic review showed that gram-negative organisms more frequently cause infections in patients with NMS. This finding prompted consensus on using preoperative prophylaxis against gram-negative pathogens, in addition to cefazolin, in Vitale and colleagues's[19] BPG for high-risk patients. This recommendation will represent a substantial change in practice, given that only 32% of 37 US children's hospitals[22] and only 47.1% of surveyed POSNA/SRS members[4] used gram-negative antimicrobials in patients with NMS before the BPG.

Additional grade B evidence has revealed that inappropriate timing, dosage, or redosing also increases SSI risk.[17] This finding prompted recommendation for monitoring adherence to perioperative antimicrobial regimens in Vitale and colleagues's[19] BPG. As Khoshbin and colleagues[25] found that compliance with antibiotic prophylaxis significantly reduced the SSI rate in pediatric surgery by 30%, improving the compliance rate in spine surgery should clearly be a focus at all institutions to reduce the SSI rate.

VANCOMYCIN POWDER

The adjunctive use of vancomycin powder in bone graft or topically in the surgical wound before closure continues to increase. The goal of intrawound use is to achieve therapeutic local concentrations while minimizing adverse effects from systemic distribution. Studies in adults have shown statistically significant decreases in infection rates with no adverse clinical effects after using topical vancomycin.[26–33] However, the data in pediatric spine patients are limited. Gans and colleagues[34] reviewed 87 consecutive patients who received 500 mg of local vancomycin powder during spine surgery, with IV cephalosporin prophylaxis. Postoperatively, there were no clinically significant changes in creatinine level; systemic vancomycin levels were undetectable with no adverse clinical effects, thus, supporting the safety of vancomycin powder in pediatric patients.

In 2014, Armaghani and colleagues[35] also analyzed the use of vancomycin powder in pediatric patients. A total of 1 g of topical powder was applied after instrumented posterior spinal fusion in 25 patients, with IV cefazolin prophylaxis. Postoperative serum levels averaged 2.5 µg/mL on postoperative day (POD) 0, 1.9 µg/mL on POD 1, and 1.1 µg/mL on POD 2. Local vancomycin levels obtained from subfascial drains were 403 µg/mL on POD 0, 251 µg/mL on POD 1, and 115 µg/mL on POD 2. There were no antibiotic-related complications and no deep infections. Given that the serum levels never reached therapeutic levels (15–20 µg/mL), although intrawound levels far exceeded this threshold, it was determined that local application of vancomycin is safe and provides local antibiotic concentrations that are supratherapeutic for at least 2 days postoperatively. Although additional studies are needed to assess the clinical efficacy in pediatric patients, the use of vancomycin powder seems to be safe in children and may contribute to decreased rates of SSI.

DIAGNOSIS

Early detection of wound infections is critical so that appropriate treatment can be initiated. Clinical symptoms of infection include back pain, localized swelling, erythema, and wound drainage. Although postoperative fever can be an indicator of infection, Blumstein and colleagues[36] showed that 72% of pediatric spinal fusion patients experience postoperative fever with temperature greater than 38°C after surgery, whereas 9% reach temperature greater than 39°C. There was no correlation between fever and positive blood or urine cultures, pneumonia, or SSI. This information demonstrates that fever is an unreliable parameter and may reassure families and health care providers in the postoperative setting.

With clinical suspicion for infection, the initial diagnostic step most often consists of obtaining appropriate laboratory tests. White blood count (WBC) with differential, erythrocyte sedimentation rate, and C-reactive protein (CRP) are important biomarkers of inflammation but often remain elevated for several weeks after surgery, which can complicate the ability to distinguish inflammatory response and SSI.[37–39] However, these laboratory test results can be trended serially for diagnosis and response to treatment.

Plasma procalcitonin (PCT) is a relatively new test that may be more specific in its ability to differentiate systemic inflammation from acute bacterial SSI. Syvanen and colleagues[37] performed a prospective study of 50 adolescent patients undergoing scoliosis surgery and found that CRP, WBC, and body temperature remained elevated for the first week after surgery, whereas all plasma PCT values except for 2 remained less than the infection threshold (0.5 ng/mL). Although there were no SSIs in this cohort, there were 2 cases of severe postoperative pneumonia in the patients with NMS; elevated PCT levels correlated with infection. The use of PCT as a marker of bacterial infection will likely continue to increase in future years.

CAUSATIVE ORGANISMS

Identification of the most common causative organisms is crucial for guiding antibiotic prophylaxis protocols and individualized treatment regimens. Acute SSIs have traditionally been caused by gram-positive organisms, such as methicillin-sensitive *Staphylococcus aureus* and MRSA,[5,6,40] whereas low virulent skin flora, including *Propionibacterium acnes* and *Staphylococcus epidermidis*, cause most of the delayed SSIs.[3,9,40–43]

Patients with NMS are more prone to polymicrobial infections that contain gram-negative bacteria, such as *Escherichia coli*, *Pseudomonas*, and *Enterobacter*.[14,17,40] This propensity may be due to contamination in the early postoperative period from bowel and bladder incontinence, gastrointestinal ostomies, tracheostomies, or shunts in these medically complex patients. Recent studies have confirmed this propensity, as Ramo and colleagues[15] found near-equal distribution of gram-positive and gram-negative organisms. Mackenzie and colleagues[6] found that gram-positive organisms accounted for 57.1% of all bacteria identified in 71 culture-positive SSIs. At 25%, *S aureus* was the most common organism. A noteworthy finding was that 46.5% of SSIs contained one or more gram-negative organisms, with patients with nonidiopathic scoliosis accounting for 97% of these.

DELAYED INFECTION

Although the CDC has defined a deep SSI as occurring within the first 90 days after surgery,[1,2] delayed infections can develop with severe adverse consequences. Mackenzie and colleagues[6] found that 33% of 78 spinal SSIs occurred after the first 30 days from surgery, whereas 10% were identified after the first 6 months. Furthermore, Ramo and colleagues[15] found that 43% of infections occur after 3 months from surgery and 27% after 12 months. Risk factors for delayed infections include comorbid medical conditions, blood transfusions, increased operative time, higher implant bulk, and not using a postoperative drain, although a more unique risk factor for delayed infection is metallurgic reaction from stainless steel resulting in a higher risk than titanium implants.[3,17,43–46]

One important, though often overlooked, risk factor for delayed infection in the pediatric population is back acne. In 2013, Nandyala and Schwend[47] performed a retrospective review of intraoperative cultures obtained from 114 pediatric patients with spinal deformity. Twenty-three percent of all cultures were positive, and 69% of these revealed *P acnes*, an established bacterial cause of delayed infection in pediatric spinal deformity surgery.[3,9,40–42] In Nandyala and Schwend's[47] study, *P acnes* was only seen in children 11 years or older and only in patients with back acne. That institution, therefore, now refers adolescents with back acne to dermatology for treatment before surgical clearance and also recommends preoperative antibacterial wash around the incision to hold the iodine-impregnated adhesive drape in place and topical antibiotics.[47] The role of back acne as a modifiable risk factor clearly requires further investigation, as preoperative treatment could prove to be an easy target to substantially reduce the rate of delayed SSI in adolescents.

TREATMENT

Treatment of SSI varies based on the acuity of onset and type of infection. Acute deep SSI (<3 months) is typically treated with aggressive debridement, retention of implants, and long-term antibiotic therapy.[3,48,49] Removal of instrumentation before fusion is avoided if possible because of concern for deformity progression. If implants are removed before fusion, then reimplantation can be considered after resolution of infection. Glotzbecker and colleagues recently presented unpublished data (Michael P. Glotzbecker, MD, Jaime A. Gomez, MD, Patricia Miller, MS, personal communication, 2015) evaluating the treatment of 101 acute (<3 months) SSIs, in which 79.2% of patients were treated successfully without recurrent infection. Seventy percent underwent serial debridement with implant retention; 7.9% required acute implant exchange; and 1 patient cleared infection after removal of instrumentation (Glotzbecker, personal communication, 2015).

Delayed SSI, however, is generally treated with implant removal after confirmation of fusion mass. Organisms colonize and form biofilm on the implants, which prohibits successful treatment of infection without removal.[3,43,49,50] Hedequist and colleagues[3] showed that no patient with delayed SSI (n = 26) cleared infection successfully without complete spinal implant removal, despite multiple debridements and aggressive antibiotic therapy. The number of operations, length of hospitalization, and cost were proportionate to the timing of removal. After implant removal, antibiotics were transitioned to oral once WBC and CRP returned to normal.

Although implant removal seems necessary for eradication of delayed infection, there is a risk of deformity progression after removal. In Hedequist and colleagues's[3] study, 23% of patients required revision for deformity progression, at an average of 16 months after implant removal. Cahill and colleagues[5] found that deformity progresses 30.3° when implants are removed 4 to 12 months from index surgery, versus 20.1° when removed greater than 1 year from index fusion. Likewise, Alpert and colleagues[42] found an average deformity progression of 33.8° after implant removal for infection. Thus, all patients with SSIs require close clinical and radiographic follow-up to assess the response to treatment and maintenance of deformity correction.

SUMMARY

SSIs complicating pediatric spine surgery incur high costs and morbidity, but the lack of quality literature in this topic has contributed to substantial surgeon practice variability. Renewed interest into the identification of risk factors as targets for infection prevention led to Vitale and colleague's[19] 2013 BPG. Notable features include preoperative chlorhexidine skin wash, nutritional assessment, use of vancomycin powder in the bone graft and/or surgical site, and both IV cefazolin and gram-negative bacilli antimicrobial prophylaxis. Although the BPG were created by expert consensus agreement for high-risk patients, it is hoped that these guidelines will direct research efforts and contribute to improved preventative protocols for all pediatric patients with spinal deformity. Long-term, high-quality studies are clearly needed to further assess the efficacy of infection prevention tactics and treatment strategies to reduce SSIs in pediatric spine patients.

REFERENCES

1. Centers for Disease Control (CDC). Surgical site infection (SSI) event. Available at: http://www.cdc.gov/nhsn/PDFs/pscManual/9pscSSIcurrent.pdf?agree=yes&next=Accept. Accessed April 1, 2015.
2. Horan TC, Andrus M, Dudeck MA. CDC/NHSN surveillance definition of health care-associated infection and criteria for specific types of infections in the acute care setting. Am J Infect Control 2008; 36(5):309–32.
3. Hedequist D, Haugen A, Hresko T, et al. Failure of attempted implant retention in spinal deformity delayed surgical site infections. Spine (Phila Pa 1976) 2009;34(1):60–4.
4. Glotzbecker MP, Vitale MG, Shea KG, et al. Surgeon practices regarding infection prevention for pediatric spinal surgery. J Pediatr Orthop 2013;33(7):694–9.
5. Cahill PJ, Warnick DE, Lee MJ, et al. Infection after spinal fusion for pediatric spinal deformity: thirty years of experience at a single institution. Spine (Phila Pa 1976) 2010;35(12):1211–7.
6. Mackenzie WG, Matsumoto H, Williams BA, et al. Surgical site infection following spinal instrumentation for scoliosis: a multicenter analysis of rates, risk factors, and pathogens. J Bone Joint Surg Am 2013;95(9):800–6. S801-2.
7. Smith JS, Shaffrey CI, Sansur CA, et al. Rates of infection after spine surgery based on 108,419 procedures: a report from the Scoliosis Research Society Morbidity and Mortality Committee. Spine (Phila Pa 1976) 2011;36(7):556–63.
8. Ryan SL, Sen A, Staggers K, et al. A standardized protocol to reduce pediatric spine surgery infection: a quality improvement initiative. J Neurosurg Pediatr 2014;14(3):259–65.
9. Aleissa S, Parsons D, Grant J, et al. Deep wound infection following pediatric scoliosis surgery: incidence and analysis of risk factors. Can J Surg 2011;54(4):263–9.
10. Croft LD, Pottinger JM, Chiang HY, et al. Risk factors for surgical site infections after pediatric spine operations. Spine (Phila Pa 1976) 2015;40(2):E112–9.
11. Divecha HM, Siddique I, Breakwell LM, et al. Complications in spinal deformity surgery in the United Kingdom: 5-year results of the annual British Scoliosis Society National Audit of Morbidity and Mortality. Eur Spine J 2014;23(Suppl 1):S55–60.
12. Martin CT, Pugely AJ, Gao Y, et al. Incidence and risk factors for early wound complications after spinal arthrodesis in children: analysis of 30-day follow-up data from the ACS-NSQIP. Spine (Phila Pa 1976) 2014;39(18):1463–70.
13. Mohamed Ali MH, Koutharawu DN, Miller F, et al. Operative and clinical markers of deep wound infection after spine fusion in children with cerebral palsy. J Pediatr Orthop 2010;30(8):851–7.

14. Sponseller PD, Shah SA, Abel MF, et al. Infection rate after spine surgery in cerebral palsy is high and impairs results: multicenter analysis of risk factors and treatment. Clin Orthop Relat Res 2010; 468(3):711–6.

15. Ramo BA, Roberts DW, Tuason D, et al. Surgical site infections after posterior spinal fusion for neuromuscular scoliosis: a thirty-year experience at a single institution. J Bone Joint Surg Am 2014;96(24): 2038–48.

16. Heffernan MJ, Seehausen DA, Andras LM, et al. Comparison of outcomes after posterior spinal fusion for adolescent idiopathic and neuromuscular scoliosis: does the surgical first assistant's level of training matter? Spine (Phila Pa 1976) 2014;39(8): 648–55.

17. Glotzbecker MP, Riedel MD, Vitale MG, et al. What's the evidence? Systematic literature review of risk factors and preventive strategies for surgical site infection following pediatric spine surgery. J Pediatr Orthop 2013;33(5):479–87.

18. Subramanyam R, Schaffzin J, Cudilo EM, et al. Systematic review of risk factors for surgical site infection in pediatric scoliosis surgery. Spine J 2015; 15(6):1422–31.

19. Vitale MG, Riedel MD, Glotzbecker MP, et al. Building consensus: development of a best practice guideline (BPG) for surgical site infection (SSI) prevention in high-risk pediatric spine surgery. J Pediatr Orthop 2013;33(5):471–8.

20. Vitale M, Wang K, Pace G. The wisdom of crowds. J Pediatr Orthop 2015;35(5 Suppl 1):S55–60.

21. Ballard MR, Miller NH, Nyquist AC, et al. A multidisciplinary approach improves infection rates in pediatric spine surgery. J Pediatr Orthop 2012;32(3):266–70.

22. McLeod LM, Keren R, Gerber J, et al. Perioperative antibiotic use for spinal surgery procedures in US children's hospitals. Spine (Phila Pa 1976) 2013; 38(7):609–16.

23. Bratzler DW, Dellinger EP, Olsen KM, et al. Clinical practice guidelines for antimicrobial prophylaxis in surgery. Am J Health Syst Pharm 2013;70(3):195–283.

24. Linam WM, Margolis PA, Staat MA, et al. Risk factors associated with surgical site infection after pediatric posterior spinal fusion procedure. Infect Control Hosp Epidemiol 2009;30(2):109–16.

25. Khoshbin A, So JP, Aleem IS, et al. Antibiotic prophylaxis to prevent surgical site infections in children: a prospective cohort study. Ann Surg 2014;19.

26. Sweet FA, Roh M, Sliva C. Intrawound application of vancomycin for prophylaxis in instrumented thoracolumbar fusions: efficacy, drug levels, and patient outcomes. Spine (Phila Pa 1976) 2011;36(24): 2084–8.

27. O'Neill KR, Smith JG, Abtahi AM, et al. Reduced surgical site infections in patients undergoing posterior spinal stabilization of traumatic injuries using vancomycin powder. Spine J 2011;11(7):641–6.

28. Theologis AA, Demirkiran G, Callahan M, et al. Local intrawound vancomycin powder decreases the risk of surgical site infections in complex adult deformity reconstruction: a cost analysis. Spine (Phila Pa 1976) 2014;39(22):1875–80.

29. Hill BW, Emohare O, Song B, et al. The use of vancomycin powder reduces surgical reoperation in posterior instrumented and noninstrumented spinal surgery. Acta Neurochir (Wien) 2014;156(4): 749–54.

30. Pahys JM, Pahys JR, Cho SK, et al. Methods to decrease postoperative infections following posterior cervical spine surgery. J Bone Joint Surg Am 2013;95(6):549–54.

31. Tubaki VR, Rajasekaran S, Shetty AP. Effects of using intravenous antibiotic only versus local intrawound vancomycin antibiotic powder application in addition to intravenous antibiotics on postoperative infection in spine surgery in 907 patients. Spine (Phila Pa 1976) 2013;38(25):2149–55.

32. Martin JR, Adogwa O, Brown CR, et al. Experience with intrawound vancomycin powder for spinal deformity surgery. Spine (Phila Pa 1976) 2014; 39(2):177–84.

33. Bakhsheshian J, Dahdaleh NS, Lam SK, et al. The use of vancomycin powder in modern spine surgery: systematic review and meta-analysis of the clinical evidence. World Neurosurg 2015;83(5): 816–23.

34. Gans I, Dormans JP, Spiegel DA, et al. Adjunctive vancomycin powder in pediatric spine surgery is safe. Spine (Phila Pa 1976) 2013;38(19): 1703–7.

35. Armaghani SJ, Menge TJ, Lovejoy SA, et al. Safety of topical vancomycin for pediatric spinal deformity: nontoxic serum levels with supratherapeutic drain levels. Spine (Phila Pa 1976) 2014;39(20): 1683–7.

36. Blumstein GW, Andras LM, Seehausen DA, et al. Fever is common postoperatively following posterior spinal fusion: infection is an uncommon cause. J Pediatr 2015;166(3):751–5.

37. Syvanen J, Peltola V, Pajulo O, et al. Normal behavior of plasma procalcitonin in adolescents undergoing surgery for scoliosis. Scand J Surg 2014; 103(1):60–5.

38. Takahashi J, Ebara S, Kamimura M, et al. Early-phase enhanced inflammatory reaction after spinal instrumentation surgery. Spine (Phila Pa 1976) 2001;26(15):1698–704.

39. Mok JM, Pekmezci M, Piper SL, et al. Use of C-reactive protein after spinal surgery: comparison with erythrocyte sedimentation rate as predictor of early postoperative infectious complications. Spine (Phila Pa 1976) 2008;33(4):415–21.

40. Farley FA, Li Y, Gilsdorf JR, et al. Postoperative spine and VEPTR infections in children: a case-control study. J Pediatr Orthop 2014;34(1):14–21.

41. Rihn JA, Lee JY, Ward WT. Infection after the surgical treatment of adolescent idiopathic scoliosis: evaluation of the diagnosis, treatment, and impact on clinical outcomes. Spine (Phila Pa 1976) 2008; 33(3):289–94.

42. Alpert HW, Farley FA, Caird MS, et al. Outcomes following removal of instrumentation after posterior spinal fusion. J Pediatr Orthop 2014;34(6):613–7.

43. Di Silvestre M, Bakaloudis G, Lolli F, et al. Late-developing infection following posterior fusion for adolescent idiopathic scoliosis. Eur Spine J 2011; 20(Suppl 1):S121–7.

44. Soultanis KC, Pyrovolou N, Zahos KA, et al. Late postoperative infection following spinal instrumentation: stainless steel versus titanium implants. J Surg Orthop Adv 2008;17(3):193–9.

45. Ho C, Sucato DJ, Richards BS. Risk factors for the development of delayed infections following posterior spinal fusion and instrumentation in adolescent idiopathic scoliosis patients. Spine (Phila Pa 1976) 2007;32(20):2272–7.

46. Shen J, Liang J, Yu H, et al. Risk factors for delayed infections after spinal fusion and instrumentation in patients with scoliosis. Clinical article. J Neurosurg Spine 2014;21(4):648–52.

47. Nandyala SV, Schwend RM. Prevalence of intraoperative tissue bacterial contamination in posterior pediatric spinal deformity surgery. Spine (Phila Pa 1976) 2013;38(8):E482–6.

48. Bachy M, Bouyer B, Vialle R. Infections after spinal correction and fusion for spinal deformities in childhood and adolescence. Int Orthop 2012;36(2):465–9.

49. Li Y, Glotzbecker M, Hedequist D. Surgical site infection after pediatric spinal deformity surgery. Curr Rev Musculoskelet Med 2012;5(2):111–9.

50. Maruo K, Berven SH. Outcome and treatment of postoperative spine surgical site infections: predictors of treatment success and failure. J Orthop Sci 2014;19(3):398–404.

Complications After Surgical Treatment of Adolescent Idiopathic Scoliosis

CrossMark

Rodrigo Góes Medéa de Mendonça, MD[a],
Jeffrey R. Sawyer, MD[b],*, Derek M. Kelly, MD[b]

KEYWORDS

- Complications • Surgical treatment • Adolescent idiopathic scoliosis

KEY POINTS

- With current instrumentation and techniques, including intraoperative neuromonitoring, neurologic complications are relatively infrequent (<1%), and most new neurologic deficits resolve without treatment.
- Infection is perhaps the most frequent reason for unanticipated repeat surgery after primary spinal fusion for adolescent idiopathic scoliosis; whether implant removal is necessary remains controversial.
- The most common areas of pseudarthrosis are at the thoracolumbar junction and at the distally fused segment.
- Curve progression (the adding-on phenomenon) and the crankshaft phenomenon occur primarily in younger patients; their effect on clinical outcomes is unclear.
- Proximal junctional kyphosis is more common in adults than in adolescents with idiopathic scoliosis; it seems to have little or no effect on functional outcomes.

Adolescent idiopathic scoliosis (AIS) is the most extensively investigated pediatric deformity, with numerous studies reporting surgical complications and reoperation rates.[1–7] The frequency of complications after AIS surgery is affected by many variables, and existing information in the literature on surgical complications remains limited because of small numbers of patients, focus on a single procedure or complication, outdated surgical techniques, and confinement to a single surgeon or center experience. Understanding the potential complications of surgical treatment of pediatric spinal deformity is essential for surgical decision making.[3,4]

Although current instrumentation and techniques produce good long-term surgical outcomes in most patients, complications do occur. Complications can be broadly categorized as neurologic or nonneurologic, with reported frequencies ranging from 7% to 15% for nonneurologic complications and generally less than 1% for neurologic complications, which are the most devastating.[1–11]

NEUROLOGIC COMPLICATIONS

Although much less frequent than nonneurologic complications, neurologic complications (eg,

[a] Santa Casa de Sao Paulo Hospital Central Sao Paulo, Rua Dr Cesario Motta Jr, 112, Vila Buarque, Sao Paulo, Brasil; [b] University of Tennessee-Campbell Clinic, Department of Orthopaedic Surgery & Biomedical Engineering, Le Bonheur Children's Hospital, 1400 South Germantown Road, Germantown, TN 38138, USA
* Corresponding author. University of Tennessee - Campbell Clinic, Department of Orthopaedic Surgery & Biomedical Engineering, Le Bonheur Children's Hospital, 1400 South Germantown Road, Germantown, TN 38138, USA.
E-mail address: jsawyer@campbellclinic.com

Orthop Clin N Am 47 (2016) 395–403
http://dx.doi.org/10.1016/j.ocl.2015.09.012
0030-5898/16/$ – see front matter © 2016 Elsevier Inc. All rights reserved.

orthopedic.theclinics.com

nerve root, cauda equina, spinal cord deficit) are the most feared, because they can result in complete or partial paralysis, peripheral nerve deficits, or rarely death. Causes of neurologic complications include extrinsic compression of the spinal cord by implants, an epidural hematoma or abscess, or iatrogenic injury to neural elements; distraction of the spinal cord during correction; and ischemic injury that results in reduced blood supply to the spinal cord.[9,10]

A 2011 report from the Scoliosis Research Society (SRS) Morbidity and Mortality Committee identified neurologic complications in 0.8% of 11,227 patients with AIS, most commonly incomplete spinal cord deficits and nerve root deficits; complete spinal cord deficits were rare and there were no cauda equina deficits. All nerve root deficits and complete spinal cord deficits had complete or partial recovery; only 1 of 41 incomplete spinal cord deficits had no recovery.[5] A metaanalysis including 1136 patients with AIS treated with instrumented posterior spinal fusion found neurologic complications in only 2 patients (0.17%), both of whom had complete recovery.[4]

Reported risk factors for neurologic complications in AIS surgery include vertebral osteotomies, kyphosis correction, a Cobb angle of more than 90°, revision surgery, and combined anterior and posterior fusions.[5,10,12] According to the 2011 SRS report,[5] use of an osteotomy (Smith-Peterson osteotomy, pedicle subtraction osteotomy, vertebral column resection) was associated with a 2% rate of new neurologic deficits, significantly higher than the rate without osteotomy (0.9%). Compared with pedicle screw-only and hook-only constructs, wire-only and anterior screw-only constructs had significantly higher rates of new neurologic deficits.

Intraoperative neuromonitoring has become a routine part of most scoliosis surgery.[12–14] The use of both somatosensory evoked potentials (SEP) and transcranial electrical stimulation-motor evoked potentials (TES-MEP) has been recommended as the most effective method for monitoring during spinal surgery.[13,14] Combined SEP and TES-MEP monitoring has been reported to have a sensitivity of 100% and specificity of 98% for sensory motor impairment. In a series of 3436 consecutive pediatric spinal procedures reported by Thuet and colleagues,[14] 74 (2.2%) potential neurologic deficits were identified; 7 patients had neurologic deficits undetected by neuromonitoring. Use of combined SEP, TES-MEP, descending neurogenic-evoked potentials, and electromyography monitoring allowed accurate detection of permanent neurologic status in 99.6% of patients.

Schwartz and colleagues[13] defined an intraoperative "alert" or clinically relevant neurophysiologic change as a persistent (over ≥3 test trials) unilateral or bilateral loss of 65% or more of the amplitude of the TES-MEP or 50% or more of the amplitude of the SEP relative to a stable baseline. When critical changes are identified in either the SEP or TES-MEP or both, blood pressure should be elevated to a mean arterial pressure of at least 90 mm Hg, hypervolemia and blood loss should be corrected, and any operative steps that preceded the changes (eg, placement of pedicle screws, osteotomty, correction maneuver) should be reversed. The use of corticosteroids remains controversial and should be determined on a case-by-case basis. If neuromonitoring patterns return to baseline, surgery can be resumed cautiously. If amplitudes do not improve after reversal of correction and implant removal, cessation of the procedure should be considered.

Because delayed-onset neurologic deficits can occur, careful neurologic monitoring of upper and lower extremity function should be continued for 48 hours after surgery. Delayed neurologic complications may be caused by progressive spinal cord ischemia secondary to traction or to the development of an epidural hematoma. Blood pressure should be monitored carefully and mean arterial blood pressure should be maintained at greater than 80 mm Hg to help maintain spinal cord perfusion; vasopressors may be required. Hemoglobin levels should be checked and corrected, and temperature should be maintained above 36.5°C (97.7°F). Unless their acquisition would substantially delay a return to surgery, computed tomography or MRI scans are helpful in delineating the cause of the deficit.

NONNEUROLOGIC COMPLICATIONS

The reported prevalence of nonneurologic complications after correction of AIS ranges from 0% to 30%.[1,5,8] Nonneurologic complications can be categorized as perioperative (intraoperative and postoperative complications occurring during the first week after surgery), early postoperative complications (occurring between postoperative weeks 2 and 4), or late postoperative complications (occurring after postoperative week 4). Carreon and colleagues[8] listed the most common nonneurologic complications in their 702 patients as respiratory complications, excessive bleeding, wound infections, and wound-related complications (eg, hematoma, seroma, dehiscence).

Infection

The reported prevalence of infection after AIS surgery ranges from 0% to 10%.[15–20] Although infection is much less frequent after AIS surgery than after treatment of nonidiopathic scoliosis, it is a well-recognized complication and is one of the most common reasons for unanticipated repeat surgery after primary spinal fusion for AIS.[21–23] In a 2011 report from the SRS Morbidity and Mortality Committee, the rate of wound infection in 11,741 patients with AIS was 1.4%.[5] A metaanalysis that included 721 patients with AIS reported an almost 4% infection rate, the lowest rate with pedicle screw constructs and the highest with Harrington rods.[4] In their analysis of 277 patients with surgical correction of scoliosis, Aleissa and colleagues[15] found the lowest rate of deep wound infections in patients with AIS (1.5%) and the highest rate in those with neuromuscular scoliosis (14%); however, Ho and colleagues,[17] in a series of 53 patients with infections after scoliosis surgery, found that the type of scoliosis was not a significant predictor of the development of infection.

Suggested risk factors for postoperative infection, other than a diagnosis of nonidiopathic scoliosis, include prolonged duration of surgery, higher volume of instrumentation, the use of an allograft, and combined anterior–posterior procedures.[15] The use of instrumentation has been suggested to increase the risk of infection because of the increase in operative time and surgical exposure, the bulk of the implants, an inflammatory reaction. Aleissa and colleagues[15] reported infection rates of 5% in patients with posterior-only surgery and 17% in those with anterior–posterior procedures. The frequency of infection was 16% with allografts and 1.4% without, although this finding has been contradicted by other studies. Blood loss, the use of perioperative medications to decrease blood loss, duration of surgery, preoperative Cobb angle, and number of levels fused were not found to be significant risk factors. Both underweight[24] and overweight have been linked to the development of postoperative infections.[25] First-generation stainless steel implants seem to increase the risk of delayed infection compared with newer generation titanium implants.[16]

Delayed infection (>1 year after surgery) also can occur, with *Staphylococcus aureus, S epidermis,* and *Propionibacterium acnes* the most frequently reported infecting organisms (**Fig. 1**).[26–28] These infections are believed to result from direct seeding of the surgical field during the index procedure, followed by a latent period and then activation at some later time.[26,27] Di Silvestre and colleagues[27] reported 15 (2.77%) delayed infections at an average of 70 months (range, 15–95) after posterior-only fusion in 540 patients with AIS. Of the 14 deep wound infections reported by Aleissa and colleagues,[15] 6 developed early (within 3 weeks) and 8 at a later time (average, 37 weeks; range, 5–72). Ho and colleagues[17] described 21 infections after treatment of AIS, 11 of which were early and 10 were late infections, and Rihn and colleagues[19] reported that of 7 infections (3%) in 236 patients, 1 was acute (17 days after surgery) and 6 were delayed (average 34 months after surgery).

The treatment of infections after AIS surgery remains an area of controversy, with some authors recommending implant removal[17,27] and others suggesting that implants should be retained to

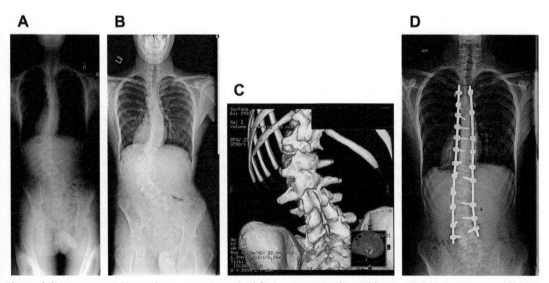

Fig. 1. (*A*) A 14-year-old boy whose posterior spinal fusion was complicated by *Staphylococcus aureus* infection, which was treated with implant removal and antibiotic therapy. (*B*) Six months later the patient had pain and curve progression was noted. (*C*) Computed tomography scan showed a pseudarthrosis at T12-L1. (*D*) Revision arthrodesis was done with pedicle screw instrumentation.

prevent progression of the deformity.[23,26,27,29] Aleissa and colleagues[15] described treatment of 8 infections with serial debridements and vacuum-assisted closure, all of which resolved without removal of implants. Two other studies support the use of vacuum-assisted closure, with none of the patients in those studies requiring implant removal.[30,31] The duration of antibiotic administration necessary for infection eradication also is debatable. Earlier studies recommended a minimum of 6 weeks of intravenous antibiotics, whereas more recent studies have concluded that a much shorter course (48–72 hours of IV antibiotics, followed by 7–14 days of oral antibiotics) is just as effective.[17,26,32]

A number of measures have been recommended for prevention of infection after AIS surgery, including preoperative administration of cefazolin, with the addition of gentamicin in high-risk groups. Myung and colleagues[18] described 2 simple changes in their protocol that result in a 10-fold reduction in infections after posterior fusion for AIS: (1) vancomycin and ceftazidime were added to cefazolin for routine antibiotic prophylaxis, and (2) pulse lavage irrigation replaced bulb syringe irrigation intraoperatively. The use of vancomycin powder has been shown to reduce significantly the frequency of surgical site infections in adult patients[33]; however, Martin and colleagues[34] found no difference in the rates of infection with and without vancomycin in 306 patients with AIS. Gans and colleagues[35] reported 3 infections (3.4%) in 87 patients in whom vancomycin powder was used; no patient experienced nephrotoxicity or red man syndrome. A systematic review found insufficient evidence to recommend prophylaxis with intravenous vancomycin or the use of vancomycin or gentamicin powder in the surgical site or graft.[16] An expert panel of pediatric spine surgeons and infectious disease specialists developed a Best Practice Guideline with 14 recommendations for preventing infection after pediatric spine surgery,[32] although Glotzbecker and colleagues[16] found insufficient evidence to recommend most of these. Aleissa and colleagues also suggested limiting the use of allograft where possible and irrigation with a betadine solution before application of the bone graft.

The clinical ramifications of postoperative infection are unclear. Several reports have noted no loss of correction or progression of deformity after implant removal.[19,36,37] Rihn and colleagues[19] found no differences in pain, function, self-image, satisfaction, or total SRS 24 scores between patients who developed an infection and those who did not.

Pseudarthrosis

Improvements in surgical techniques and instrumentation, the inclusion of intraarticular fusion, and meticulous dissection around the transverse processes have decreased the pseudarthrosis rate to approximately 1% in patients with AIS. A systematic review of the literature in identified a 22.7% frequency of symptomatic pseudarthrosis, most commonly after noninstrumented fusion, and a 2% to 7% frequency in instrumented fusions.[1,4,7,22] A metaanalysis of 1565 instrumented posterior spinal fusions, found pseudarthroses in 2%, more frequent with Harrington rods (3%) than with Cotrel-Dubosset constructs (2%); no pseudarthroses occurred in 254 patients with all-pedicle screw fixation.[4] The most common areas of pseudarthrosis are at the thoracolumbar junction and at the distally fused segment. With more rigid and stronger implants, pseudarthrosis may not be apparent for years. Pseudarthrosis may be identified by oblique radiographs, computed tomography, or bone scan (**Fig. 2**); however, pseudarthrosis can be confirmed definitively only by surgical exploration. If a pseudarthrosis does not cause pain or loss of correction, surgery may not be necessary. If surgery is indicated, the pseudarthrosis is treated as any other joint to be fused: the edges are freshened and decorticated, autogenous bone graft is inserted, and instrumentation is applied.

Curve Progression

After infection and pseudarthrosis, curve progression is the most common cause of reoperation, with a rate of approximately 1%. In their series of 1057 fusions for AIS, Luhmann and colleagues[22] reported reoperations in 4% of patients, most of which were for infection (34%) or pseudarthrosis (26%); 17% of reoperations (approximately 2% of total patients) were required because of curve progression of the adjacent unfused spine. Progression of the curve below the level of spinal fusion has been described as the "adding-on" phenomenon[38–40] and is reported to occur in from 2% to as many of 5% of patients (**Fig. 3**). Wang and colleagues[40] reported adding-on in 23 patients with AIS and identified several risk factors: age 14 years and younger, stable vertebra minus lowest instrumented vertebra difference of more than 1 level, and preoperative deviation of the first level distal to the lowest instrumented vertebra of more than 10 mm. Cho and colleagues[38] found age and Risser grade to be significant predictors for adding-on, suggesting that patients with more growth potential may be at increased risk of curve progression below the

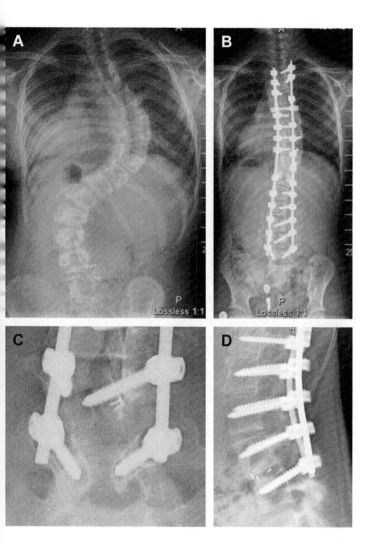

Fig. 2. After a long spinal fusion for scoliosis (*A*), this patient developed a pseudarthrosis at L4-L5 with windshield wipering of the distal screws (*B*). A 360° fusion was done, with revision of her distal fixation and posterior lumbar interbody fusion (*C* and *D*).

fusion. They also emphasized the difference between the 2 subtypes of Lenke 1A curves: adding-on was twice as likely in curves with a right L4 tilt than in those with a left L4 tilt. Schlechter and colleagues[41] also cited younger age and lower Risser grade, as well as lower weight, as risk factors.

The clinical effects of adding-on remain unclear, but unsatisfactory clinical outcomes and frequent need for reoperation have been described.[42,43] Progression of the initial lumbar curve can result in decompression of coronal balance and unsatisfactory results.

Crankshaft Phenomenon

The crankshaft phenomenon was relatively frequent with earlier posterior instrumentation systems (**Fig. 4**), but has markedly decreased in frequency in recent years, primarily owing to the use of growth-friendly techniques.[3,4,44] It may

occur when significant growth remains after posterior spinal fusion because of continued anterior growth. This complication is more likely to occur in younger children (<10 years of age) with an open triradiate cartilage and a Risser sign of 0 or 1 and is relatively infrequent in adolescents, who are closer to skeletal maturity.[3,4] Clinical and animal studies have shown no occurrence of this phenomenon when segmental pedicle-screw constructs were used.[44–47] Surgery may be postponed in younger patients, and for those who are at high risk for crankshaft phenomenon, anterior fusion may be considered.

Decompensation and Sagittal Deformity (Flatback Deformity)

With the introduction of current generation spine instrumentation, decompensation and flatback deformity are much less frequent than they were

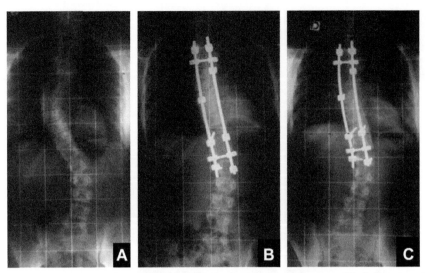

Fig. 3. Adding-on phenomenon. After correction of a single right thoracic curve (*A*), follow-up at 1.5 months showed deviation of L1 of 33 mm from center sacral vertical line and Cobb angle of 13° (*B*). The deviation and angle had progressed to 38 mm and 19°, respectively, at the 8-month follow-up (*C*). (*From* Lakhal W, Loret JE, de Bodman C, et al. The progression of lumbar curves in adolescent Lenke 1 scoliosis and the distal adding-on phenomenon. Orthop Traumatol Surg Res 2014;100(4 Suppl):S250; with permission.)

with the use of Harrington rods.[6] Risk factors associated with decompensation include failure to identify the curve pattern, failure to select proper fusion levels, derotation, lumbar curve progression after selective thoracic fusion, overcorrection of the thoracic curve, rigid lumbosacral hemicurve, crankshaft phenomenon, and adding-on proximal or distal to the fused spine[48] (**Fig. 5**). Depending on the amount of growth remaining, decompensation can be managed by

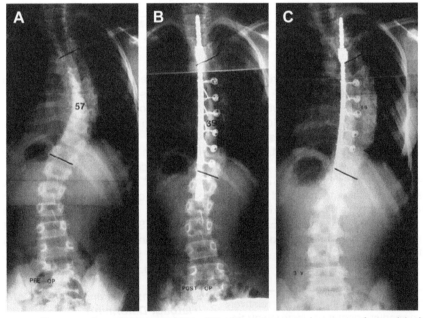

Fig. 4. Three years after correction of 57° curve (*A*) to 39° with instrumented posterior fusion (*B*), the deformity recurred because of the crankshaft phenomenon (*C*). (*From* Warner WC, Sawyer JR, Kelly DM. Scoliosis and kyphosis. In: Canale ST, Beaty JH, editors. Campbell's operative orthopaediics. 12th edition. Philadelphia: Elsevier; 2013; with permission.)

A
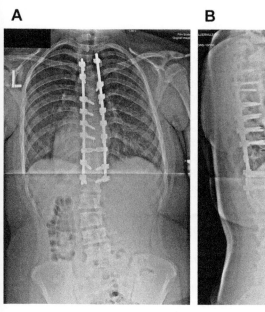

B
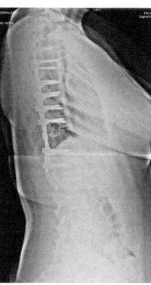

Fig. 5. (*A*) Posterior-anterior and (*B*) lateral radiographs show flatback deformity after posterior spinal fusion and instrumentation for adolescent idiopathic scoliosis because of an inability to achieve normal thoracic kyphosis at the time of surgery.

extension of the fusion (insufficient growth remaining) or with an orthosis (sufficient growth remaining).[3,4]

Proximal Junctional Kyphosis

Proximal junctional kyphosis (PJK) is a radiographic phenomenon in the sagittal plane seen after instrumented fusion for spinal deformity.[4,49,50] In pediatric patients, PJK often appears as a kyphotic change in the disk space above the fusion. The reported incidence of junctional kyphosis ranges from 17% to 39%, depending on the method used to define it. Reported risk factors include type of instrumentation, older age at surgery, surgical correction of thoracic kyphosis of more than 50°, and fusion to the sacrum. Helgeson and colleagues[51] evaluated 283 patients with AIS and found the frequency of PJK to be 0% with hooks-only instrumentation, 2.5% with hybrid instrumentation, 8% with all-screws constructs, and 5.6% with screws/proximal hooks.

PJK most often is identified 12 to 24 months after surgery.[50,52] Despite its radiographic frequency, PJK seems to have little or no effect on clinical outcome.[49,51]

SUMMARY

Even with current techniques and instrumentation, complications can occur after operative treatment of AIS. The most dreaded complications—neurologic deficits—are relatively infrequent, occurring in 1% or less of patients. Nonneurologic deficits,

such as infection, pseudarthrosis, curve progression, and PJK, are more frequent, but are much less likely to require reoperation or to cause poor functional outcomes. Understanding the potential complications of surgical treatment of pediatric spinal deformity is essential for surgical decision making.

REFERENCES

1. Divecha HM, Siddique I, Breakwell LM, et al. Complications in spinal deformity surgery in the United Kingdom: 5-year results of the annual British Scoliosis Society National Audit of Morbidity and Mortality. Eur Spine J 2014;23(Suppl 1):S55–60.
2. Ibrahim KN, Newton PO, Sucato DJ. Safety and outcome in the surgery of adolescent idiopathic scoliosis. Spine Deform, in press. Available at: http://www.spine-deformity.org/article/S2212-134X %2812%2900013-5/abstract. Accessed October 12, 2015.
3. Lykissas MG, Crawford AH, Jain VV. Complications of surgical treatment of pediatric spinal deformities. Orthop Clin North Am 2013;44:357–70.
4. Lykissas MG, Jain VV, Nathan ST, et al. Mid- to long-term outcomes in adolescent idiopathic scoliosis after instrumented posterior spinal fusion: a meta-analysis. Spine (Phila Pa 1976) 2013;38:E113–9.
5. Reames DL, Smith JS, Fu KG, et al. Complications in the surgical treatment of 19,360 cases of pediatric scoliosis. A review of the Scoliosis Research Society Morbidity and Mortality Database. Spine (Phila Pa 1976) 2011;36:1484–91.

6. Unnikrishnan R, Renjitkumar J, Menon VK. Adolescent idiopathic scoliosis: retrospective analysis of 235 surgically treated cases. Indian J Orthop 2010;44:35–41.

7. Weiss HR, Goodall D. Rate of complications in scoliosis surgery—a systematic review of the Pub Med literature. Scoliosis 2008;3:9.

8. Carreon LY, Puno RM, Lenke LG, et al. Non-neurologic complications following surgery for adolescent idiopathic scoliosis. J Bone Joint Surg Am 2007;89: 2427–32.

9. Hamilton DK, Smith JS, Sansur CA, et al. Rates of new neurological deficit associated with spine surgery based on 108,419 procedures: a report of the Scoliosis Research Society Morbidity and Mortality Committee. Spine (Phila Pa 1976) 2011;36:1218–28.

10. Pahys JM, Guille JT, D'Andrea LP, et al. Neurologic injury in the surgical treatment of idiopathic scoliosis: guidelines for assessment and management. J Am Acad Orthop Surg 2009;17:426–34.

11. Seo HJ, Kim HJ, Ro YJ, et al. Non-neurologic complications following surgery for scoliosis. Korean J Anesthesiol 2013;64:40–6.

12. Pastorelli F, Di Silvestre M, Plasmati R, et al. The prevention of neural complications in the surgical treatment of scoliosis: the role of the neurophysiological intraoperative monitoring. Eur J Spine 2011; 20(Suppl 1):S104–14.

13. Schwartz DM, Auerbach JD, Dormans JP, et al. Neurophysiological detection of impending spinal cord injury during scoliosis surgery. J Bone Joint Surg Am 2007;89:2240–9.

14. Thuet ED, Winscher JC, Padberg AM, et al. Validity and reliability of intraoperative monitoring in pediatric spinal deformity surgery: a 23-year experience of 3436 cases. Spine (Phila Pa 1976) 2010;35: 1880–6.

15. Aleissa S, Parsons D, Grant J, et al. Deep wound infection following pediatric scoliosis surgery: incidence and analysis of risk factors. Can J Surg 2011;54:263–9.

16. Glotzbecker MP, Riedel MD, Vitale MG, et al. What's the evidence? Systematic literature review of risk factors and preventive strategies for surgical site infection following pediatric spine surgery. J Pediatr Orthop 2013;33:479–87.

17. Ho C, Skaggs DL, Weiss JM, et al. Management of infection after instrumented posterior spine fusion in pediatric scoliosis. Spine (Phila Pa 1976) 2007; 32:2739–44.

18. Myung KS, Glassman DM, Tolo VT, et al. Simple steps to minimize spine infections in adolescent idiopathic scoliosis. J Pediatr Orthop 2014;34:29–33.

19. Rihn JA, Lee JY, Ward WT. Infection after the surgical treatment of adolescent idiopathic scoliosis. Evaluation of the diagnosis, treatment, and impact on clinical outcomes. Spine (Phila Pa 1976) 2008; 33:289–94.

20. Smith JS, Shaffrey CI, Sansur CA, et al. Rates of infection after spine surgery based on 108,419 procedures: a report from the Scoliosis Research Society Morbidity and Mortality Committee. Spine (Phila Pa 1976) 2011;36:556–63.

21. Li Z, Shen J, Qiu G, et al. Unplanned reoperation within 30 days of fusion surgery for spinal deformity. PLoS One 2014;9:e87172.

22. Luhmann SJ, Lenke LG, Bridwell KH, et al. Revision surgery after primary spine fusion for idiopathic scoliosis. Spine (Phila Pa 1976) 2009;34:2191–7.

23. Sponseller PD. Pediatric revision spinal deformity surgery: issues and complications. Spine (Phila Pa 1976) 2010;35:2205–10.

24. Tarrant RC, Nugent M, Nugent AP, et al. Anthropometric characteristics, high prevalence of undernutrition and weight loss: impact on outcomes in patients with adolescent idiopathic scoliosis after spinal fusion. Eur Spine J 2015;24:281–9.

25. Basques BA, Bohl DD, Golinvaux NS, et al. Patient factors are associated with poor short-term outcomes after posterior fusion for adolescent idiopathic scoliosis. Clin Orthop Relat Res 2015;473: 286–94.

26. Clark CE, Shufflebarger HL. Late-developing infection in instrumented idiopathic scoliosis. Spine (Phila Pa 1976) 1999;18:1909–12.

27. Di Silvestre M, Bakaloudis G, Lolli F, et al. Late-developing infection following posterior fusion for adolescent idiopathic scoliosis. Eur Spine J 2011; 20(Suppl 1):S121–7.

28. Richards BS, Emara KM. Delayed infections after posterior TSRH spinal instrumentation for idiopathic scoliosis. Spine (Phila Pa 1976) 2001;26:1990–6.

29. Hedequist D, Haugen A, Hresko T, et al. Failure of attempted implant retention in spinal deformity delayed surgical site infections. Spine (Phila Pa 1976) 2009;34:60–4.

30. Canavese F, Kraibich JI. Use of vacuum assisted closure in instrumented spinal deformities for children with postoperative deep infections. Indian J Orthop 2010;44:177–83.

31. van Rhee MA, de Klerk LW, Verhaar JA. Vacuum-assisted wound closure of deep infections after instrumented spinal fusion in six children with neuromuscular scoliosis. Spine J 2007;7:596–600.

32. Vitale MG, Riedel MD, Glotzbecker MP, et al. Building consensus: development of a Best Practice Guideline (BPG) for surgical site infection (SSI) prevention in high-risk pediatric spine surgery. J Pediatr Orthop 2013;33:471–8.

33. Sweet FA, Roh M, Silva C. Intrawound application of vancomycin for prophylaxis in instrumented thoracolumbar fusions: efficacy, drug levels, and

patient outcomes. Spine (Phila Pa 1976) 2011;36:
2084–8.

34. Martin JR, Adogwa O, Brown CR, et al. Experience
with intrawound vancomycin powder for spinal
deformity surgery. Spine (Phila Pa 1976) 2014;39:
177–84.

35. Gans I, Dormans JP, Spiegel DA, et al. Adjunctive
vancomycin powder in pediatric spine surgery is
safe. Spine (Phila Pa 1976) 2013;38:1703–7.

36. Muschik M, Lück W, Schlenzka D. Implant removal
for late-developing infection after instrumented posterior fusion for scoliosis: reinstrumentation reduces
loss of correction. A retrospective analysis of 45
cases. Eur Spine J 2004;13:645–51.

37. Rathjen K, Wood M, McClung A, et al. Clinical and
radiographic results after implant removal in idiopathic scoliosis. Spine (Phila Pa 1976) 2007;32:
2184–8.

38. Cho RH, Yaszay B, Bartley C, et al. Which Lenke 1A
curves are at the greatest risk for adding on... and
why? Spine (Phila Pa 1976) 2012;37:1384–90.

39. Lakhal W, Loret JE, de Bodman C, et al. The progression of lumbar curves in adolescent Lenke 1
scoliosis and the distal adding-on phenomenon.
Orthop Traumatol Surg Res 2014;100(4 Suppl):
S249–54.

40. Wang Y, Hansen ES, Høy K, et al. Distal adding-on
phenomenon in Lenke 1A scoliosis: risk factor identification and treatment strategy comparison. Spine
(Phila Pa 1976) 2011;36:1113–22.

41. Schlechter J, Newton PO, Vidyadhar V, et al. Risk factors for distal adding-on identified: what to watch out
for. Present at the 43rd Annual Meeting of the Scoliosis
Research Society. Salt Lake City (UT), September 10–
13, 2008. Available at: www.srs.org/professionals/
meetings/am08/doc/oral_abstracts.pdf. Accessed
August 27, 2015.

42. Lehman Ra Jr, Lenke LG, Keeler KA, et al. Operative treatment of adolescent idiopathic scoliosis
with posterior pedicle screw-only constructs: minimum three-year follow-up on one hundred fourteen
cases. Spine 2008;33:1598–604.

43. Suk SI, Lee SM, Chung ER, et al. Selective thoracic
fusion with segmental pedicle screw fixation in the
treatment of thoracic idiopathic scoliosis: more
than 5-year follow-up. Spine 2005;30:1602–9.

44. Tao F, Zhao Y, Wu Y, et al. The effect of differing spinal fusion instrumentation on the occurrence of postoperative crankshaft phenomenon in adolescent
idiopathic scoliosis. J Spinal Disord Tech 2010;23:
e75–80.

45. Burton DC, Ahser MA, Lai SM. Scoliosis correction
maintenance in skeletally immature patients with
idiopathic scoliosis: is anterior fusion really necessary? Spine (Phila Pa 1976) 2000;25:61–8.

46. Kioschos HC, Asher MA, Lark RG, et al. Overpower-
ing the crankshaft mechanism: the effect of posterior
spinal fusion with and without stiff transpedicular fixation on anterior spinal column growth in immature
canines. Spine (Phila Pa 1976) 1996;21:1168–73.

47. Sarlak AY, Atmaca H, Buluc L, et al. Juvenile idiopathic scoliosis treated with posterior arthrodesis
and segmental pedicel screw instrumentation
before the age of 9 years: a 5-year follow-up. Scoliosis 2009;4:1.

48. Wood KB. Postsurgical sagittal and coronal
plane decompensation in deformity surgery. In:
Vacarro AR, Regan JJ, Crawford AH, et al, editors.
Complications of pediatric and adult spinal surgery.
Boca Raton (FL): Taylor & Francis Group; 2004. p.
687–708.

49. Cho SK, Kim YJ, Lenke LG. Proximal junctional
kyphosis following spinal deformity surgery in the
pediatric patient. J Am Acad Orthop Surg 2015;23:
408–14.

50. Kim HJ, Lenke LG, Shaffrey CI, et al. Proximal junctional kyphosis (PJK) as a distinct form of adjacent
segment pathology (ASP) following spinal deformity
surgery: a systematic review. Spine (Phila Pa 1976)
2012;37(Suppl 22):S144–64.

51. Helgeson MD, Shah SA, Newton PO, et al. Evaluation of proximal junctional kyphosis in adolescent
idiopathic scoliosis following pedicle screw, hook,
or hybrid instrumentation. Spine (Phila Pa 1976)
2010;35(2):177–81.

52. Hollenbeck SM, Glattes RC, Asher MA, et al. The
prevalence of increased proximal junctional flexion
following posterior instrumentation and arthrodesis
for adolescent idiopathic scoliosis. Spine (Phila Pa
1976) 2008;33:1675–81.

Complications Related to the Treatment of Slipped Capital Femoral Epiphysis

John Roaten, MD, David D. Spence, MD*

KEYWORDS

- Slipped capital femoral epiphysis • Complications • Osteonecrosis • Chondrolysis • Impingement
- Osteoarthritis

KEY POINTS

- Because the natural history of nonoperative treatment of slipped capital femoral epiphysis is slip progression and subsequent hip deformity, surgical stabilization is required.
- The current rate of osteonecrosis after surgical treatment of slipped capital femoral epiphysis is approximately 20%, and, because it appears to be related to the stability of the slip, it may not be avoidable, regardless of treatment, in unstable slips.
- The overall incidence at chondrolysis is estimated to be approximately 7% (range 0% to 55%). Pin penetration into the joint is the most frequently cited cause, but this has been contradicted by several studies.
- Other complications, such as slipped capital femoral epiphysis–induced impingement, fixation failure, growth arrest, and development of a bilateral slip are less frequent but can cause significant morbidity if not promptly diagnosed and appropriately treated.
- Although some complications may be inevitable despite best treatment practices, most stable slips have good outcomes with few complications.

INTRODUCTION

Slipped capital femoral epiphysis (SCFE) is a condition of the young hip in which mechanical overload of the proximal femoral physis results in anterior and superior displacement of the femoral metaphysis relative to the epiphysis. A varus and external rotation deformity usually results, although a valgus deformity may be present in up to 10%.[1] Although the incidence in the United States is approximately 10 in 100,000 people, variations by region have been reported.[2] The cause of SCFE is often multifactorial, including both biochemical and biomechanical forces acting at the physis of the proximal femur in a susceptible individual. SCFE has been classified as either stable, in which the patient can walk with or without an assistive device, or unstable, in which walking is not possible.[3] The natural history of untreated SCFE is slip progression and subsequent hip deformity, which can lead directly to adjacent cartilage damage and degenerative changes of the hip joint.[4,5] The treatment of SCFE requires surgical stabilization of the proximal femoral epiphysis, but the optimal technique and timing of care remain controversial. Although the goal of treatment is to minimize complications, the overall complication rate of SCFE remains high. The purpose of this article is to review those

Funding Sources: No funding was received in support of this study.
Conflict of Interest: None.
Department of Orthopaedic Surgery & Biomedical Engineering, University of Tennessee-Campbell Clinic, 1211 Union Avenue, Suite 510, Memphis, TN 38104, USA
* Corresponding author.
E-mail address: dspence@campbellclinic.com

Orthop Clin N Am 47 (2016) 405–413
http://dx.doi.org/10.1016/j.ocl.2015.09.013

complications. Among the more reported complications are osteonecrosis (ON) of the femoral head, chondrolysis, SCFE-induced impingement with associated articular cartilage damage and labral injury, fixation failure and deformity progression, growth arrest, and development of bilateral disease.

OSTEONECROSIS

ON is perhaps the most feared complication related to SCFE and is associated with poorer outcomes (**Fig. 1**). The etiology of ON is not entirely elucidated, but is likely related to a combination of direct damage of the retinacular vessels that supply the femoral head and an intracapsular tamponade caused by hemorrhage. Loder and colleagues[3] established a relationship between unstable slips and ON in their series of 55 patients treated with internal fixation: 47% (14 of 30) of unstable slips developed ON. Twenty years later, in a review of the literature, Loder[6] reported an overall incidence of 21% (88 of 417) of ON in unstable slips.

In a separate retrospective study of 240 patients evaluating the factors influencing the development of ON, all 21 hips (8.75%) that had ON were classified as unstable at presentation, whereas none of those classified as stable had ON, regardless of severity. Although the slip severity had no effect in the stable group, the risk of ON in the unstable group increased with increasing slip severity.[7] ON is related to the stability of the slip and, thus, may not be avoidable, regardless of treatment; however, methods to minimize the rate of ON have been developed. In an attempt to determine a cause of ON, 5 unstable slips in Loder's later study were evaluated with angiography, which found kinking of the epiphyseal vessels, with 1 of 3 hips having a return of the blood supply after a reduction maneuver.[6] In contrast, intracapsular

pressure measurements showed an increase from 48 mm Hg to 75 mm Hg after reduction maneuver, which is significantly higher than a normal unaffected hip measurement of 23 mm Hg. After capsulotomy, this pressure decreased significantly to 17 mm Hg.[8] In the presence of chronic changes, a forceful manipulation of an unstable SCFE can cause cessation of flow through the posterior physeal retinacular vessels as they become stretched over posterior callous at the head and neck junction resulting in higher rates of ON.[9]

It remains controversial whether reduction is protective against, promoting of, or neutral for ON. In contrast to Loder's[6] perfusion findings, Kitano and colleagues[10] found reduction, whether purposeful or inadvertent, to be related to the risk of ON and recommended against such treatment in unstable or acute SCFE. For this reason, they also cautioned against the use of a fracture table. In a comparative study of intracapsular cuneiform osteotomy and in-situ pinning for unstable slips, Walton and colleagues[11] showed the 2 groups had ON rates of 25% and 42%, respectively. In the in situ pinning group, further analysis found a protective role for incomplete rather than complete reduction, with a decrease in the ON rate from 80% to 33%. Partial reduction, to the point at which it was before the acute component of the slip, through an open approach for hip joint decompression (Parsch method) on a regular operating table, has produced rates of ON of less than 10% at 5 years.[12]

Other techniques for anatomic reduction have been described, such as the modified Dunn technique, which allows for resection of posterior callus and reorientation and fixation of the femoral epiphysis via a safe surgical dislocation approach,[13] and have produced rates of ON as low as 8% in some reports,[11] whereas in other reports the incidence of ON with the modified Dunn is as high as

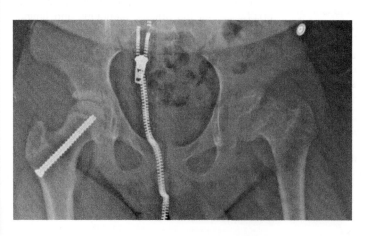

Fig. 1. Osteonecrosis of the left hip in a 12-year-old girl after surgical treatment of an unstable SCFE.

30%.[14–16] Other recommendations to minimize the risk of complications include the use of the modified Dunn procedure at specialty centers where a higher-volume surgeon experienced with the procedure can be available in the operating room.[17] These investigators also suggested that the modified Dunn be done urgently (<24 hours) only for acute, severe (slip angle >50°) slips with only mild metaphyseal remodeling. Further investigation with randomized, matched groups of unstable slips will be helpful in determining the best treatment for unstable slips to obtain the lowest rate of ON possible.

CHONDROLYSIS

Chondrolysis is suspected if the patient complains of pain and stiffness in the hip and has more than 50% joint space reduction of the involved hip or a joint space measuring less than 3 mm in bilateral cases.[2] The etiology of chondrolysis is unknown, is likely multifactorial, and can occur with or without treatment. The overall incidence of chondrolysis is estimated at 7%, depending on the series but has ranged from 0% to 55%.[18] Persistent pin penetration into the joint surface is most frequently cited as the cause, with a frequency of 88% in a study of 17 hips with a diagnosis of chondrolysis.[2,19] In contrast, in a series of 14 hips with transient penetration of the joint by a guide pin, screw, or both that was recognized and corrected during the surgical procedure, no patient had chondrolysis at 2-year follow-up.[20] Additionally, in a retrospective review, Dendane[21] did not find transient intra-articular pin penetration to be a risk factor. Moreover, Dendane[21] found that obesity and delay in diagnosis of more than

60 days was significantly associated with the development of chondrolysis after SCFE. An immune reaction has also been suggested as a possible cause based on joint aspirations,[18] but further study is required to validate this hypothesis.

Regardless of its cause, chondrolysis is thought to have better outcomes than the complication of ON. In a long-term (average 14 years) follow-up study, Tudisco and colleagues[21] noted diminishing pain and radiographic restoration of the joint space by 10 months; however, all of their patients had decreased range of motion at final follow-up. Patients with the worst outcomes had severe slippage or ON. Treatment for chondrolysis is aimed at pain reduction and maintenance of range of motion.[21] Patients should be placed on limited activities with diminished weight bearing and started on range-of-motion physical therapy. Surgical interventions such as hinged distraction, periosteal patches, and osteochondral allografts have been performed but require further investigation.[22,23]

SLIPPED CAPITAL FEMORAL EPIPHYSIS–INDUCED IMPINGEMENT

The true incidence of degenerative joint disease (DJD) after SCFE is unclear but is thought to be most closely associated with SCFE-induced impingement. The characteristic deformity produced by SCFE results in cam morphology of the hip and creates a potential geometric conflict between the femoral head and neck and the acetabulum that can lead to femoroacetabular impingement (FAI) (**Fig. 2**). Acetabular retroversion may be present before the slip and also

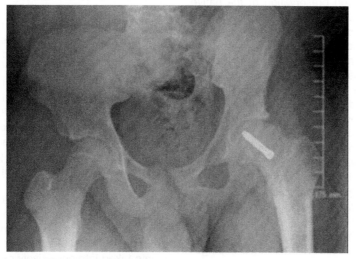

Fig. 2. Femoroacetabular impingement after SCFE.

may contribute to a combined (cam and pincer) FAI. Radiographic assessment of even mild cases of SCFE has found loss of normal head/neck ratios and significant increases in the α angle as measured on the Dunn lateral view.[24] In their series of 121 hips with stable SCFE treated with in situ fixation, Castañeda and colleagues[25] found signs of DJD in all; clinical and radiographic signs of FAI were present in 79% of hips that were followed up for a minimum of 20 years after mild SCFE (grade I, II, or III). A direct correlation was identified between the degree of deformity and the presence of DJD in early adulthood. In a study comparing post-SCFE hips and those with primary osteoarthritis at the time of joint arthroplasty, patients with post-SCFE deformity were 11 years younger than those who had primary osteoarthritis.[26] This finding was attributed to the loss of head/neck offset, abnormal rotation of the femoral head resulting in reorientation of the articular cartilage on the femoral head typical of the abnormal SCFE hips in this study.

Milder slips have been treated with in situ pinning with low rates of complications; however, impingement-related articular damage, regardless of slip severity, has been reported.[24,27,28] Lee and colleagues[29] found that osteoarthritis rates after SCFE ranged from 24% at 11 years to 92% at 28 years. The long-term natural history of untreated, stable slips includes decreased Iowa Hip Ratings scores with increased slip severity; mild slips are distinct from moderate to severe slips in that the incidence of DJD is only 36% in contrast to 100% in more severe slips.[30]

Surgical treatment of SCFE-induced impingement has increased over the last 10 years and has been focused on preservation of the native joint as an alternative to hip arthroplasty.[31] The decision to operate on a young hip with structural impingement before degenerative symptoms occur remains controversial. Of 89 hips treated with surgical hip dislocation for prearthritic hip disease, Beaulé and colleagues[32] had only 6 hips (7%) that required total joint arthroplasty at 7-year follow-up; however, 38% of these patients required removal of internal fixation hardware, and the authors concluded that less-invasive approaches to the treatment of this condition should be considered. With the treatment evolving for FAI related to SCFE, open surgical hip dislocation remains the gold standard. With improving techniques and further research, arthroscopy may supplant this open technique, especially for the treatment of mild cases of prearthritic impingement after SCFE.

FIXATION FAILURE AND SLIP PROGRESSION

Fixation failure also is a known complication associated with the treatment of SCFE and can lead to hardware-related symptoms or be directly related to slip progression. Smooth pins and cannulated screws are the most common hardware used for fixation, regardless of the procedure chosen. Although smooth pins allow for easier removal and the potential for added growth, pin migration and breakage have been reported.[33–35] As a result, fixation with 1 or 2 cannulated screws has become the standard fixation at most centers. Multiple clinical studies have shown satisfactory results with single screw constructs, even in higher-grade slips[36–40]; however, most of these studies evaluated stable slips of varying degrees of severity and acuity and did not specifically address the challenge presented by an unstable slip. An in vitro study simulating unstable slips in porcine models used single- and double-screw constructs in varying configurations to treat the simulated slips and then tested them mechanically for failure. The investigators did not find a difference in configuration patterns but did find added strength and stiffness in the 2-screw models. Additionally, at degrees of displacement of more than 2 mm, they found significantly higher failure loads in the 2-screw compared with the singe screw-model.[41] Orientation to the physis of those screws, whether perpendicular or oblique, was not found to significantly affect resistance to shear forces. Whether the loads produced in this study can be naturally reproduced in vivo is uncertain. Karol and colleagues[42] found only 33% improved stiffness in a double-screw bovine model and argued that such gain did not outweigh the risk associated with placement of the additional screw. Although 2 screws may be stronger biomechanically, there are risks associated with the placement of a second screw. Another study found that a single screw was adequate in mild slips and avoided the risks associated with additional screws.[43] Blanco and colleagues[44] found a direct correlation between an increasing number of pins and increased rates of complications without a significant difference in time to closure of the proximal femoral physis. Based on these findings, the authors concluded that single-pin or screw fixation provided dependable physeal closure and minimized implant-related complications.

Intra-articular placement of a screw can occur as a result of trying to obtain maximal fixation within the epiphysis. Additionally, determining appropriate screw length based on measurements taken intraoperatively can be a challenge.

Although it is desirable to obtain maximal purchase in the epiphysis, it is equally important to avoid intra-articular penetration of the screw tip. Careful measurements of the screw length, use of fluoroscopy in multiple planes during placement, and consideration of the spherical shape of the femoral head will help avoid this complication. A screw that is seen to be too long at insertion can potentially be left prominent on the anterolateral surface of the proximal femur, but a prominence of more than 1.5 cm has been associated with a "windshield wiper" loosening effect caused by the forces exerted on the screw head from the overlying soft tissues.[45] Additionally, placement of the screw tip eccentric to a center-center position can allow for inadequate fixation and further migration of the capital epiphysis.[46]

GROWTH ARREST

Epiphysiodesis prevents further slippage of the epiphysis on the metaphysis and, thus, has become the goal of most surgical SCFE treatments. The average age of most patients with SCFE is 12 years, and with the goal of epiphysiodesis, the expectation is that 3 mm a year of limb growth from the proximal femoral physis will be lost. Cessation of proximal femoral physeal growth has several potential consequences, particularly in younger patients, such as creation of unequal leg lengths and altered femoral growth parameters, such as a shortened femoral neck and relative trochanteric overgrowth, extra-articular impingement, coxa vara, and resultant altered gait patterns. In younger patients, in whom a larger discrepancy might be expected, other methods of growth-sparing fixation may be considered. Physeal closure typically occurs by 5 to 6 months. Evidence is conflicting as to whether this is influenced by the number of screws or pins used, but some evidence shows that more implants spanning the physis lead to earlier closure.[44,47,48] Threaded pins or screws that cross the physis can lead to closure of the physis,[49] which may not be desirable in very young patients. If continued growth is desired, avoiding implants with threads on both sides of the physis should be considered. There is evidence that the type of implant used can affect this outcome, including early closure of the physis and shortening of the femoral neck.

In a study aimed at evaluating continued physeal growth, Laplaza and Burke[50] showed evidence of the epiphysis "growing off" threaded Steinman and Knowles pins in 29% and 18% of cases, respectively. No hips stabilized with a cannulated screw continued to grow after surgery, however, and the authors recommended use of these implants. Originally designed for adult hip fractures, a hook device developed by Hansson uses a smooth-barreled pin and a hook that is deployed after insertion into the epiphysis. This pin and hook provides stable fixation in both the metaphysis and the epiphysis, as well as continued growth, and can be removed at a later date. In his report of the use of this device for the treatment of SCFE, Hansson[51] found no tendency toward premature physeal closure in asymptomatic hips that were pinned prophylactically or in 73% of unilateral slips at 1 to 6 years of follow-up. The growth of the femoral neck also was found to be similar to that of the asymptomatic hip. Further development of growth-sparing techniques and implants that still allow for stable fixation may have a benefit in patients with significant growth remaining.

DEVELOPMENT OF BILATERAL DISEASE

Presentation of a unilateral SCFE should prompt evaluation for the presence of bilateral disease. While a contralateral slip is not technically a complication of the initial slip, the risk of a contralateral slip is significant, and a delay in diagnosis may have grave consequences. The incidence of contralateral slips that are not diagnosed at the initial slip but are present and asymptomatic also is unclear and difficult to determine,[52] as only a small percent of missed slips in the contralateral hip are symptomatic.[53] The risk of contralateral slip development in patients who are first seen with a unilateral slip has been reported to be 2335 times higher than the risk of the initial slip[54]; however, prophylactic treatment of the contralateral hip in a patient who presents with unilateral disease remains controversial. The incidence of bilateral disease development is often cited as between 20% and 40% but has been reported to be as high as 80% in some series, which many authors use as an argument for pinning of the contralateral, asymptomatic hip. Schultz and colleagues,[54] analyzing pooled data from the literature, assessed the probability of developing a contralateral slip at varying time intervals, comparing these findings with the outcomes of hips that were pinned prophylactically. They concluded that prophylactic pinning, overall, is beneficial to the long-term outcome of that hip. They also noted that sound clinical judgment with respect to the age, sex, and endocrine status of the patient is essential.

Other authors have presented evidence to the contrary. In a large meta-analysis including 325 articles from 1931 to 1998, Castro and colleagues[55] determined the risk of contralateral slip to be greatly elevated, but, based on the outcomes from the included studies, they concluded that most bilateral cases that developed after the initial pinning were diagnosed early and treated appropriately; therefore, close follow-up and not prophylactic pinning was most supported by the literature. Yildirim and colleagues[56] presented data in support of pinning of the contralateral hip. These investigators followed up with 227 patients who presented with unilateral disease and noted that 36% had a contralateral slip at a mean of 6.5 months. Of these patients, 5 (6%) had either ON or chondrolysis. Because of the high prevalence of a subsequent contralateral slip and the complications associated with the second slip, they concluded that prophylactic pinning of the contralateral hip in a patient with unilateral SCFE is safer than and preferable to observation and symptomatic treatment.

Determining the risk of a contralateral slip is paramount; however, no gold standard for forecasting this event exists. Evaluating the posterior slope angle (**Fig. 3**) has shown promise as a predictor of the risk of development of a contralateral slip, but obtaining standard frog-lateral radiographs for comparison can be difficult. A larger posterior slope angle reflects a more vertical orientation of the capital femoral physis, which can result in increased shear forces on the physis. Research has found that a range of 12° to 15° as measured on the contralateral hip indicates an increased risk for development of

bilateral disease.[57–59] In a clinical study by Phillips and colleagues,[58] when a value of 14° was used as an indication for prophylactic pinning, 83% of the contralateral slips would have been prevented, 21% would have been pinned unnecessarily, and the number needed to treat to prevent one subsequent contralateral slip was 1.79.

The modified Oxford bone age score also has been reported to be a predictor of the risk of development of a contralateral SCFE in patients presenting with a unilateral slip but is not widely used in clinical practice.[60] Scoring the degree of ossification of the calcaneal apophysis also has been described but requires additional foot radiographs.[61] Other clinical factors associated with increased risk of contralateral slip reported in one study are remaining obese (body mass index higher than the 95th percentile) after treatment of the initial slip and having an acute initial slip. Interestingly, reduction in body mass index to less than the 95th percentile was protective in that study.[62] Other risk factors for contralateral SCFE include young age (girls younger than 10 years, boys younger than 12 years) at primary diagnosis,[63,64] skeletal immaturity,[65] female sex,[53,65] endocrine disorders such as adiposogenital dystrophy,[66–69] the angle of the slip at primary diagnosis,[53] an increased slope angle of the physis,[70] and an open triradiate cartilage (23% progression if open).[71]

It is important that the clinician evaluating a unilateral slipped capital epiphysis be aware that the contralateral hip may be initially involved or may become so. He or she must also be aware of the described risk factors and use these as part of the clinical, radiographic, and social background to come to a decision about prophylactically pinning the contralateral hip.

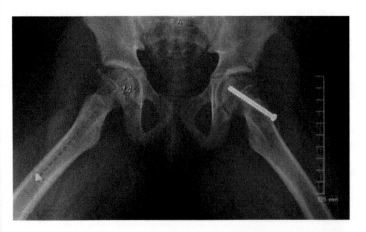

Fig. 3. Posterior slope angle: angle between a line along the plane of the physis and one perpendicular to the femoral neck-diaphyseal axis. An angle of 12° to 15° is considered a risk factor in the development of bilateral slips.

SUMMARY

Slipped capital femoral epiphysis is a common hip disorder and is associated with a high complication rate. Although some complications may be unavoidable, minimizing complications, particularly those related to treatment, may further improve patient outcomes. Although the optimal treatment of SCFE remains controversial, the goal of treatment should include stable fixation performed in a careful manner with minimal residual deformity without additional insult to the epiphyseal vascularity. Further study is required to determine the most appropriate timing of intervention and which techniques and implants will result in the best outcomes. Improved awareness and recognition of early and late complications, as well as techniques to treat them, are imperative in the management of patient with SCFE.

REFERENCES

1. Koczewski P. Valgus slipped capital femoral epiphysis: subcapital growth plate orientation analysis. J Pediatr Orthop B 2013;22:548–52.
2. Aronsson DD, Loder RT, Weinstein SL, et al. Slipped capital femoral epiphysis: current concepts. J Am Acad Orthop Surg 2006;14:666–79.
3. Loder RT, Richards BS, Shapiro PS, et al. Acute slipped capital femoral epiphysis: the importance of physeal stability. J Bone Joint Surg Am 1993;75:1134–40.
4. Novais EN, Hill MK, Carry PM, et al. Modified Dunn procedure is superior to in situ pinning for short-term clinical and radiographic improvement in severe stable SCFE. Clin Orthop Relat Res 2014;473:2108–17.
5. Novais EN, Millis MB. Slipped capital femoral epiphysis: prevalence, pathogenesis, and natural history. Clin Orthop Relat Res 2012;470:3432–8.
6. Loder RT. What is the cause of avascular necrosis in unstable slipped capital femoral epiphysis and what can be done to lower the rate? J Pediatr Orthop 2013;33(Suppl 1):S88–91.
7. Tokmakova KP, Stanton RP, Mason DE. Factors influencing the development of osteonecrosis in patients treated for slipped capital femoral epiphysis. J Bone Joint Surg Am 2003;85:798–801.
8. Herrera-Soto JA, Duffy MF, Birnbaum MA, et al. Increased intracapsular pressures after unstable slipped capital femoral epiphysis. J Pediatr Orthop 2008;28:723–8.
9. Wenger DR, Bomar JD. Acute, unstable, slipped capital femoral epiphysis: is there a role for in situ fixation? J Pediatr Orthop 2014;34(Suppl 1):S11–7.
10. Kitano T, Nakagawa K, Wada M, et al. Closed reduction of slipped capital femoral epiphysis: high-risk factor for avascular necrosis. J Pediatr Orthop B 2015;24:281–5.
11. Walton RD, Martin E, Wright D, et al. The treatment of an unstable slipped capital femoral epiphysis by either intracapsular cuneiform osteotomy or pinning in situ: a comparative study. Bone Joint J 2015;97:412–9.
12. Parsch K, Weller S, Parsch D. Open reduction and smooth Kirschner wire fixation for unstable slipped capital femoral epiphysis. J Pediatr Orthop 2009;29:1–8.
13. Dunn DM. The treatment of adolescent slipping of the upper femoral epiphysis. J Bone Joint Surg Br 1964;46:621–9.
14. Huber H, Dora C, Ramseier LE, et al. Adolescent slipped capital femoral epiphysis treated by a modified Dunn osteotomy with surgical hip dislocation. J Bone Joint Surg Br 2011;93:833–8.
15. Madan SS, Cooper AP, Davies AG, et al. The treatment of severe slipped capital femoral epiphysis via the Ganz surgical dislocation and anatomical reduction: a prospective study. Bone Joint J 2013;95:424–9.
16. Slongo T, Kakaty D, Krause F, et al. Treatment of slipped capital femoral epiphysis with a modified Dunn procedure. J Bone Joint Surg Am 2010;92:2898–908.
17. Upasani VV, Matheney TH, Spencer SA, et al. Complications after modified Dunn osteotomy for the treatment of adolescent slipped capital femoral epiphysis. J Pediatr Orthop 2014;34:661–7.
18. Lubicky JP. Chondrolysis and avascular necrosis: complications of slipped capital femoral epiphysis. J Pediatr Orthop B 1996;5:162–7.
19. Jofe MH, Lehman W, Ehrlich MG. Chondrolysis following slipped capital femoral epiphysis. J Pediatr Orthop B 2004;13:29–31.
20. Zionts LE, Simonian PT, Harvey JP Jr. Transient penetration of the hip joint during in situ cannulated-screw fixation of slipped capital femoral epiphysis. J Bone Joint Surg Am 1991;73:1054–60.
21. Tudisco C, Caterini R, Farsetti P, et al. Chondrolysis of the hip complicating slipped capital femoral epiphysis: long-term follow-up of nine patients. J Pediatr Orthop B 1999;8:107–11.
22. Millis MB, Zaltz I. Current perspectives on the pediatric hip: selected topics in hip dysplasia, Perthes disease, and chondrolysis: synopsis of the hip subspecialty session at the POSNA Annual Meeting, May 1, 2013, Toronto. J Pediatr Orthop 2014;34(Suppl 1):S36–43.
23. Thacker MM, Feldman DS, Madan SS, et al. Hinged distraction of the adolescent arthritic hip. J Pediatr Orthop 2005;25:178–82.
24. Fraitzl CR, Kafer W, Nelitz M, et al. Radiological evidence of femoroacetabular impingement in mild

slipped capital femoral epiphysis: a mean follow-up of 14.4 years after pinning in situ. J Bone Joint Surg Br 2007;89:1592–6.

25. Castañeda P, Ponce C, Villareal G, et al. The natural history of osteoarthritis after a slipped capital femoral epiphysis/the pistol grip deformity. J Pediatr Orthop 2013;33(Suppl 1):S76–82.

26. Abraham E, Gonzalez MH, Pratap S, et al. Clinical implications of anatomical wear characteristics in slipped capital femoral epiphysis and primary osteoarthritis. J Pediatr Orthop 2007;27:788–95.

27. Larson AN, Sierra RJ, Yu EM, et al. Outcomes of slipped capital femoral epiphysis treated with in situ pinning. J Pediatr Orthop 2012;32:125–30.

28. Zilkens C, Bittersohl B, Jager M, et al. Significance of clinical and radiographic findings in young adults after slipped capital femoral epiphysis. Int Orthop 2011;35:1295–301.

29. Lee CB, Matheney T, Yen YM. Case reports: acetabular damage after mild slipped capital femoral epiphysis. Clin Orthop Relat Res 2013;471:2163–72.

30. Carney BT, Weinstein SL. Natural history of untreated chronic slipped capital femoral epiphysis. Clin Orthop Relat Res 1996;322:43–7.

31. Peters CL. Mild to moderate hip OA: joint preservation or total hip arthroplasty? J Arthroplasty 2015;30:1109–12.

32. Beaulé PE, Singh A, Poitras S, et al. Surgical dislocation of the hip for the treatment of pre-arthritic hip disease. J Arthroplasty 2015;30(9):1502–5.

33. Violas P, Chapuis M, Bracq H. Percutaneous in situ pin fixation in superior femoral epiphysiolysis. Rev Chir Orthop Reparatrice Appar Mot 1998;84:617–22.

34. Kruger DM, Herzenberg JE, Viviano DM, et al. Biomechanical comparison of single- and double-pin fixation for acute slipped capital femoral epiphysis. Clin Orthop Relat Res 1990;259:277–81.

35. Belkoff SM, Millis DL, Probst CW. Biomechanical comparison of 1-screw and 2-divergent pin internal fixations for treatment of slipped capital femoral epiphysis, using specimens obtained from immature dogs. Am J Vet Res 1993;54:1770–3.

36. Aronson DD, Carlson WE. Slipped capital femoral epiphysis. A prospective study of fixation with a single screw. J Bone Joint Surg Am 1992;74:810–9.

37. Aronson DD, Loder RT. Slipped capital femoral epiphysis in black children. J Pediatr Orthop 1992;12:74–9.

38. de Sanctis N, Di Gennaro G, Pempinello C, et al. Is gentle manipulative reduction and percutaneous fixation with a single screw the best management of acute and acute-on-chronic slipped capital femoral epiphysis? A report of 70 patients. J Pediatr Orthop B 1996;5:90–5.

39. Gonzalez-Moran G, Carsi B, Abril JC, et al. Results after preoperative traction and pinning in slipped capital femoral epiphysis: K wires versus cannulated screws. J Pediatr Orthop B 1998;7:53–8.

40. Herman MJ, Dormans JP, Davidson RS, et al. Screw fixation of grade III slipped capital femoral epiphysis. Clin Orthop Relat Res 1996;322:77–85.

41. Kishan S, Upasani V, Mahar A, et al. Biomechanical stability of single-screw versus two-screw fixation of an unstable slipped capital femoral epiphysis model: effect of screw position in the femoral neck. J Pediatr Orthop 2006;26:601–5.

42. Karol LA, Doane RM, Cornicelli SF, et al. Single versus double screw fixation for treatment of slipped capital femoral epiphysis: a biomechanical analysis. J Pediatr Orthop 1992;12:741–5.

43. Schmitz MR. Biomechanical testing of unstable slipped capital femoral epiphysis screw fixation: worth the risk of a second screw? J Pediatr Orthop 2015;35:496–500.

44. Blanco JS, Taylor B, Johnston CE 2nd. Comparison of single pin versus multiple pin fixation in treatment of slipped capital femoral epiphysis. J Pediatr Orthop 1992;12:384–9.

45. Maletis GB, Bassett GS. Windshield-wiper loosening: a complication of in situ screw fixation of slipped capital femoral epiphysis. J Pediatr Orthop 1993;13:607–9.

46. Herring JA, editor. Tachdjian's pediatric orthopedics. 4th edition. Philadelphia: Saunders-Elsevier; 2008. p. 839–94.

47. Emery RJ, Todd RC, Dunn DM. Prophylactic pinning in slipped upper femoral epiphysis. Prevention of complications. J Bone Joint Surg Br 1990;72:217–9.

48. Seller K, Raab P, Wild A, et al. Risk-benefit analysis of prophylactic pinning in slipped capital femoral epiphysis. J Pediatr Orthop B 2001;10:192–6.

49. Hansson G, Nathorst-Westfelt J. Management of the contralateral hip in patients with unilateral slipped upper femoral epiphysis: to fix or not to fix – consequences of two strategies. J Bone Joint Surg Br 2012;94:596–602.

50. Laplaza FJ, Burke SW. Epiphyseal growth after pinning of slipped capital femoral epiphysis. J Pediatr Orthop 1995;15:357–61.

51. Hansson LI. Osteosynthesis with the hook-pin in slipped capital femoral epiphysis. Acta Orthop Scand 1982;53:87–96.

52. Jerre R, Billing L, Hansson G, et al. Bilaterality in slipped capital femoral epiphysis: importance of a reliable radiographic method. J Pediatr Orthop B 1996;5:80–4.

53. Jerre R, Billing L, Hansson G, et al. The contralateral hip in patients primarily treated for unilateral slipped upper femoral epiphysis. Long-term follow-up of 61 hips. J Bone Joint Surg Br 1994;76:563–7.

54. Schultz WR, Weinstein JN, Weinstein SL, et al. Prophylactic pinning of the contralateral hip in slipped capital femoral epiphysis: evaluation of long-term outcome for the contralateral hip with use of decision analysis. J Bone Joint Surg Am 2002;84:1305–14.

55. Castro FP Jr, Bennett JT, Doulens K. Epidemiological perspective on prophylactic pinning in patients with unilateral slipped capital femoral epiphysis. J Pediatr Orthop 2000;20:745–8.

56. Yildirim Y, Bautista S, Davidson RS. Chondrolysis, osteonecrosis, and slip severity in patients with subsequent contralateral slipped capital femoral epiphysis. J Bone Joint Surg Am 2008;90:485–92.

57. Bellemore JM, Carpenter EC, Yu NY, et al. Biomechanics of slipped capital femoral epiphysis: evaluation of the posterior sloping angle. J Pediatr Orthop 2015. [Epub ahead of print].

58. Phillips PM, Phadnis J, Willoughby R, et al. Posterior sloping angle as a predictor of contralateral slip in slipped capital femoral epiphysis. J Bone Joint Surg Am 2013;95:146–50.

59. Barrios C, Blasco MA, Blasco MC, et al. Posterior sloping angle of the capital femoral physis: a predictor of bilaterality in slipped capital femoral epiphysis. J Pediatr Orthop 2005;25:445–9.

60. Popejoy D, Emara K, Birch J. Prediction of contralateral slipped capital femoral epiphysis using the modified Oxford bone age score. J Pediatr Orthop 2012;32:290–4.

61. Nicholson AD, Huez CM, Sanders JO, et al. Calcaneal scoring as an adjunct to modified Oxford hip scores: prediction of contralateral slipped capital femoral epiphysis. J Pediatr Orthop 2015. [Epub ahead of print].

62. Nasreddine AY, Heyworth BE, Zurakowski D, et al. A reduction in body mass index lowers risk for bilateral slipped capital femoral epiphysis. Clin Orthop Relat Res 2013;471:2137–44.

63. Riad J, Bajelidze G, Gabos PG. Bilateral slipped capital femoral epiphysis: predictive factors for contralateral slip. J Pediatr Orthop 2007;27:411–4.

64. Bidwell TA, Susan Stott N. Sequential slipped capital femoral epiphyses: who is at risk for a second slip? ANZ J Surg 2006;76:973–6.

65. Koenig KM, Thomson JD, Anderson KL, et al. Does skeletal maturity predict sequential contralateral involvement after fixation of slipped capital femoral epiphysis? J Pediatr Orthop 2007;27:796–800.

66. Blethen SL, Rundle AC. Slipped capital femoral epiphysis in children treated with growth hormone. A summary of the National Cooperative Growth Study experience. Horm Res 1996;46:113–6.

67. Ogden JA, Southwick WO. Endocrine dysfunction and slipped captial femoral epiphysis. Yale J Biol Med 1977;50:1–16.

68. Moorefield WG Jr, Urbaniak JR, Ogden WS, et al. Acquired hypothyroidism and slipped capital femoral epiphysis. Report of three cases. J Bone Joint Surg Am 1976;58:705–8.

69. Nixon JR, Douglas JF. Bilateral slipping of the upper femoral epiphysis in end-stage renal failure. A report of two cases. J Bone Joint Surg Br 1980;62:18–21.

70. Zenios M, Ramachandran M, Axt M, et al. Posterior sloping angle of the capital femoral physis: interobserver and intraobserver reliability testing and predictor of bilaterality. J Pediatr Orthop 2007;27:801–4.

71. Billing L, Severin E. Slipping epiphysis of the hip; a roentgenological and clinical study based on a new roentgen technique. Acta Radiol Suppl 1959;174:1–76.

Upper Extremity

Complications of Distal Radius Fixation

Dennis S. Lee, MD[a],*, Douglas R. Weikert, MD[b]

KEYWORDS

- Complications • Tendon rupture • Distal radius fracture • Tenosynovitis

KEY POINTS

- Complications following fixation of distal radius fractures remain prevalent despite advances in fixation technology.
- Volar locked plating, dorsal plating, dorsal bridge plating, fragment-specific fixation, external fixation, and percutaneous pinning confer fixation-specific risks as well as complications common to all treatment modalities.
- Understanding of the complications associated with various fixation options is essential to informed decision making and optimizing patient outcome.

BACKGROUND

Distal radius fractures are common upper extremity injuries, with an annual incidence of 16.2 fractures per 10,000 persons,[1] or more than 640,000 cases per year.[2] Prior studies have highlighted the significant variation in treating these injuries owing to regionality, patient age, sex, race, and whether a hand surgeon is the treating provider.[3–5] Regardless, the burden of distal radius fractures is expected to increase as the US population ages, concomitant with a trend toward more widespread use of internal fixation.[6]

Fixation strategies for distal radius fractures have undergone a rapid shift toward open treatment since the introduction of volar locked plating (VLP), particularly among younger US orthopedic surgeons.[7] In addition to VLP, there exists a myriad of other fixation options, including percutaneous pinning, external fixation (bridging and nonbridging), dorsal plating, dorsal bridge plating, and fragment-specific fixation.[8]

VLP seems to be trending as the most popular choice of fixation,[7] but enthusiasm for this option should be tempered by an understanding of its complications compared with other methods. A recent meta-analysis by Li-Hai and colleagues[9] showed similar complication rates between external fixation and VLP at 30.9% and 23.9%, respectively, but also found a significantly higher rate of reoperation caused by complications in the latter. In a randomized controlled trial with 5-year follow-up, Williksen and colleagues[10] found that the incidence of secondary operations for complications was 31% in patients treated with VLP, which was significantly greater than the 17% incidence in those treated with external fixation and percutaneous pinning. Arora and colleagues[11] reported an overall complication rate of 27%, with flexor and extensor tendon injury being the most frequent complications (57%). The risk of complications may also be higher in elderly patients undergoing VLP, as suggested by a randomized controlled trial by Arora and colleagues[12]

Disclosures: The authors report no potential conflicts of interest.
[a] Orthopaedic Surgery and Rehabilitation, Vanderbilt University Medical Center, 1215 21st Avenue South, Medical Center East, South Tower, Suite 4200, Nashville, TN 37232, USA; [b] Orthopaedic Surgery and Rehabilitation, Hand and Upper Extremity Center, Vanderbilt University Medical Center, 1215 21st Avenue South, Medical Center East, South Tower, Suite 3200, Nashville, TN 37232, USA
* Corresponding author.
E-mail address: dennis.lee@vanderbilt.edu

that found a 36% complication rate in patients older than 65 years of age. Lutz and colleagues[13] reported similar findings.

There is a vast but largely inconclusive body of evidence[14–17] regarding the ideal fixation for distal radius fractures. With the resultant lack of definitive evidence-based guidelines[18] and overall complication rates exceeding 30%,[11,19] familiarity with the complications of various methods of distal radius fixation can better equip practicing surgeons in making informed decisions on a case-by-case basis.

POSTOPERATIVE INFECTION

Infection is an ever-present risk following distal radius fixation because of violation of the integument. *Staphylococcus aureus* remains the most common isolated microbe, followed by mixed flora.[20] Methicillin-resistant *S aureus* is also increasingly being cultured from hand and wrist infections and should be considered as a causative organism.[21]

Pin-track or superficial infections following external fixation represent the most common type of postoperative infection following distal radius fixation. A 2007 Cochrane Systematic Review found a 25% overall incidence,[14] with smaller series reporting even higher rates in excess of 50% to 67%.[22,23] Percutaneous pinning has a lower, albeit still present, risk of pin-track or superficial infection, with another 2007 Cochrane Review finding a range from 0% to 10%.[17] A more recent meta-analysis of 7 randomized controlled trials by Chaudhry and colleagues[24] revealed an 8.2% incidence. Other smaller series report ranges from 2% to 34%.[25–27] Pins left outside the skin are associated with a significantly greater infection rate than those buried deep to the skin.[25] Nearly all of these studies reported infection resolution with oral antibiotics with or without pin removal.

In contrast, open reduction and internal fixation (ORIF) with volar and/or dorsal plating results in lower infection rates, ranging from 0% to 3%.[11,24,28,29] Open fractures of the distal radius clearly increase the risk of postoperative infection, regardless of fixation, with the largest series reporting a 44% incidence, of which 68% were soft tissue infections and 32% were caused by osteomyelitis.[30]

EXTENSOR TENDON INJURY
Percutaneous Pinning and External Fixation

Percutaneous pinning places several of the extensor tendons at risk. Chia and colleagues[31]

delineated specific tendinous structures that may be injured by Kirschner wires (K wires) placed in various trajectories. Their findings are summarized in **Table 1**. Injury to the abductor pollicis longus or extensor pollicis brevis from radial styloid pinning was avoided by ensuring that the starting point was either dorsal or volar to the first dorsal compartment. The investigators recommended making small incisions to facilitate direct visualization and protection of underlying structures, as well as avoiding placement of K wires more than 5 mm ulnar to the Lister tubercle, because this places the extensor digitorum communis (EDC) tendons at risk.

Despite the anatomic risk of extensor tendon penetration with percutaneous pinning, the incidence of clinically relevant tendon injury or rupture is low. Karantana and colleagues[32] found 1 instance of extensor pollicis longus (EPL) rupture from a cohort of 64 patients. More recently, Chaudhry and colleagues[24] documented 6 cases of tendon rupture from percutaneous pinning in their meta-analysis of 875 patients pooled from 7 randomized trials for an incidence of 0.7%. Rates of extensor tendon injury from external fixator pin placement are also low,[14] probably in part because of the generally accepted surgical technique that encourages a formal incision and blunt dissection down to bone when placing pins.[33]

Volar Plating

Extensor tendon injury, particularly EPL rupture, is a well-documented complication of volar plating or any hardware placed in a volar-to-dorsal trajectory.[34,35] This injury is typically caused by drill bit penetration or prominent dorsal screw tips (**Fig. 1**).[36] The incidence of this complication is

Table 1
Structures at risk with percutaneous pinning

Pin Trajectory	Structures at Risk
Volar styloid	SRN branches
Dorsal styloid	SRN branches
Transverse radial	APL, SRN trunk and branches
Dorsal rim	EPL, EDC
Dorsoulnar	EDM

Abbreviations: APL, abductor pollicis longus; EDC, extensor digitorum communis; EDM, extensor digit minimi; EPL, extensor pollicis longus; SRN, superficial radial nerve.

Data from Chia B, Catalano LW 3rd, Glickel SZ, et al. Percutaneous pinning of distal radius fractures: an anatomic study demonstrating the proximity of K wires to structures at risk. J Hand Surg Am 2009;34(6):1014–20.

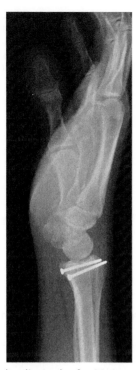

Fig. 1. Lateral radiograph of a 36-year-old man with prominent dorsal tip of the proximal screw, which led to EPL rupture.

significant, with a series of 35 patients by Al-Rashid and colleagues[37] reporting an 8.6% rate of EPL rupture following VLP fixation. Arora and colleagues[11] examined a larger cohort of 114 patients and found a lower incidence of 1.8%. More recently, Zenke and colleagues[38] examined a series of 286 patients and found a rate of 2.1%.

Symptoms that may herald impending EPL rupture include tenderness and swelling over the course of the tendon.[39] Once rupture has occurred, management is usually in the form of transfer of the extensor indicis proprius (EIP) tendon (**Fig. 2**) or reconstruction with an intercalary tendon graft. In addition, other extensor tendons can be injured by prominent dorsal screw tips, as shown by reports of EIP and EDC tendon rupture,[40] as well as intersection syndrome.[41]

Short of rupture, prominent dorsal screw tips from volar plating can also lead to tenosynovitis of the extensor tendons. Published studies report incidences ranging from 0% to 14%.[11,12,41–44] This problem is typically addressed with removal of hardware to avoid tendon rupture.

Dorsal Plating

Extensor tendon rupture and tenosynovitis following dorsal plating have historically been troublesome

complications dating back to the 1980s with the use of 3.5-mm stainless steel T plates.[45–49] Lower profile plates, like the 2.5-mm Synthes π plate (Synthes, Paoli, PA) were then introduced in an effort to minimize extensor tendon irritation. However, the π plate produced persistent extensor tendon complications, with multiple investigators reporting unacceptably high rates ranging from 18% to 48%.[50,51]

Newer-generation dorsal plates, which incorporate precontoured, ultra–low-profile designs and recessed screw holes with or without locking technology, seem to have reduced the rate of extensor tendon complications. Carter and colleagues[52] described their experience with the low-profile Forte plate (Zimmer, Warsaw, IN) and found no extensor tendon ruptures, but did remove the plate in 10% of patients because of radial wrist extensor tendon irritation. Simic and colleagues[53] reported no extensor tendon complications in their series of 60 distal radius fractures treated with the LoCon-T dorsal plate (Wright Medical, Arlington, TN). Jupiter and Marent-Huber[54] examined their experience with fragment-specific 2.4-mm locking plates (Synthes, Paoli, PA) and found no extensor tendon complications caused by dorsally placed plates. However, they did report 9 out of 125 patients with extensor tenosynovitis, and an additional 2 patients with tendon rupture caused by prominent dorsal screw tips from volar hardware. Rozental and colleagues[51] reported no cases of extensor tenosynovitis or rupture in the 9 patients who underwent low-profile dorsal plating. Compared with VLP, Yue and colleagues[55] found no significant difference in tendon irritation or rupture.

Dorsal Bridge Plating

Dorsal bridge plating as described by Hanel[56] seems to have a lower incidence of extensor tendon complications, with the most recent study of 18 patients by Lauder and colleagues[29] reporting no cases of tenosynovitis or rupture. Other investigators with larger series report more complications, such as Ruch and colleagues[57] (3 of 22 with extensor lag), Hanel and colleagues[58] (2 of 134 with extensor tendon adhesions, 1 of 134 with EPL rupture), and Hanel and colleagues[56] (1 of 62 with extensor carpi radialis longus rupture).

Nonoperative Treatment

Practicing surgeons should also be aware of the risk of EPL tendon rupture following fractures treated nonoperatively, and may consider it as a manifestation of the natural history of certain distal

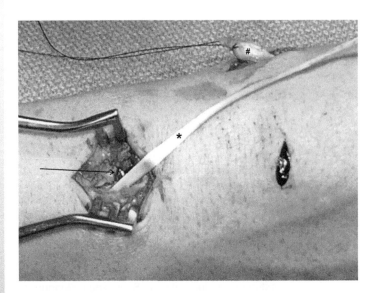

Fig. 2. Intraoperative view of the patient from **Fig. 1** with prominent dorsal screw tip (*arrow*), harvested EIP tendon (*asterisk*), and distal stump of ruptured EPL tendon (#).

radius fractures. Engkvist and Lundborg[59] postulated that the EPL tendon in the region of Lister's tubercle has poor intrinsic vascularity, and that hematoma formation in the third dorsal compartment interferes with tendon nutrition, ultimately leading to delayed rupture. Other investigators hypothesize tear propagation following partial tearing, crush ischemia, and cumulative attrition along callus or the extensor retinaculum as possible causes.[60] Irrespective of treatment modality, attention to patient reports of pain or swelling along the extensor tendons, or extensor lag, should alert surgeons to the possibility of tenosynovitis or rupture.

FLEXOR TENDON INJURY

Flexor tendon injury following fixation of distal radius fractures is less common than extensor tendon injury.[39,60] Orbay and Touhami[61] stressed the importance of the watershed line, which is the bony transverse ridge found along the volar distal edge of the radius that marks the distal extent of the concave-shaped pronator fossa. The flexor tendons approach bone at the watershed line, and thus plates placed with their distal edges at or distal to this landmark are at risk of irritating the overlying flexor tendons, resulting in tenosynovitis or rupture.

A systematic review of 21 studies from 1973 to 2013 by Asadollahi and Keith[62] found a total of 47 cases of flexor tendon rupture. The mean age of patients was 61 years, with a median interval between surgery and rupture of 9 months. The flexor pollicis longus (FPL) was the most frequently ruptured tendon, followed by the index flexor digitorum profundus. The flexor carpi radialis

tendon can also become irritated from volar plate fixation.[44]

In 2 separate series, Arora and colleagues[11] reported 9 out of 114 and 4 out of 36 [12] cases of flexor tenosynovitis that were treated with implant removal. They also documented 2 cases of FPL rupture caused by abrasion from prominent distal screw heads that had become disengaged.[11] Other case reports similarly confirm instances of FPL rupture following application of volar plates at or distal to the watershed line.[63–65] Chronic steroid use has also been implicated in FPL rupture following volar plate fixation.[66] In addition, FPL rupture can occur at any point following volar plate fixation, with 1 case report occurring 10 years after the patient's index surgery.[67] Some investigators advocate repair of the pronator quadratus as a preventative measure, which provides a protective tissue layer between volar hardware and the flexor tendons[61,68]

CARPAL TUNNEL SYNDROME AND MEDIAN NEUROPATHY

Carpal tunnel syndrome is a known complication of distal radius fractures regardless of treatment method, and can occur acutely, subacutely, or in delayed fashion.[39,69] The condition is typically caused by increased carpal tunnel pressure,[39] with nerve transaction or entrapment being less common causes.

In a matched cohort study comparing nonoperative versus VLP fixation in elderly patients, Lutz and colleagues[13] found median neuropathy to be the most common complication in both operative and nonoperative groups, reporting an overall incidence of 8.5%. The operative and nonoperative groups each had incidences of 6.2% and 11%, respectively. Arora and colleagues[11] reported a lower incidence of 2.6% following VLP fixation.

A Cochrane Review comparing percutaneous pinning with conservative treatment found comparable rates ranging from 0% to 8%.[17] Another Cochrane Review examining external fixation reported incidences of 5% to 7%.[14] Other studies report similar rates, with a trend toward a higher incidence in patients undergoing volar plating compared with other methods of fixation.[32,34,70,71] More recently, a 2015 analysis of the Swedish National Patient Registry by Navarro and colleagues[72] found the incidence of carpal tunnel release following plate fixation to be 8.7 per 10,000 person-years. This incidence was significantly higher than in those who underwent external fixation (1.6 per 10,000 person-years) or percutaneous pinning (0.9 per 10,000 person-years).

Given the common occurrence of this complication, some surgeons advocate empiric carpal tunnel release in all distal radius fractures undergoing fixation,[73] whereas others suggest a more selective approach limited to patients with preexisting or acute signs of carpal tunnel syndrome.[69,74] Regardless of approach, focused history taking and physical examination remain crucial at all time points during the treatment period.

SUPERFICIAL RADIAL NERVE INJURY

Superficial radial nerve (SRN) palsy from isolated volar plating is rare,[69] but is documented following fragment-specific fixation, with a series by Benson and colleagues[75] reporting 10 out of 81 patients with numbness in the SRN distribution. Direct injury to the SRN is more of a concern with percutaneous pinning and external fixation. In addition, both of these modalities are often used for provisional fixation during application of plates and therefore confer a transient risk of intraoperative injury in these instances.

A cadaveric study by Chia and colleagues[31] found that volar and dorsal radial styloid pins were on average 1.5 mm and 0.35 mm away, respectively, from the closest branches of the SRN. The investigators also showed that transverse radial pins were on average 1.1 mm away from the trunk or branches of the SRN (see **Table 1**).

Clinically, Glanvill and colleagues[76] reported a 13% incidence of SRN injury with radial styloid pinning. A 2007 Cochrane Review found rates ranging from 0% to 13% using only percutaneous pinning. Glickel and colleagues[77] documented 1 case of SRN neuropraxia in their series of 54

patients who underwent percutaneous pinning. Karantana and colleagues[32] reported 10 transient SRN palsies out of 64 patients treated with percutaneous pins. Roh and colleagues[35] found 2 out of 38 patients with SRN injury after being treated with external fixation and percutaneous pinning. Kumbaraci and colleagues[70] reported 2 out of 35 patients who sustained SRN injury following similar fixation. A 2007 Cochrane Review found rates ranging from 4% to 13% using both external fixation and percutaneous pinning.[17]

As shown by Glickel and colleagues,[77] the risk of neural and tendon injury can be minimized with the use of small incisions to facilitate direct visualization and soft tissue protectors (syringe tips, blunt large-gauge needles). Because percutaneous pinning remains an integral part of both provisional and definitive fixation of distal radius fractures, awareness of the various structures at risk with different pin configurations is important in minimizing the chance of iatrogenic injury.

COMPLEX REGIONAL PAIN SYNDROME

Complex regional pain syndrome (CRPS) has been associated with distal radius fractures treated both operatively and conservatively. Characterized by unexplained pain, swelling, vasomotor instability, and joint stiffness, 2 types are recognized: type I, which occurs secondary to a noxious event (formerly known as reflex sympathetic dystrophy); and type II, also known as causalgia, which is caused by direct peripheral nerve injury.[78]

CRPS has been reported following all types of fixation, with rates ranging from 3% to 25%.[14,16,17,34,35,70,71,79] Given its broad spectrum of presentations, CRPS remains difficult to treat, and efforts are largely directed toward prevention and prompt diagnosis. However, prevention and diagnosis are also difficult given several different diagnostic criteria set forth by various investigators.[80]

The pathogenesis of type I CRPS remains a topic of debate, but 2 randomized controlled trials by Zollinger and colleagues[81,82] showed that vitamin C reduced the risk of developing CRPS following distal radius fractures. Based on these findings, the investigators recommended a daily dose of 500 mg for 50 days. The American Academy of Orthopaedic Surgeons clinical practice guidelines support this regimen with a moderate recommendation but also state that the 2 trials by Zollinger and colleagues[81,82] have significant limitations because of the lack of diagnostic standardization, and no validated method to assess outcome after CRPS.[18]

A subsequent double-blinded randomized controlled trial by Ekrol and colleagues[80] showed no difference in the incidence of CRPS between their vitamin C–treated and control groups. Although the evidence on the benefit of vitamin C in the prevention of CRPS remains equivocal, many surgeons choose to recommend its supplementation given the low side effect profile. Once CRPS has developed, prompt institution of therapy and multimodal pain control agents are the cornerstones of initial management.

LOSS OF REDUCTION

Loss of reduction is a major complication following all forms of distal radius fixation and typically occurs as a result of dorsal collapse from excessive dorsal tilt, loss of radial length, or loss of reduction of the lunate facet.[69] Percutaneous pinning in particular is often criticized as being unable to maintain the immediate postoperative reduction. In their Swedish registry analysis, Navarro and colleagues[72] reported a reoperation rate because of reduction loss of 122 per 10,000 person-years with percutaneous pinning, compared with 93 per 10,000 person-years with external fixation, and 60 per 10,000 person-years with plating. The investigators also found that reoperation for reduction loss occurred earlier in the postoperative period with external fixation or percutaneous pinning compared with plating. In contrast, in a series of 54 patients, Glickel and colleagues[77] reported no significant differences between measurements from immediate postoperative and final follow-up radiographs, and no cases of reoperation.

External fixation and plating can also be prone to loss of reduction. Farah and colleagues[83] reported a 48.5% secondary displacement rate in their series of 35 distal radius fractures treated with external fixation. Leung and colleagues [84] reported loss of reduction in 5 out of 75 fractures treated with external fixation and percutaneous pinning, with 4 requiring reoperation. In addition, 5 out of 70 fractures treated with plate fixation lost reduction, with 2 requiring reoperation. Rozental and Blazar[44] reported a 9.8% incidence of loss of reduction with fracture collapse in their series of 41 patients treated with VLP. Fok and colleagues[42] reported 2 out of 101 intra-articular fractures with loss of reduction, of which 1 required reoperation.

Despite a significant rate of reduction loss, plating seems to maintain radiographic parameters better than other fixation methods. Esposito and colleagues[28] pooled data from 5 studies and found plating to be associated with a significantly smaller ulnar variance, suggesting that radial length was better restored with this method than with external fixation. Wei and colleagues[85] performed a meta-analysis of 12 trials comparing external fixation with ORIF and found that the latter restored anatomic volar tilt better, but cautioned against generalizing from this result because of substantial heterogeneity of the data.

Examining VLP specifically, Roh and colleagues[35] showed superior radiologic outcome in terms of ulnar variance compared with external fixation, but this did not influence functional outcomes at 1-year follow-up. Karantana and colleagues[32] found VLP to be better at restoring volar tilt and radial height compared with percutaneous pinning, but this did not translate to better function. Williksen and colleagues[71] also found less radial and ulnar shortening with VLP compared with external fixation.

The lunate facet merits special consideration because this fragment is prone to losing reduction when attempting fixation with VLP alone.[86] Specifically, in volar shear patterns with less than 15 mm of lunate facet available for fixation or greater than 5 mm of initial lunate subsidence, Beck and colleagues[87] recommend supplementing VLP with additional fixation (extensions, pins, wire forms, suture, miniscrews) to maintain reduction of the small volar lunate facet fragments.

Regarding other forms of plate fixation, Jupiter and Marent-Huber[54] reported loss of reduction in 2 out of 150 patients using 2.4-mm locking plates in fragment-specific fashion. Ruch and Papadonikolakis[41] documented volar collapse in 5 out of 20 patients treated with standard dorsal plating, whereas Simic and colleagues[53] reported no loss of reduction with low-profile dorsal plating in 60 fractures. Rozental and colleagues[51] reported no instances of loss of reduction in their series of 28 patients treated with either a π plate or low-profile dorsal plate. Loss of reduction remains an inherent risk with any form of distal radius fixation, and attention to reduction technique, mechanically advantageous hardware placement, and meticulous scrutiny of intraoperative radiographs helps to minimize the occurrence of this complication.

NONUNION

Nonunion is rare following distal radius fixation, with various studies documenting incidences of less than 1%.[88] More recently, Lutz and colleagues[13] reported 1 nonunion out of 129 operatively treated elderly patients. Hanel and colleagues[58] reported 1 nonunion out of 144 fractures treated with dorsal bridge plating. When indicated, management is typically in the form of revision plate fixation with structural autogenous bone graft.

POSTTRAUMATIC ARTHRITIS

Regardless of treatment modality, radiocarpal arthritis is a known potential radiographic finding following distal radius fractures, particularly in intra-articular patterns with residual step-off and gap displacement.[89–91] Seminal work by Knirk and Jupiter[90] reported a radiographic prevalence of 65% in patients with intra-articular fractures followed for a mean period of 6.7 years.

Arora and colleagues[12] documented a 44% rate of radiographically evident radiocarpal arthritis in elderly patients treated with volar locking plates, compared with 62% in those treated conservatively. No patients had pain associated with their radiographic changes, but follow-up in this study was limited to 1 year. Leung and colleagues[84] reported significantly less severe radiographic arthritic grades in those treated with plating versus external fixation and percutaneous pinning. Jupiter and Marent-Huber[54] reported a 27% prevalence of radiographically apparent signs of arthritis by 2 years after fragment-specific fixation. At an average follow-up of 15 years, Goldfarb and colleagues[92] noted radiocarpal arthritis in 13 of 16 wrists that underwent open reduction and fixation with either plates or pins.

Despite clear evidence of radiographic radiocarpal arthritis following distal radius fractures, such findings do not seem to correlate with patient symptoms or functional impairment.[93,94] Forward and colleagues[95] reported a 68% incidence of patients with intra-articular fractures who developed radiographic evidence of arthritis at a mean follow-up of 38 years. However, functional outcome was no different compared with population norms. Patients should be counseled on the long-term risk of developing radiographic arthritic changes following distal radius fixation, but that such changes may have minimal overall functional and symptomatic impact.

SUMMARY

Complications following any form of distal radius fixation remain prevalent. With an armamentarium of fixation options available to practicing surgeons, familiarity with the risks of newer plate technology as it compares with other conventional methods is crucial to maximizing surgical outcome and managing patient expectations. Given the heterogeneity of fracture patterns and patient-specific factors, there is unlikely to be a single ideal fixation method. Future work is needed to

better delineate which fixation option is better suited for which cases, with consideration of the potential complications playing a key role.

REFERENCES

1. Karl JW, Olson PR, Rosenwasser MP. The epidemiology of upper extremity fractures in the United States, 2009. J Orthop Trauma 2015;29(8):e242–4.
2. Chung KC, Spilson SV. The frequency and epidemiology of hand and forearm fractures in the United States. J Hand Surg Am 2001;26(5):908–15.
3. Fanuele J, Koval KJ, Lurie J, et al. Distal radial fracture treatment: what you get may depend on your age and address. J Bone Joint Surg Am 2009; 91(6):1313–9.
4. Chung KC, Shauver MJ, Yin H. The relationship between ASSH membership and the treatment of distal radius fracture in the United States Medicare population. J Hand Surg Am 2011;36(8):1288–93.
5. Chung KC, Shauver MJ, Yin H, et al. Variations in the use of internal fixation for distal radial fracture in the United States Medicare population. J Bone Joint Surg Am 2011;93(23):2154–62.
6. Shauver MJ, Yin H, Banerjee M, et al. Current and future national costs to Medicare for the treatment of distal radius fracture in the elderly. J Hand Surg Am 2011;36(8):1282–7.
7. Koval KJ, Harrast JJ, Anglen JO, et al. Fractures of the distal part of the radius. The evolution of practice over time. Where's the evidence? J Bone Joint Surg Am 2008;90(9):1855–61.
8. Brogan DM, Richard MJ, Ruch D, et al. Management of severely comminuted distal radius fractures. J Hand Surg Am 2015;40(9):1905–14.
9. Li-hai Z, Ya-nan W, Zhi M, et al. Volar locking plate versus external fixation for the treatment of unstable distal radial fractures: a meta-analysis of randomized controlled trials. J Surg Res 2015;193(1): 324–33.
10. Williksen JH, Husby T, Hellund JC, et al. External fixation and adjuvant pins versus volar locking plate fixation in unstable distal radius fractures: a randomized, controlled study with a 5-year follow-up. J Hand Surg Am 2015;40(7):1333–40.
11. Arora R, Lutz M, Hennerbichler A, et al. Complications following internal fixation of unstable distal radius fracture with a palmar locking-plate. J Orthop Trauma 2007;21(5):316–22.
12. Arora R, Lutz M, Deml C, et al. A prospective randomized trial comparing nonoperative treatment with volar locking plate fixation for displaced and unstable distal radial fractures in patients sixty-five years of age and older. J Bone Joint Surg Am 2011;93(23):2146–53.
13. Lutz K, Yeoh KM, MacDermid JC, et al. Complications associated with operative versus nonsurgical

treatment of distal radius fractures in patients aged 65 years and older. J Hand Surg Am 2014;39(7): 1280–6.

14. Handoll HH, Huntley JS, Madhok R. External fixation versus conservative treatment for distal radial fractures in adults. Cochrane Database Syst Rev 2007;(3):CD006194.

15. Handoll HH, Huntley JS, Madhok R. Different methods of external fixation for treating distal radial fractures in adults. Cochrane Database Syst Rev 2008;(1):CD006522.

16. Handoll HH, Madhok R. Surgical interventions for treating distal radial fractures in adults. Cochrane Database Syst Rev 2003;(3):CD003209.

17. Handoll HH, Vaghela MV, Madhok R. Percutaneous pinning for treating distal radial fractures in adults. Cochrane Database Syst Rev 2007;(3):CD006080.

18. Lichtman DM, Yeoh KM, MacDermid JC, et al. American Academy of Orthopaedic Surgeons clinical practice guideline on: the treatment of distal radius fractures. J Bone Joint Surg Am 2011;93(8):775–8.

19. Cooney WP 3rd, Dobyns JH, Linscheid RL. Complications of Colles' fractures. J Bone Joint Surg Am 1980;62(4):613–9.

20. Houshian S, Seyedipour S, Wedderkopp N. Epidemiology of bacterial hand infections. Int J Infect Dis 2006;10(4):315–9.

21. Gaston RG, Kuremsky MA. Postoperative infections: prevention and management. Hand Clin 2010;26(2): 265–80.

22. Anderson JT, Lucas GL, Buhr BR. Complications of treating distal radius fractures with external fixation: a community experience. Iowa Orthop J 2004;24: 53–9.

23. Hutchinson DT, Bachus KN, Higgenbotham T. External fixation of the distal radius: to predrill or not to predrill. J Hand Surg Am 2000;25(6):1064–8.

24. Chaudhry H, Kleinlugtenbelt YV, Mundi R, et al. Are volar locking plates superior to percutaneous K-wires for distal radius fractures? A meta-analysis. Clin Orthop Relat Res 2015;473(9):3017–27.

25. Hargreaves DG, Drew SJ, Eckersley R. Kirschner wire pin tract infection rates: a randomized controlled trial between percutaneous and buried wires. J Hand Surg Br 2004;29(4):374–6.

26. Lakshmanan P, Dixit V, Reed MR, et al. Infection rate of percutaneous Kirschner wire fixation for distal radius fractures. J Orthop Surg (Hong Kong) 2010; 18(1):85–6.

27. Subramanian P, Kantharuban S, Shilston S, et al. Complications of Kirschner-wire fixation in distal radius fractures. Tech Hand Up Extrem Surg 2012; 16(3):120–3.

28. Esposito J, Schemitsch EH, Saccone M, et al. External fixation versus open reduction with plate fixation for distal radius fractures: a meta-analysis of randomised controlled trials. Injury 2013;44(4):409–16.

29. Lauder A, Agnew S, Bakri K, et al. Functional outcomes following bridge plate fixation for distal radius fractures. J Hand Surg Am 2015;40(8):1554–62.

30. Rozental TD, Beredjiklian PK, Steinberg DR, et al. Open fractures of the distal radius. J Hand Surg Am 2002;27(1):77–85.

31. Chia B, Catalano LW 3rd, Glickel SZ, et al. Percutaneous pinning of distal radius fractures: an anatomic study demonstrating the proximity of K-wires to structures at risk. J Hand Surg Am 2009;34(6):1014–20.

32. Karantana A, Downing ND, Forward DP, et al. Surgical treatment of distal radial fractures with a volar locking plate versus conventional percutaneous methods: a randomized controlled trial. J Bone Joint Surg Am 2013;95(19):1737–44.

33. Payandeh JB, McKee MD. External fixation of distal radius fractures. Orthop Clin North Am 2007;38(2): 187–92, vi.

34. Gradl G, Gradl G, Wendt M, et al. Non-bridging external fixation employing multiplanar K-wires versus volar locked plating for dorsally displaced fractures of the distal radius. Arch Orthop Trauma Surg 2013; 133(5):595–602.

35. Roh YH, Lee BK, Baek JR, et al. A randomized comparison of volar plate and external fixation for intra-articular distal radius fractures. J Hand Surg Am 2015;40(1):34–41.

36. Benson EC, DeCarvalho A, Mikola EA, et al. Two potential causes of EPL rupture after distal radius volar plate fixation. Clin Orthop Relat Res 2006;451:218–22.

37. Al-Rashid M, Theivendran K, Craigen MA. Delayed ruptures of the extensor tendon secondary to the use of volar locking compression plates for distal radial fractures. J Bone Joint Surg Br 2006;88(12):1610–2.

38. Zenke Y, Sakai A, Oshige T, et al. Extensor pollicis longus tendon ruptures after the use of volar locking plates for distal radius fractures. Hand Surg 2013; 18(2):169–73.

39. Davis DI, Baratz M. Soft tissue complications of distal radius fractures. Hand Clin 2010;26(2):229–35.

40. Grewal R, MacDermid JC, King GJ, et al. Open reduction internal fixation versus percutaneous pinning with external fixation of distal radius fractures: a prospective, randomized clinical trial. J Hand Surg Am 2011; 36(12):1899–906.

41. Ruch DS, Papadonikolakis A. Volar versus dorsal plating in the management of intra-articular distal radius fractures. J Hand Surg Am 2006;31(1):9–16.

42. Fok MW, Klausmeyer MA, Fernandez DL, et al. Volar plate fixation of intra-articular distal radius fractures: a retrospective study. J Wrist Surg 2013;2(3): 247–54.

43. Orbay JL, Fernandez DL. Volar fixation for dorsally displaced fractures of the distal radius: a preliminary report. J Hand Surg Am 2002;27(2):205–15.

44. Rozental TD, Blazar PE. Functional outcome and complications after volar plating for dorsally displaced,

unstable fractures of the distal radius. J Hand Surg Am 2006;31(3):359–65.

45. Axelrod TS, McMurtry RY. Open reduction and internal fixation of comminuted, intraarticular fractures of the distal radius. J Hand Surg Am 1990; 15(1):1–11.

46. Fernandez DL, Geissler WB. Treatment of displaced articular fractures of the radius. J Hand Surg Am 1991;16(3):375–84.

47. Fitoussi F, Ip WY, Chow SP. Treatment of displaced intra-articular fractures of the distal end of the radius with plates. J Bone Joint Surg Am 1997; 79(9):1303–12.

48. Jupiter JB, Lipton H. The operative treatment of in-traarticular fractures of the distal radius. Clin Orthop Relat Res 1993;(292):48–61.

49. Tavakolian JD, Jupiter JB. Dorsal plating for distal radius fractures. Hand Clin 2005;21(3):341–6.

50. Ring D, Jupiter JB, Brennwald J, et al. Prospective multicenter trial of a plate for dorsal fixation of distal radius fractures. J Hand Surg Am 1997; 22(5):777–84.

51. Rozental TD, Beredjiklian PK, Bozentka DJ. Functional outcome and complications following two types of dorsal plating for unstable fractures of the distal part of the radius. J Bone Joint Surg Am 2003;85-A(10):1956–60.

52. Carter PR, Frederick HA, Laseter GF. Open reduction and internal fixation of unstable distal radius fractures with a low-profile plate: a multicenter study of 73 fractures. J Hand Surg Am 1998;23(2):300–7.

53. Simic PM, Robison J, Gardner MJ, et al. Treatment of distal radius fractures with a low-profile dorsal plating system: an outcomes assessment. J Hand Surg Am 2006;31(3):382–6.

54. Jupiter JB, Marent-Huber M. Operative management of distal radial fractures with 2.4-millimeter locking plates. A multicenter prospective case series. J Bone Joint Surg Am 2009;91(1):55–65.

55. Yu YR, Makhni MC, Tabrizi S, et al. Complications of low-profile dorsal versus volar locking plates in the distal radius: a comparative study. J Hand Surg Am 2011;36(7):1135–41.

56. Hanel DP, Lu TS, Weil WM. Bridge plating of distal radius fractures: the Harborview method. Clin Orthop Relat Res 2006;445:91–9.

57. Ruch DS, Ginn TA, Yang CC, et al. Use of a distraction plate for distal radial fractures with metaphyseal and diaphyseal comminution. J Bone Joint Surg Am 2005;87(5):945–54.

58. Hanel DP, Ruhlman SD, Katolik LI, et al. Complications associated with distraction plate fixation of wrist fractures. Hand Clin 2010;26(2):237–43.

59. Engkvist O, Lundborg G. Rupture of the extensor pollicis longus tendon after fracture of the lower end of the radius–a clinical and microangiographic study. Hand 1979;11(1):76–86.

60. Stern PJ, Derr RG. Non-osseous complications following distal radius fractures. Iowa Orthop J 1993; 13:63–9.

61. Orbay JL, Touhami A. Current concepts in volar fixed-angle fixation of unstable distal radius fractures. Clin Orthop Relat Res 2006;445:58–67.

62. Asadollahi S, Keith PP. Flexor tendon injuries following plate fixation of distal radius fractures: a systematic review of the literature. J Orthop Trauma 2013;14(4):227–34.

63. Cross AW, Schmidt CC. Flexor tendon injuries following locked volar plating of distal radius fractures. J Hand Surg Am 2008;33(2):164–7.

64. Klug RA, Press CM, Gonzalez MH. Rupture of the flexor pollicis longus tendon after volar fixed-angle plating of a distal radius fracture: a case report. J Hand Surg Am 2007;32(7):984–8.

65. Koo SC, Ho ST. Delayed rupture of flexor pollicis longus tendon after volar plating of the distal radius. Hand Surg 2006;11(1–2):67–70.

66. Bell JS, Wollstein R, Citron ND. Rupture of flexor pollicis longus tendon: a complication of volar plating of the distal radius. J Bone Joint Surg Br 1998;80(2): 225–6.

67. Monda MK, Ellis A, Karmani S. Late rupture of flexor pollicis longus tendon 10 years after volar buttress plate fixation of a distal radius fracture: a case report. Acta Orthop Belg 2010;76(4):549–51.

68. Cho CH, Lee KJ, Song KS, et al. Delayed rupture of flexor pollicis longus after volar plating for a distal radius fracture. Clin Orthop Surg 2012;4(4):325–8.

69. Berglund LM, Messer TM. Complications of volar plate fixation for managing distal radius fractures. J Am Acad Orthop Surg 2009;17(6):369–77.

70. Kumbaraci M, Kucuk L, Karapinar L, et al. Retrospective comparison of external fixation versus volar locking plate in the treatment of unstable intra-articular distal radius fractures. Eur J Orthop Surg Traumatol 2014;24(2):173–8.

71. Williksen JH, Frihagen F, Hellund JC, et al. Volar locking plates versus external fixation and adjuvant pin fixation in unstable distal radius fractures: a randomized, controlled study. J Hand Surg Am 2013; 38(8):1469–76.

72. Navarro CM, Pettersson HJ, Enocson A. Complications after distal radius fracture surgery: results from a Swedish nationwide registry study. J Orthop Trauma 2015;29(2):e36–42.

73. Gwathmey FW Jr, Brunton LM, Pensy RA, et al. Volar plate osteosynthesis of distal radius fractures with concurrent prophylactic carpal tunnel release using a hybrid flexor carpi radialis approach. J Hand Surg Am 2010;35(7):1082–8.e4.

74. Lattmann T, Dietrich M, Meier C, et al. Comparison of 2 surgical approaches for volar locking plate osteosynthesis of the distal radius. J Hand Surg Am 2008; 33(7):1135–43.

75. Benson LS, Minihane KP, Stern LD, et al. The outcome of intra-articular distal radius fractures treated with fragment-specific fixation. J Hand Surg Am 2006; 31(8):1333–9.

76. Glanvill R, Boon JM, Birkholtz F, et al. Superficial radial nerve injury during standard K-wire fixation of uncomplicated distal radial fractures. Orthopedics 2006;29(7):639–41.

77. Glickel SZ, Catalano LW, Raia FJ, et al. Long-term outcomes of closed reduction and percutaneous pinning for the treatment of distal radius fractures. J Hand Surg Am 2008;33(10):1700–5.

78. Stanton-Hicks M. Complex regional pain syndrome (type I, RSD; type II, causalgia): controversies. Clin J Pain 2000;16(2 Suppl):S33–40.

79. Shukla R, Jain RK, Sharma NK, et al. External fixation versus volar locking plate for displaced intra-articular distal radius fractures: a prospective randomized comparative study of the functional outcomes. J Orthop Trauma 2014;15(4):265–70.

80. Ekrol I, Duckworth AD, Ralston SH, et al. The influence of vitamin C on the outcome of distal radial fractures: a double-blind, randomized controlled trial. J Bone Joint Surg Am 2014;96(17):1451–9.

81. Zollinger PE, Tuinebreijer WE, Breederveld RS, et al. Can vitamin C prevent complex regional pain syndrome in patients with wrist fractures? A randomized, controlled, multicenter dose-response study. J Bone Joint Surg Am 2007;89(7):1424–31.

82. Zollinger PE, Tuinebreijer WE, Kreis RW, et al. Effect of vitamin C on frequency of reflex sympathetic dystrophy in wrist fractures: a randomised trial. Lancet 1999;354(9195):2025–8.

83. Farah N, Nassar L, Farah Z, et al. Secondary displacement of distal radius fractures treated by bridging external fixation. J Hand Surg Eur Vol 2014;39(4):423–8.

84. Leung F, Tu YK, Chew WY, et al. Comparison of external and percutaneous pin fixation with plate fixation for intra-articular distal radial fractures. A randomized study. J Bone Joint Surg Am 2008;90(1): 16–22.

85. Wei DH, Poolman RW, Bhandari M, et al. External fixation versus internal fixation for unstable distal radius fractures: a systematic review and meta-analysis of comparative clinical trials. J Orthop Trauma 2012;26(7):386–94.

86. Harness NG, Jupiter JB, Orbay JL, et al. Loss of fixation of the volar lunate facet fragment in fractures of the distal part of the radius. J Bone Joint Surg Am 2004;86-A(9):1900–8.

87. Beck JD, Harness NG, Spencer HT. Volar plate fixation failure for volar shearing distal radius fractures with small lunate facet fragments. J Hand Surg Am 2014;39(4):670–8.

88. Prommersberger KJ, Fernandez DL. Nonunion of distal radius fractures. Clin Orthop Relat Res 2004;(419):51–6.

89. Baratz ME, Des Jardins JD, Anderson DD, et al. Displaced intra-articular fractures of the distal radius: the effect of fracture displacement on contact stresses in a cadaver model. J Hand Surg Am 1996;21(2):183–8.

90. Knirk JL, Jupiter JB. Intra-articular fractures of the distal end of the radius in young adults. J Bone Joint Surg Am 1986;68(5):647–59.

91. Trumble TE, Schmitt SR, Vedder NB. Factors affecting functional outcome of displaced intra-articular distal radius fractures. J Hand Surg Am 1994;19(2):325–40.

92. Goldfarb CA, Rudzki JR, Catalano LW, et al. Fifteen-year outcome of displaced intra-articular fractures of the distal radius. J Hand Surg Am 2006;31(4): 633–9.

93. Gruber G, Zacherl M, Giessauf C, et al. Quality of life after volar plate fixation of articular fractures of the distal part of the radius. J Bone Joint Surg Am 2010;92(5):1170–8.

94. Ng CY, McQueen MM. What are the radiological predictors of functional outcome following fractures of the distal radius? J Bone Joint Surg Br 2011;93(2): 145–50.

95. Forward DP, Davis TR, Sithole JS. Do young patients with malunited fractures of the distal radius inevitably develop symptomatic post-traumatic osteoarthritis? J Bone Joint Surg Br 2008;90(5):629–37.

Complications of Carpal Tunnel Release

John W. Karl, MD, MPH, Stephanie M. Gancarczyk, MD, Robert J. Strauch, MD*

KEYWORDS

- Carpal tunnel syndrome • Complications • Revision • Median nerve • Release

KEY POINTS

- Complications of carpal tunnel release are rare and include intraoperative technical errors, postoperative infection and pain, and persistent or recurrent symptoms.
- Evaluation should include a detailed history and physical examination in addition to electrodiagnostic examination and other imaging.
- A course of nonoperative management including splinting, injections, occupational therapy, and desensitization should be considered.
- Revision carpal tunnel release may be indicated if symptoms fail to improve and electrodiagnostic results worsen compared with preoperative values.

INTRODUCTION

Carpal tunnel syndrome is the most common peripheral compression neuropathy and one of the most frequent disorders of the hand, affecting 4.9% to 7.1% of the population.[1,2] It was originally described in 1854 and has been treated surgically since Learmonth's[3] description of release of the transverse carpal ligament in 1933.[4] Today, carpal tunnel release (CTR) surgery is among the most common hand procedures. The number of CTRs performed in the United States increased 38% from 360,000 per year in 1996 to 577,000 in 2006.[5]

Although this surgery has been shown to be reliably safe and effective, complications do occur.[6,7] These complications include intraoperative injury to nerves, vessels, and tendons; postoperative complications, such as infection, pain syndromes, and wrist instability; and treatment failures. The ability to competently evaluate and manage these complications is an essential part of hand surgery.

REVIEW OF ANATOMY

An understanding of the normal anatomy of the carpal tunnel as well as the common variants guide incision placement and operative technique for CTR and can help prevent iatrogenic injury.

The carpal tunnel is defined by the curved carpus dorsally and the transverse carpal ligament volarly, which runs from the scaphoid tuberosity and medial ridge of the trapezium to the hook of the hamate and the pisiform (**Fig. 1**). It is narrowest at the level of the hook of the hamate where the tunnel is only 20 mm wide and 10 mm deep.[8] This constriction is 2.0 to 2.5 cm distal to the start of the canal and is caused by prominence of the capitate, increased thickness of the transverse carpal ligament, and the position of the hamate. This area often corresponds to the hourglass deformity of the median nerve seen in cases of severe carpal tunnel syndrome.

The authors have no conflicts of interest related to this topic.
Department of Orthopaedic Surgery, Columbia University Medical Center, 622 West 168th Street, PH-1130, New York, NY 10032, USA
* Corresponding author.
E-mail address: robertjstrauch@hotmail.com

Orthop Clin N Am 47 (2016) 425–433
http://dx.doi.org/10.1016/j.ocl.2015.09.015
0030-5898/16/$ – see front matter © 2016 Elsevier Inc. All rights reserved.

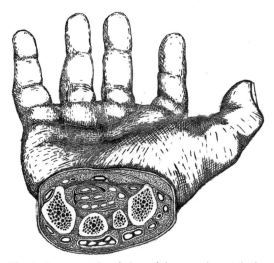

Fig. 1. A cross-sectional view of the carpal tunnel. The fibro-osseous tunnel is defined by the carpus dorsally, the transverse carpal ligament volarly, the scaphoid and trapezium medially, and the pisiform and hamate laterally. It is narrowest at the level of the hook of the hamate. The carpal tunnel contains the flexor digitorum superficialis, flexor digitorum profundus, and flexor pollicis longus tendons and the median nerve. (*Courtesy of* E.P. Trupia, MD, New York, NY.)

The carpal tunnel contains 10 structures: 4 flexor digitorum superficialis (FDS) and 4 flexor digitorum profundus (FDP) tendons, the flexor pollicis longus tendon, and the median nerve. The nerve is the most superficial structure and overlies the FDS and FDP tendons to the index finger.

The median nerve gives off 2 branches in the vicinity of the carpal tunnel that may be injured during release. The palmar cutaneous branch provides sensory innervation to the thenar eminence and arises from the radial side of the median nerve an average of 6 cm proximal to the transverse carpal ligament.[9] The nerve then pierces the antebrachial fascia proximal to the wrist and travels in the subcutaneous tissue into the palm before branching out. The palm may also be innervated by transverse palmar branches that leave the ulnar nerve in the Guyon canal and course radially across the hand.[10]

The thenar branch of the median nerve innervates the thenar muscles and generally branches off after the carpal tunnel but can branch within the tunnel and continue with the main nerve (subligamentous) or perforate the transverse carpal ligament (transligamentous).[11] The thenar branch generally stems from the radial side of the nerve, but anomalous branches from the ulnar aspect that cross over the top of the nerve have been described.[12]

Although there are usually no major vessels in the carpal tunnel proper, there are several nearby that may be injured during release. The ulnar artery runs through the Guyon canal with the ulnar nerve and is usually ulnar to the hook of the hamate but is often found radial to the hamate, putting it at risk. The superficial palmar arch is the transverse anastomosis between the ulnar and superficial radial arteries in the palm and lies in a fat pad 5 mm distal to the edge of the transverse carpal ligament.[10] There may also be an anomalous persistent median artery that travels with the median nerve.

INTRAOPERATIVE COMPLICATIONS

The normal anatomy and common anatomic variants of the volar palm and wrist have been well described, and this understanding contributes to the overall low rates of intraoperative complications. Permanent injury to the palmar cutaneous branch, thenar branch, and common digital nerves occur in only 0.03%, 0.01%, and 0.12% of cases, respectively. Injury to the median nerve proper occurs in 0.06% of cases.[13] Risk of nerve injury has been found to be higher in patients undergoing endoscopic CTR compared with open, though most are temporary neurapraxias.[14]

The palmar cutaneous branch of the median nerve may be injured during superficial skin dissection or while releasing the proximal portion of the transverse carpal ligament with scissors or an endoscopic device. Nerve injury can lead to persistent paresthesias or painful neuroma formation.

If surgical dissection is taken too far distally, the common digital nerves may be injured. Similar to the palmar cutaneous branch, damage to these nerves can result in persistent paresthesias or the formation of painful neuromas. In addition, innervation to the first and second lumbricals may be compromised, potentially leading to weakened metacarpophalangeal flexion and interphalangeal extension of the index and long fingers.

The thenar branch may be damaged by surgical dissection distal to the carpal tunnel or may be encountered proximally beneath the transverse carpal ligament, piercing the ligament, or crossing the carpal tunnel in the case of a subligamentous, transligamentous, or ulnar-originating variant.[10] Loss of function of the thenar branch causes weakness of thumb abduction and apposition, leading to markedly decreased grip strength and loss of hand function. Careful distinction must be made, however, between preexisting thenar atrophy from carpal tunnel syndrome and new or worsening dysfunction after iatrogenic injury.

Injury to the median nerve proper may occur during incision of the transverse carpal ligament, as it is the most superficial structure within the carpal tunnel. The nerve is mixed, containing both motor and sensory fibers, so injury may present with a variable pattern of deficit. The nerve may also be damaged during intraneural dissection while attempting to release fascicles from an area of internal scarring. In addition to direct injury, this procedure may lead to recurrence of more severe scarring and should not be done routinely.[15]

While attempting to avoid the branches of the median nerve, which usually reside on the radial side of the carpal tunnel, surgeons may err to the ulnar side of the tunnel, increasing the risk of injury to the contents of the Guyon canal. The ulnar nerve is inured in 0.03% of cases.[13] Injury to the deep motor branch may occur, leading to loss of innervation to most of the intrinsic muscles of the hand. These muscles include the ulnar 2 lumbricals, the dorsal and palmar interosseous muscles, the abductor digiti minimi, the opponens digiti minimi, and the flexor digiti minimi. Loss of the intrinsic musculature can result in ulnar clawing with hyperextension of the metacarpophalangeal joints and flexion of the interphalangeal joints of the fourth and fifth digits. Patients may also have weakened or absent finger abduction.

Also within or superficial to the Guyon canal, the ulnar artery may be damaged by an incision placed too far ulnarly. If patients have an incomplete arch and, thus, no collateral circulation from the radial artery, loss of the ulnar artery would lead to ischemia of the ulnar side of the hand. In either case, damage to the artery could result in serious bleeding. Furthermore, the injury might not be appreciated until after the wound was closed if a tourniquet is used, complicating its diagnosis and management.

As the superficial palmar arch lies just distal to the transverse carpal ligament and is obscured in fat, it is vulnerable to injury and is damaged in 0.1% of CTRs.[13] Damage to the arch is unlikely to cause ischemia but again may cause significant bleeding when the tourniquet is released.

Injury to flexor tendons occurs in 0.1% of cases and generally involves a partial tenotomy as opposed to a complete transection.[13] This injury may leave the flexor tendons more prone to rupture in the future and may also lead to adhesions and triggering.

POSTOPERATIVE COMPLICATIONS

In the absence of technical errors during the surgery, patients may still have complications after CTR, including infection, postoperative pain, and tendon problems. As with most soft tissue surgeries of the hand, postoperative wound infection is rare after CTR, occurring in only 0.36% of cases.[16] Most of these are superficial, with only 0.13% of cases having deep infections.

After CTR, some patients may develop pain in the area of the scar that can be invoked by pressure or light touch. Scar tenderness is less common after endoscopic release compared with open and more common in patients with depressive symptoms.[14,17] Although most of these resolve spontaneously within a few months, some patients do have more persistent pain.[18] This pain may be due to a failure to protect the crossing cutaneous nerve branches or from adhesions to the median nerve.[19,20]

Patients may also develop pain in the thenar and/or hypothenar eminence that is worse with pressure or grasping. The cause of this so-called pillar pain is unknown but may be due to postoperative swelling or temporary instability of the insertions of the thenar and hypothenar musculature on the transverse carpal ligament.[19,21] Nearly all cases resolve spontaneously in 6 to 9 months. There is no difference in the rates of pillar pain between patients undergoing open or endoscopic release.[14]

Postoperative hypothenar pain that does not resolve may localize to the pisotriquetral joint. The pisiform is stabilized by the flexor carpi ulnaris and abductor digiti minimi ulnarly and the transverse carpal ligament radially and may be destabilized after transection of the ligament in certain patients with preexisting chondromalacia or subluxation of pisotriquetral joint, causing pain.[22] The pain will intensify with pressure on pisotriquetral joint and flexion, extension, or ulnar deviation of the wrist. Patients will experience temporary pain relief with intra-articular anesthetic injection. Surgical excision of the pisiform can provide permanent relief.[22–24]

Complex regional pain syndrome (formerly known as causalgia and reflex sympathetic dystrophy) may rarely occur after CTR without any clear predisposing factors. Patients may have a constellation of sensory, motor, vasomotor, and pseudomotor complaints. Treatments include hand therapy; medications, such as gabapentin, antidepressants, and bisphosphonates; and interventions including sympathetic blocks and botulinum toxin injections.[25] Referral to a pain specialist should be considered early for these patients as well as careful evaluation for iatrogenic nerve injury.

In addition to pain, patients may have mechanical symptoms related to the flexor tendons contained in the carpal tunnel after release of the transverse carpal ligament. Damage to the tendons during release may cause inflammation and adhesions leading to triggering at the wrist. Patients may also develop triggering at the A1 pulleys, which may be due to overloading after loss of the pulley effect of the transverse carpal ligament.[26] Alternatively, this may simply be unrecognized or new-onset stenosing tenosynovitis as carpal tunnel syndrome and trigger fingers are commonly seen together.[27] Patients may also rarely have bowstringing of the flexor tendons with wrist flexion or symptomatic subluxation of the FDS to the ring and small finger over the hook of the hamate.[19]

TREATMENT FAILURE

After CTR, many patients feel immediate relief, particularly of their nocturnal symptoms. However, particularly in cases whereby the median nerve has been severely compressed for many years, symptoms of numbness may not begin to improve for 6 months and may never completely resolve. Patients need to be counseled on this possibility before CTR. If patients have no improvement in symptoms after 12 months or have initial improvement in symptoms followed by clinical deterioration, they may be considered to have failed treatment. Failure of primary CTR occurs rarely but has been reported in 7% to 25% of patients in some series with approximately 5% to 12% requiring secondary surgery.[28–31] Causes of treatment failure can be thought of in 3 categories: incomplete release, recurrent compression, and incorrect diagnosis.

Incomplete release of the transverse carpal ligament proper (usually at the distal end), the flexor retinaculum distally, or the antebrachial fascia proximally can cause persistent carpal tunnel syndrome and is the most common reason for reoperation.[32] Although there has been controversy about different surgical techniques, a recent meta-analysis found no difference in the rates of persistent symptoms between patients undergoing open or endoscopic release.[14]

Some patients may have good improvement of their symptoms initially, only to have them recur in the months after surgery. This pattern accounts for nearly 20% of revision surgeries and is more common in patients with diabetes and hypertension.[33,34] Early recurrence may be due to incomplete release as the unreleased structure becomes a new site of nerve compression. Late recurrence is thought to be due to dense scar formation from the cut ligament ends that can entrap the intact nerve.[7,20,35] The nerve itself is uninjured but is encased in fibrous tissue for the length of the ligament and, occasionally, proximally into the forearm.[15] This extraneural scarring impedes gliding of and blood flow to the nerve, in addition to mechanical compression (**Fig. 2**). To avoid this, some authors recommend splinting the wrist in slight extension after CTR to keep the nerve seated in the tunnel and away from the cut ligament ends.[15,36]

Incomplete release and nerve entrapment in scar may occur together as well. In a study by Jones and colleagues,[37] 58% of patients with continued median nerve compression were noted to have incomplete release and 100% of patients had circumferential fibrosis of the median nerve.

In addition to persistent or recurrent nerve compression, continued neurologic symptoms after CTR may be due to an alternate diagnosis. This diagnosis may include previous nerve injury leading to intraneural scarring, other sites or sources

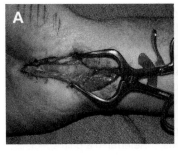 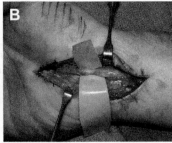

Fig. 2. This patient is a 51-year-old man who underwent right CTR 2 months before presentation with initial improvement in nighttime pain, which was his main complaint. He then rapidly lost sensation in his median nerve distribution and developed thenar atrophy. Repeat electromyography showed markedly worsened conduction of the median nerve compared with the preoperative study with absent motor signals. (A) On exploration, a firm scar tissue structure resembling the transverse carpal ligament was found to be compressing the nerve. The entire structure was released from the distal third of the forearm to the level of the superficial palmar arch. (B) Marked constriction of the median nerve at the proximal end of the carpal tunnel in an hourglass configuration was noted. Internal neurolysis of the nerve was then performed using a microscope; all of the fascicles were seen to be intact from the distal forearm to beyond the division of the motor branch.

of nerve compression, or other medical conditions that mimic the symptoms of carpal tunnel syndrome.

The median nerve may be compressed inside or outside of the carpal tunnel by ganglion cysts, arterial aneurysms, gouty tophi, sarcoidosis, or other space-occupying lesions, leading to a CTS-like picture that is not relieved by release of the tunnel.[32] Similarly, the nerve may rarely be compressed more proximally in the arm by the ligament of Struthers, the tendinous arch formed by superficial and deep heads of the pronator teres, the fibrous edge of the proximal flexor digitorum superficialis, the bicipital aponeurosis, or muscular anomalies, such as the Gantzer's muscle, palmaris profundus, or flexor carpi radialis brevis.[31,38]

The neural elements that become the median nerve may be compressed by cervical stenosis, tumor, or syringomyelia while in the spinal cord or while exiting the spinal foramina in the setting of cervical radiculopathy.[39] Brachial plexopathy and thoracic outlet syndrome may mimic carpal tunnel syndrome. This injury is the so-called double-crush injury whereby the nerve is compressed in the carpal tunnel as well as another location, making release of only the carpal tunnel insufficient to improve symptoms.

Systemic disease or other neurologic conditions may mimic symptoms of carpal tunnel syndrome, leading to inappropriate surgery. Although diabetes is associated with the development of true carpal tunnel syndrome, diabetic peripheral neuropathy may present with hand numbness in the absence of median nerve compression. Similarly, patients with multiple sclerosis or other demyelinating central or peripheral neuropathies can produce a clinical picture easily mistaken for carpal tunnel syndrome.[39]

EVALUATION

In evaluating patients with complications following CTR, a detailed history is the first step. Careful delineation and documentation of patients' current complaints must be compared with their preoperative symptoms. Patients with incomplete release of the carpal tunnel will likely have continued or recurrent symptoms similar to those they experienced before surgery. Patients with perineural scarring, however, often have a longer period of relief after surgery, followed by gradually worsening scar sensitivity, pain, in addition to numbness.[32] Consideration must also be given to other clues in the history that suggest systemic disease or other cause of median mononeuropathy.

Thorough physical examination may also help to elucidate the cause of treatment failure. Patients

with recurrent symptoms due to compression of the released nerve in scar may have an amplified Tinel sign because the nerve is more superficial after surgery. They may also have a negative Phalen test because the proximal edge of the transverse carpal ligament is no longer intact to compress the flexed wrist.[15]

Patients with damage to the palmar cutaneous branch or digital branch will have anesthesia of the thenar eminence or digits, respectively, and may have a painful neuroma at the site of injury. Those with thenar branch damage will have weakness of the thenar musculature on thumb abduction and apposition. Again, it is important to differentiate persistent preoperative weakness from new-onset weakness. Patients with injury to the deep motor branch of the ulnar nerve will have intrinsic weakness.

Relief of symptoms with corticosteroid injections into the carpal tunnel is useful in diagnosis and prediction of success after primary CTR.[40] Particularly when combined with provocative examination maneuvers, steroid injection is also a good indicator of success of revision carpal tunnel surgery.[28,30]

Electrodiagnostic testing is useful in the evaluation of patients with continued symptoms after CTRs. However, though electromyography (EMG) results may improve somewhat after successful CTR, they often do not normalize for a prolonged period of time, if ever.[41] Therefore, EMG results need to be considered in the context of the patients. It may also be useful to review in detail the preoperative electrodiagnostic testing for suggestions of other neuropathic conditions or compression at other sites.[39]

Imaging should be considered to evaluate patients with recurrent or persistent symptoms after CTR. Plain radiographs of the wrist can identify fractures, dislocations, or progressive arthritis contributing to compression of the median nerve. More advanced imaging, such as MRI, may be useful in identifying perineural scar formation or space-occupying lesions in the wrist or elsewhere in the arm.[42]

TREATMENT

Intraoperative complications that are recognized should be treated as quickly as possible. Nerve injuries that result in dense motor or sensory defects require immediate exploration and, if indicated, nerve repair. Similarly, iatrogenic flexor tendon lacerations should be repaired at the time of initial surgery if recognized. If unrecognized initially, plans for elective repair should be made as quickly as possible.

If an injury to the median nerve proper occurs that alters the internal architecture of the nerve, a median nerve neuroma in-continuity may form, disrupting the function of the nerve even though the external structure seems intact.[43,44] In this case, an internal neurolysis may be indicated. The internal and external epineurium layers are incised, and the offending neuroma is removed. The perineurium is preserved as the blood-nerve barrier and defect is filled with nerve autograft from the anterior branch of the medial antebrachial cutaneous nerve, lateral antebrachial cutaneous nerve, sural nerve, or terminal anterior interosseous nerve.[31] Some investigators advocate internal neurolysis in most of the secondary CTRs, though this is not widely accepted.[15,31]

Yamamoto and colleagues[44] described an anterolateral thigh flap with vascularized lateral femoral cutaneous nerve for reconstruction after neuroma excision. An anterolateral thigh flap is transferred to the wrist and the median nerve gap repaired using the vascularized lateral femoral cutaneous nerve. The lateral circumflex femoral vessels are used as the pedicle from the thigh and are anastomosed to the radial artery in an end-to-side fashion. Their concomitant veins are anastomosed to available cutaneous veins using an end-to-end technique.

Suspected injury to the palmar cutaneous branch of the median nerve can be treated by exploration and primary repair, if identified early, or by neuroma excision, followed by neurolysis and transposition between deep and superficial layers of the flexor muscles, if identified late.[31] The nerve is then transposed between the deep and superficial layers of the flexor muscles to provide a healthy bed for healing as far away as possible from the overlying skin and scar. Injury to the superficial palmar arch may be of little consequence if recognized early but if not addressed may lead to large hematoma and increased risk of infection and palmar skin necrosis, requiring flap coverage.

Infection after CTR is exceedingly rare. When present, draining wounds may require an irrigation and debridement, followed by the appropriate course of antibiotics. Because of the close proximity of the flexor tendons and median nerve, if soft tissue defects remain, immediate coverage with a local, regional, or free flap may be indicated.[45]

For patients with persistent or recurrent median nerve compression symptoms, a course of nonoperative management including splinting, injections, occupational therapy, and desensitization should be attempted. If symptoms fail to improve and EMG results worsen, revision CTR may be required.

In order to expose normal anatomy and identify tissue planes, the incision for revision CTR should extend both proximal and distal from the previous incision.[46,47] Care should be taken to avoid crossing the wrist crease perpendicularly to decrease the risk postoperative contracture. The transverse carpal ligament is identified and released in its entirety, and then the median nerve should be carefully dissected and explored, freeing it from surrounding scar. Often it is found adhered to the radial undersurface of the transverse carpal ligament.[31,46]

After the nerve is explored and released, the tissue bed surrounding the median nerve should be evaluated for healing potential, as simple repeat neurolysis is often ineffective unless the cause is incomplete release.[48] If there is substantial scarring or poor vascularity for healing, surgical treatment must provide improved soft tissue coverage to promote vascularity and decrease scar reformation. Several local flaps have been described for this purpose, including the hypothenar fat pad, abductor digiti minimi, synovial, pronator quadratus, and palmaris brevis flaps.[49] In addition, a variety of regional and free flaps have been proposed, including radial forearm, omentum, and lateral arm flaps. Vein grafts and synthetic substitutes are also increasing in popularity.

The hypothenar fat pad is used most commonly because the donor tissue is local and the technique is straightforward (**Fig. 3**). An incision is made just lateral to the hypothenar eminence and the superficial plane is developed between

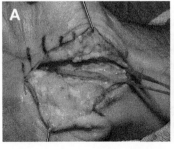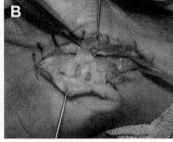

Fig. 3. (*A*) After exploration and release of the median nerve, the hypothenar fat pad can be visualized at the ulnar margin of the incision. (*B*) The fat pad is dissected from the skin superficially and the thenar musculature below is left attached on the ulnar side. The tissue is then brought radially and sutured in place to cover and protect the injured median nerve.

the dermis of the hypothenar skin and underlying fat, taking care not to devascularize the overlying skin.[50] The superficial dissection is continued ulnarly to the dermal insertion of the palmaris brevis. The deep dissection is between the adipose layer and hypothenar muscles. The ulnar neurovascular structures are identified and protected in the Guyon canal. The fat pad is elevated and mobilized to lay between the median nerve and released transverse carpal ligament and is sutured to the radial wall of the carpal tunnel, adjacent to the flexor pollicis longus. A similar dissection has been described for mobilization of the palmaris brevis turnover flap.[43]

When using the omental free flap, adipose tissue is harvested with the gastroepiploic artery and vein and the omentum is wrapped around the neurolysed median nerve. The radial artery and cephalic vein are exposed approximately 7 cm proximal to the wrist crease through an extended carpal tunnel incision, and the artery and vein are anastomosed in an end-to-side and end-to-end fashion, respectively.[51] A split-thickness skin graft may be needed to cover the donor tissue in order to minimize any venous constriction.

A pronator quadratus flap can also be used to provide a more favorable healing environment for the median nerve more proximally in the wrist. Working though ulnar and radial windows in the volar wrist, the muscle is mobilized on its neurovascular pedicle.[52] The flap is then elevated superficially to augment the bed of the nerve.

Nerve wrapping has also been described as an alternative technique of minimizing postoperative scar formation and fibrosis. The reverse radial artery fascial flap is created by incising the volar forearm fascia and dissecting along a plane just superficial to the epimysium of the forearm muscles, preserving vascular connections to the radial vessels.[53] Next, the radial artery and vein are divided proximally and the fascial flap is turned distally to wrap around the median nerve and serve as a limit to scar formation.

Venous grafting has also been described, using autologous vein graft to protect the healing nerve from recurrent scar formation. Varitimidis and colleagues[54] showed promising results with harvest of the greater saphenous vein for this purpose.

OUTCOMES

Reported outcomes after failed CTR vary widely with little high-level data or consistency in the literature, and outcomes vary widely with the cause of treatment failure and with the method of treatment. Historically, those treated for incomplete release have been thought to fare better than those revised for scar formation and fibrosis.[49] However, some studies have shown that incomplete release does not correlate with final symptoms or satisfaction after revision CTR.[28,29]

In a retrospective review by Beck and colleagues,[28] they found that although complete relief after revision CTR is often delayed when compared with outcomes of primary CTR, there are minimal differences in disability long-term. In a study by Cobb and colleagues,[29] the mean time to regular employment after reoperation was approximately 7.8 weeks and the mean time to resumption of normal recreational activities was approximately 8 weeks. Of the 116 patients that underwent reoperation for carpal tunnel, 38 rated the surgical procedure as completely successful and 52 stated that the operation greatly improved quality of life, whereas only 14 patients rated the surgery as completely unsuccessful, with 21 stating that there was little to no improvement in quality of life. In a subanalysis, patients that filed claims, including worker's compensation, private disability insurance, Social Security disability income, or supplemental security income, had worse symptoms than those who had not filed for compensation.

Strasberg and colleagues[55] evaluated 45 patients who had secondary carpal tunnel surgery. They found that 53% of patients reported significant improvement of their symptoms, 29% had no change in their symptoms, and 18% reported worsening symptoms. Of the 39 unemployed workers, 28% returned to work. A patient's chance of a successful outcome was significantly less in the worker's compensation population. Overall, there was no correlation between patient outcomes and surgical findings or the procedure performed.

Patients undergoing revision surgery with hypothenar fat pad transposition seem to do well. Craft and colleagues[46] evaluated 28 such patients and found that pain completely disappeared in 83% of patients and 2-point discrimination improved by about 1 mm. Those with recurrent symptoms due to incomplete release were excluded.

Strickland and colleagues[50] found that 96% of patients reported satisfactory outcomes after hypothenar fat pad grafting. Of note, even among those in the worker's compensation group, 94% had a satisfactory. In addition, they found the average time to return to work for the non–worker's compensation group was 12 weeks compared with 37 weeks for the worker's compensation group.

A small case series by Goitz and Steichen[51] studied the outcome of the omental transfer flap.

They noted 5 of 6 patients that underwent this procedure for recurrent carpal tunnel syndrome were satisfied with their results and thought that the operation improved quality of life.

Other studies have found less encouraging results with other grafting strategies. Dahlin and colleagues[56] followed 15 patients with recurrent carpal tunnel syndrome who underwent a free or pedicled flap as treatment in the revision. Of the 15 patients studied, only 3 considered themselves cured or near cured, 7 were improved, 1 was unchanged, and 3 were worse than before surgery. Patients who were thought to have a neuroma or reflex sympathetic dystrophy were excluded from evaluation.

SUMMARY

Complications of CTR are rare and include intraoperative technical errors, postoperative infection and pain, and persistent or recurrent symptoms. Evaluation should include a detailed history and physical examination, in addition to electrodiagnostic examination and other imaging. A course of nonoperative management including splinting, injections, occupational therapy, and desensitization should be considered. Revision CTR may be indicated if symptoms fail to improve and EMG results worsen compared with preoperative values. Revision surgery includes nerve exploration and repeat release and may be augmented with local or free tissue grafting. Reported outcomes after revision CTR vary widely but are overall less good than primary surgery.

REFERENCES

1. Atroshi I, Gummesson C, Johnsson R, et al. Prevalence of carpal tunnel syndrome in a general population. JAMA 1999;282(2):153–8.
2. Shiri R. The prevalence and incidence of carpal tunnel syndrome in US working populations. Scand J Work Environ Health 2014;40(1):101–2.
3. Learmonth JR. The principle of decompression in the treatment of certain diseases of peripheral nerves. Surg Clin North Am 1933;13:905–13.
4. Lo SL, Raskin K, Lester H, et al. Carpal tunnel syndrome: a historical perspective. Hand Clin 2002; 18(2):211–7, v.
5. Fajardo M, Kim SH, Szabo RM. Incidence of carpal tunnel release: trends and implications within the United States ambulatory care setting. J Hand Surg 2012;37(8):1599–605.
6. Kulick MI, Gordillo G, Javidi T, et al. Long-term analysis of patients having surgical treatment for carpal tunnel syndrome. J Hand Surg 1986;11(1):59–66.
7. Phalen GS. The carpal-tunnel syndrome. Seventeen years' experience in diagnosis and treatment of six hundred fifty-four hands. J Bone Joint Surg Am 1966;48(2):211–28.
8. Cobb TK, Dalley BK, Posteraro RH, et al. Anatomy of the flexor retinaculum. J Hand Surg 1993;18(1): 91–9.
9. Martin CH, Seiler JG 3rd, Lesesne JS. The cutaneous innervation of the palm: an anatomic study of the ulnar and median nerves. J Hand Surg 1996;21(4):634–8.
10. Rotman MB, Donovan JP. Practical anatomy of the carpal tunnel. Hand Clin 2002;18(2):219–30.
11. Lanz U. Anatomical variations of the median nerve in the carpal tunnel. J Hand Surg 1977;2(1):44–53.
12. Entin MA. Carpal tunnel syndrome and its variants. Surg Clin North Am 1968;48(5):1097–112.
13. Boeckstyns ME, Sorensen AI. Does endoscopic carpal tunnel release have a higher rate of complications than open carpal tunnel release? An analysis of published series. J Hand Surg 1999;24(1):9–15.
14. Sayegh ET, Strauch RJ. Open versus endoscopic carpal tunnel release: a meta-analysis of randomized controlled trials. Clin Orthop Relat Res 2015; 473(3):1120–32.
15. Braun RM, Rechnic M, Fowler E. Complications related to carpal tunnel release. Hand Clin 2002; 18(2):347–57.
16. Harness NG, Inacio MC, Pfeil FF, et al. Rate of infection after carpal tunnel release surgery and effect of antibiotic prophylaxis. J Hand Surg 2010;35(2):189–96.
17. Kim JK, Kim YK. Predictors of scar pain after open carpal tunnel release. J Hand Surg 2011;36(6): 1042–6.
18. Citron ND, Bendall SP. Local symptoms after open carpal tunnel release. A randomized prospective trial of two incisions. J Hand Surg 1997;22(3): 317–21.
19. Hunt TR, Osterman AL. Complications of the treatment of carpal tunnel syndrome. Hand Clin 1994; 10(1):63–71.
20. Wadstroem J, Nigst H. Reoperation for carpal tunnel syndrome. A retrospective analysis of forty cases. Ann Chir Main 1986;5(1):54–8.
21. Eversmann WW Jr. Compression and entrapment neuropathies of the upper extremity. J Hand Surg 1983;8(5 Pt 2):759–66.
22. Seradge H, Seradge E. Piso-triquetral pain syndrome after carpal tunnel release. J Hand Surg 1989;14(5):858–62.
23. Rigoni G, Madonia F. Piso-triquetral syndrome following incision of the retinaculum flexorum. Helv Chir Acta 1992;58(4):413–7 [in German].
24. Stahl S, Stahl S, Calif E. Latent pisotriquetral arthrosis unmasked following carpal tunnel release. Orthopedics 2010;33(9):673.

25. Carroll I, Curtin CM. Management of chronic pain following nerve injuries/CRPS type II. Hand Clin 2013;29(3):401–8.

26. Mackinnon SE. Secondary carpal tunnel surgery. Neurosurg Clin N Am 1991;2(1):75–91.

27. Gancarczyk SM, Strauch RJ. Carpal tunnel syndrome and trigger digit: common diagnoses that occur "hand in hand". J Hand Surg 2013;38(8): 1635 7.

28. Beck JD, Brothers JG, Maloney PJ, et al. Predicting the outcome of revision carpal tunnel release. J Hand Surg 2012;37(2):282–7.

29. Cobb TK, Amadio PC, Leatherwood DF, et al. Outcome of reoperation for carpal tunnel syndrome. J Hand Surg 1996;21(3):347–56.

30. Neuhaus V, Christoforou D, Cheriyan T, et al. Evaluation and treatment of failed carpal tunnel release. Orthop Clin North Am 2012;43(4):439–47.

31. Tung TH, Mackinnon SE. Secondary carpal tunnel surgery. Plast Reconstr Surg 2001;107(7):1830–43 [quiz: 1844, 1933].

32. Stutz N, Gohritz A, van Schoonhoven J, et al. Revision surgery after carpal tunnel release–analysis of the pathology in 200 cases during a 2 year period. J Hand Surg 2006;31(1):68–71.

33. Schreiber JE, Foran MP, Schreiber DJ, et al. Common risk factors seen in secondary carpal tunnel surgery. Ann Plast Surg 2005;55(3):262–5.

34. Zieske L, Ebersole GC, Davidge K, et al. Revision carpal tunnel surgery: a 10-year review of intraoperative findings and outcomes. J Hand Surg 2013; 38(8):1530–9.

35. O'Malley MJ, Evanoff M, Terrono AL, et al. Factors that determine reexploration treatment of carpal tunnel syndrome. J Hand Surg 1992;17(4):638–41.

36. Tubiana R. Carpal tunnel syndrome: some views on its management. Ann Chir Main Memb Super 1990; 9(5):325–30.

37. Jones NF, Ahn HC, Eo S. Revision surgery for persistent and recurrent carpal tunnel syndrome and for failed carpal tunnel release. Plast Reconstr Surg 2012;129(3):683–92.

38. Mazurek MT, Shin AY. Upper extremity peripheral nerve anatomy: current concepts and applications. Clin Orthop Relat Res 2001;(383):7–20.

39. Witt JC, Stevens JC. Neurologic disorders masquerading as carpal tunnel syndrome: 12 cases of failed carpal tunnel release. Mayo Clin Proc 2000; 75(4):409–13.

40. Edgell SE, McCabe SJ, Breidenbach WC, et al. Predicting the outcome of carpal tunnel release. J Hand Surg 2003;28(2):255–61.

41. Kanatani T, Nagura I, Kurosaka M, et al. Electrophysiological assessment of carpal tunnel syndrome in elderly patients: one-year follow-up study. J Hand Surg 2014;39(11):2188–91.

42. Campagna R, Pessis E, Feydy A, et al. MRI assessment of recurrent carpal tunnel syndrome after open surgical release of the median nerve. AJR Am J Roentgenol 2009;193(3):644–50.

43. Rose EH. The use of the palmaris brevis flap in recurrent carpal tunnel syndrome. Hand Clin 1996; 12(2):389–95.

44. Yamamoto T, Narushima M, Yoshimatsu H, et al. Free anterolateral thigh flap with vascularized lateral femoral cutaneous nerve for the treatment of neuroma-in-continuity and recurrent carpal tunnel syndrome after carpal tunnel release. Microsurgery 2014;34(2):145–8.

45. Leslie BM, Ruby LK. Coverage of a carpal tunnel wound dehiscence with the abductor digiti minimi muscle flap. J Hand Surg 1988;13(1):36–9.

46. Craft RO, Duncan SF, Smith AA. Management of recurrent carpal tunnel syndrome with microneurolysis and the hypothenar fat pad flap. Hand 2007;2(3): 85–9.

47. Dellon AL, Chang BW. An alternative incision for approaching recurrent median nerve compression at the wrist. Plast Reconstr Surg 1992;89(3):576–8.

48. Amadio PC. Interventions for recurrent/persistent carpal tunnel syndrome after carpal tunnel release. J Hand Surg 2009;34(7):1320–2.

49. Santosa KB, Chung KC, Waljee JF. Complications of compressive neuropathy: prevention and management strategies. Hand Clin 2015;31(2):139–49.

50. Strickland JW, Idler RS, Lourie GM, et al. The hypothenar fat pad flap for management of recalcitrant carpal tunnel syndrome. J Hand Surg 1996;21(5): 840–8.

51. Goitz RJ, Steichen JB. Microvascular omental transfer for the treatment of severe recurrent median neuritis of the wrist: a long-term follow-up. Plast Reconstr Surg 2005;115(1):163–71.

52. Dellon AL, Mackinnon SE. The pronator quadratus muscle flap. J Hand Surg 1984;9(3):423–7.

53. Tham SK, Ireland DC, Riccio M, et al. Reverse radial artery fascial flap: a treatment for the chronically scarred median nerve in recurrent carpal tunnel syndrome. J Hand Surg 1996;21(5):849–54.

54. Varitimidis SE, Riano F, Vardakas DG, et al. Recurrent compressive neuropathy of the median nerve at the wrist: treatment with autogenous saphenous vein wrapping. J Hand Surg 2000;25(3):271–5.

55. Strasberg SR, Novak CB, Mackinnon SE, et al. Subjective and employment outcome following secondary carpal tunnel surgery. Ann Plast Surg 1994; 32(5):485–9.

56. Dahlin LB, Lekholm C, Kardum P, et al. Coverage of the median nerve with free and pedicled flaps for the treatment of recurrent severe carpal tunnel syndrome. Scand J Plast Reconstr Surg Hand Surg 2002;36(3):172–6.

Complications of Distal Biceps Repair

Mark Tyson Garon, MD, Jeffrey A. Greenberg, MD, MS*

KEYWORDS

- Distal biceps • Complications • Repair • Reconstruction

KEY POINTS

- Repair of distal biceps ruptures in active, healthy patients has a high satisfaction rate regardless of technique or approach.
- The total complication rate after repair of the distal biceps tendon is 15% to 35% and is independent of approach; however, anterior-only approaches increased the rate of lateral antebrachial cutaneous nerve palsy.
- The most common complication after distal biceps tendon repair is neurapraxia of the lateral antebrachial cutaneous nerve.
- Other complications include posterior interosseous nerve injury, heterotopic ossification, stiffness, weakness, wound infections, complex regional pain syndrome, re-rupture, median and ulnar nerve injuries, brachial artery injury, proximal radius fracture, and hardware failure.
- Repairs using suture anchors or transosseous screws have a higher rate of re-rupture. Chronic repairs performed with the elbow in a flexed position do not lead to an increased rate of stiffness.

ANATOMY

The biceps brachii is a diarthrodial muscle, which acts as a powerful forearm supinator. The muscle is located in the anterior compartment of the arm and is innervated by the musculocutaneous nerve. As the name implies there are 2 heads of the biceps brachii, short and long. The short head originates from the coracoid tip, whereas the long head originates from the supraglenoid tubercle and/or superior labrum. The distal biceps tendon can be found in the antecubital fossa between the brachioradialis and the pronator teres. The tendon courses distally and inserts onto the radial tuberosity 23 mm distal to the articular cartilage of the radial head. The footprint on the radial tuberosity measures 21 mm by 7 mm and is located on the posterior ulnar surface, with the short head inserting more radial and distal to the proximal and ulnar long head (**Fig. 1**).[1–3] A secondary attachment includes the lacertus fibrosis, which attaches medially to the deep fascia of the anterior compartment and may prevent retraction of the ruptured distal biceps tendon.

BACKGROUND

Ruptures of the distal attachment of the biceps brachii are a rare injury with a reported rate of 1.2 per 100,000 patients or 2.55 per 100,000 patient-years. Ruptures typically occur in the dominant arm of men in the fourth or fifth decade of life.[4,5] Patients report an eccentric extension load on a flexed elbow followed by a pop with pain, swelling, and ecchymosis in the region of the antecubital fossa. Frequently, patients present with anterior arm pain and weakness with elbow flexion and supination and a deformity secondary to retraction of the biceps.

NONOPERATIVE TREATMENT

Nonoperative treatment includes early range of motion and advancement to resistive exercises

Disclosure Statement: The authors have nothing to disclose.
Indiana Hand to Shoulder Center, 8501 Harcourt Road, Indianapolis, IN 46260, USA
* Corresponding author.
E-mail address: handdr@me.com

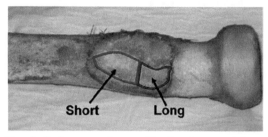

Fig. 1. Cadaver specimen with the short and long head insertions mapped out with red and blue ink. Note that the short head inserts distal to the long head and occupies a larger area. (*From* Jarrett CD, Weir DM, Stuffman ES, et al. Anatomic and biomechanical analysis of the short and long head components of the distal biceps tendon. J Shoulder Elbow Surg 2012;21:942–8; with permission.)

and functional rehabilitation within 4 weeks of injury. Nonoperative treatment leads to acceptable functional outcomes in sedentary or low-demand patients. However, active patients generally are limited by a decrease in supination strength and endurance of 21% to 55% and 86%, respectively. Elbow flexion strength is also decreased by 8% to 13%, and endurance is decreased by 62% in nonsurgically treated patients.[6–8] As a result of this decrease in function, surgical repair is commonly recommended for young active patients.[9]

OPERATIVE TREATMENT

Current indications for distal biceps repair include full-thickness tears or partial-thickness tears, which have failed conservative treatment in active, healthy, compliant patients who desire full strength and endurance. Nonanatomic and anatomic repairs have been described. Nonanatomic repairs in which the biceps is repaired to the brachialis reconstitutes the contour of the biceps muscle; however, nonanatomic repairs do not restore supination strength or biceps endurance power. Contemporary techniques utilize either 1 or 2 incisions. A variety of fixation devices have been described that facilitate strong repairs.[10–29]

Before 1961, operative treatment was fraught with complications with a rate of radial nerve injury close to 15%. In 1961, the Boyd-Anderson 2-incision technique was proposed for the anatomic repair of the distal biceps tendon in order to reduce the incidence of radial nerve palsy. This used an anterior incision to retrieve and deliver the distal biceps tendon to a posterior incision where the biceps is repaired to the exposed biceps tuberosity. Exposure of the biceps tuberosity posteriorly required subperiosteal elevation of the anconeus, which led to a

high rate of heterotopic ossification (HO) and synostosis.[6,30] Using this technique, Karunakar and colleagues[30] demonstrated that 66% recovered strength and endurance of supination and flexion with no radial nerve palsies.

Although patient satisfaction remained high, the Mayo modification of the 2-incision technique has been described to perform a muscle-splitting approach through the extensors in an attempt to prevent HO and synostosis.[15,20,31] Recently, the one-incision technique has been advocated by some surgeons.[10–13,16–18] Proponents of this technique report a decreased rate of HO and synostosis with low rates of posterior interosseous nerve (PIN) injury. Critiques of the one-incision technique include failure to anatomically restore the distal biceps attachment and an increased rate of lateral antebrachial cutaneous nerve (LABC) neuropraxia.[18,32] Although most surgeons agree that repair in active healthy patients is indicated to restore function, currently there is no consensus on whether the one- or 2-incision technique should be used. Recent studies show no difference in complication rates; however, the anterior-only approach is associated with an increased rate of LABC neuropraxia.[18]

RESULTS

Functional results of the operative treatment of distal biceps ruptures are generally favorable with high patient satisfaction rates (>90%). Most studies report greater than 80% recovery of flexion and supination strength and endurance, with some studies reporting increased strength and endurance when compared with the atraumatic contralateral side. Patients must also be counseled on the cosmetic differences between operative and nonoperative treatment. Nonoperative treatment of a retracted ruptured biceps tendon may lead to a change in contour of the anterior arm. Although the contour may be reestablished with operative treatment, scars on the anterior arm may prove to be unsightly for some patients.

GENERAL COMPLICATIONS

Overall complication following with repair of the distal biceps tendon vary, with studies reporting ranges between 0% to 50%. The total complication rate is estimated between 15 and 35%.[33–35] These common complications include neurologic injuries (10%–15%), HO (0%–50%), reruptures (1%–5%), hardware failure (0%–20%), chronic regional pain syndrome (CRPS) (2%), wound problems (2%–30%), stiffness (4%), and weakness (15%–50%), with some more rare complications being reported.[18,20,30,33,34,36] Multiple studies have shown no difference in complication rates between 2-incision and one-incision techniques; however, an anterior-only repair is associated with a higher rate of LABC palsy.[18] Several studies support an increased complication rate with the use of suture anchors or transosseous screws when compared with cortical button or transosseous suture repair[10,12,13,17,35]; however, a recent study by Banerjee and colleagues[34] suggested a higher complication rate with cortical button repair. Researchers have suggested that repair of the distal biceps tendon has a steep learning curve, suggesting that more experienced surgeons may have a lower complication rate.[29]

LATERAL ANTEBRACHIAL CUTANEOUS NERVE

The LABC is a continuation of the musculocutaneous nerve from the lateral cord of the brachial plexus and provides sensation to the radial aspect of the forearm. The anterior exposure for repair of the distal biceps often encounters the LABC as it emerges from between the biceps and brachialis and then runs laterally between the biceps and the brachioradialis where it divides into volar and dorsal branches.

Current literature reports a 5% to 57% rate of injury to the LABC.[12,14,18,20,30,33] Most injuries to the LABC are transient neurapaxias and typically result in temporary numbness along the lateral aspect of the forearm; however, some may persist for years. In the case of neurotmesis, a painful neuroma may develop and permanent numbness and dysesthesias may result.

To prevent injury to the LABC, the nerve should be identified and protected during the anterior approach, especially in the case of chronic ruptures in which adhesions must be released to allow for additional excursion of the tendon for repair. Proximal retrieval of the biceps tendon may jeopardize the nerve as it passes between the brachialis and biceps muscle bellies. In the case of partial biceps tendon attrition, some researchers advocate a posterior-only approach in order to prevent injury to the anterior structures.[21]

In the event of an injury to the LABC in which the nerve was visualized in continuity, intraoperatively, watchful waiting is generally undertaken. Although rare, an intraoperative laceration of the nerve may require repair to prevent permanent decreased sensation over the radial aspect of the forearm and neuroma formation.

POSTERIOR INTEROSSEOUS NERVE

The radial nerve arises from between the brachialis and brachioradialis muscles and gives rise to the PIN and superficial radial sensory nerve. The PIN courses between the deep and superficial heads of the supinator and then lies on the dorsal cortex of the radius proximally, innervating the muscles of the dorsal compartment of the forearm. The terminal branch of the PIN lies in the floor of the fourth dorsal compartment sending sensory branches to the wrist joint.

Injury to the PIN can occur with both the one-incision and 2-incision approach and may occur via errant drill bit placement, entrapment under a cortical button, or dissection along the proximal radius. Injury to the PIN leads to weakness with finger and thumb extension and radial deviation with attempted wrist extension. Historically, repair of the distal biceps tendon was complicated by injury to the PIN in 10% to 15% of patients.[30] More recent literature has suggested that injury to the PIN has decreased to less than 10%, with rates as low as 1%.[12,14,18,20,33,34]

Prevention of injury to the PIN is important no matter what technique is used to repair the distal biceps tendon. When using an anterior approach, the arm is supinated to protect the PIN and when passing pins or drilling. Oscillation or tapping of the slotted passing pin is recommended to prevent ensnarement of the posterior soft tissues. The PIN is also at risk during placement of transosseous sutures or a cortical button, which is seated on the posterior-lateral radius. A small posterior-lateral incision can be made to ensure that the PIN is not under the cortical button. Intraoperative fluoroscopy to ensure that the button is seated appropriately on the proximal radius with no soft tissue interposition is recommended. In either case, the cortical button should be deployed just as it exits the posterior cortex, so as to avoid soft tissue entrapment. Multiple cadaveric studies have determined the most dangerous orientation of drill bit use in the proximal forearm is distal and radially directed drilling at the radial tuberosity. This technique put the PIN at the most risk, with drill bits impaling or penetrating within 1 mm of the PIN. Drilling is recommended with the forearm in full supination with the drill directed anterior to posterior in a slightly ulnar direction.[37,38] Cadaveric studies show the cortical button to be an average of 9.3 mm from the PIN, with the closest being 7 mm when drilled anterior to posterior in full supination.[39]

When performing the posterior portion of the 2-incision approach, pronation of the forearm is important to move the PIN anterior to the surgical field. Although this may help to protect the PIN, it may also lead to compression.[40] Some researchers advocate performing the anterior approach followed by placement of a blunt instrument over and around the ulnar side of the radius. The blunt instrument is advanced through the extensor digitorum communis, and an incision is made over the now subcutaneous instrument on the posterior-lateral aspect of the elbow. When using retractors along the radius, some surgeons discourage the use of a Hohmann retractor over the radial aspect of the proximal radius to avoid injury to the PIN (**Fig. 2**). No matter what approach and instrumentation is used, if dissection within the supinator is performed, visualization of the PIN is recommended.

In the event of an observed, intraoperative injury to the PIN, standard nerve repair principles should be adhered to in order to prevent long-term functional deficits. If embarrassment of the PIN is found on the postoperative examination and the nerve was not visualized intraoperatively, early exploration with release of the offending structures or repair of the lacerated nerve should be considered. If the nerve was visualized in continuity at the end of the procedure with no impingement of hardware, a wait-and-see approach may be used, as a neurapraxic injury is most likely. Electrodiagnostic studies may be performed as early as 3 weeks in order to give a baseline status for the nerve. Exploration and nerve repair or neurolysis should be performed early if there is a lack of evidence of reinnervation on serial neurodiagnostic studies. Waiting beyond 6 months for exploration, neurolysis and/or nerve repair is likely to lead to poor results. In the case of chronic PIN injuries greater than 6 months, tendon transfers are recommended to reestablish finger extension and thumb interphalangeal joint extension.[41]

SUPERFICIAL RADIAL NERVE

The superficial radial nerve supplies sensation to the dorsoradial aspect of the hand and thumb. The nerve enters the forearm under the cover of the brachioradialis muscle and runs distally where it emerges dorsally from under the brachioradialis. Injury to the nerve is encountered in 5% to 10% of repairs and is generally a neuropraxia from aggressive lateral traction within the wound.[29,30,33] Some researchers discourage the use of lateral retractors within the wound and recommend skin hooks only in order to prevent injury to the superficial radial nerve. Observation is generally the treatment of choice as most of the numbness improves. Permanent damage and neuromas may develop, but symptomatic treatment is generally recommended.

MEDIAN NERVE

The median nerve arises from contributions of the medial and lateral cords of the brachial plexus, runs along the medial aspect of the arm, and traverses the antecubital fossa just medial to the brachial artery and biceps tendon. The nerve enters the forearm between the superficial and deep heads of the pronator teres before coming to rest between the flexor digitorum superficialis and profundus. The median nerve along with the anterior interosseous nerve innervate the thenar muscles as well as all of the volar forearm musculature with the exception of the flexor digitorum profundus to the small and ring fingers and the flexor carpi ulnaris.

Injury to the median nerve, although rare in the setting of biceps tendon repair (~4%), may lead to devastating results and was originally described in 1967.[30,33] Injury is a result of aberrant dissection and/or aggressive retraction medially on the neurovascular bundle. Injury to the median nerve at the level of the elbow affects the forearm flexor/pronator mass, anterior interosseous nerve innervated musculature, and the thenar musculature. In addition to the weakness of thumb opposition, weakness in thumb interphalangeal joint flexion, finger flexion, and wrist flexion is observed; patients also complain of numbness on the volar side of the thumb, index, middle and radial ring digits and palm. Observation is indicated for

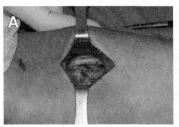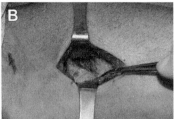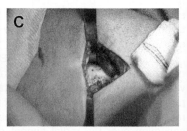

Fig. 2. Anterior approach to left arm. (*A*) Superficial branch of the radial nerve and the vascular leash of Henry can be seen. (*B*) Leading proximal edge of supinator can be seen. (*C*) PIN (not seen) is protected by a Hohmann retractor.

neurapraxic injuries. Repair versus reconstruction with tendon transfers is considered if no improvement is noted clinically or on nerve studies. Acute neurotmesis is treated with repair using modern microsurgical techniques. Chronic median nerve injuries are generally treated with tendon transfers to recover thumb opposition, finger flexion, and wrist flexion.[41]

Prevention of median nerve injuries during the repair of distal biceps tendon repairs is centered around the identification of anatomic landmarks and the avoidance of aggressive medial retraction. Wide retractors should be used to increase access to the repair site but also to dissipate the force over a large area. Medial dissection should be avoided, and dissection should be directed lateral to the brachial artery.

ULNAR NERVE

The ulnar nerve arises from the medial cord of the brachial plexus and enters the forearm posterior to the medial epicondyle through the cubital tunnel and 2 heads of the flexor carpi ulnaris. The flexor carpi ulnaris, flexor digitorum profundus to the ring and small fingers, ulnar 2 lumbricals, hypothenar muscles, interossei, and the deep head of the flexor pollicis brevis are all innervated by the ulnar nerve.

Injury to the ulnar nerve is a very rare occurrence during distal biceps repair (<2%),[30,33] given the anatomic location of the nerve as it passes into the forearm. Although the nerve is not visualized in the routine surgical approaches to the distal biceps tendon, injuries during repair have been reported. Injuries to the ulnar nerve present as weakness in the ulnar 2 fingers, inability to adduct or abduct the fingers, and ulnar clawing in more chronic cases. As in the case of median nerve injuries, dissection should not stray medially during biceps tendon retrieval, lysis of adhesions, and repair.

STIFFNESS

The functional range of motion of the elbow is 30° to 130° of flexion with 50° of pronation and supination. Early passive range of motion is necessary to reduce postoperative stiffness, and splinting should be limited to at most 3 weeks postoperatively. Some operative techniques allow for early active range of motion of the elbow; however, outcomes after early passive range of motion are similar.

On review of the Boyd-Anderson technique, 19% of patients lacked a 100° arc of forearm rotation and 5% lacked a 100° arc of elbow flexion and extension. Recent publications report good maintenance of elbow flexion and extension with stiffness in about 4% of patients. However, forearm rotation has proved to be the most difficult motion to restore, with about 12% of patients reporting a decrease in range of motion.[30] Most patients are able to regain functional elbow and forearm motion postoperatively; elbows in which the tendon was repaired in flexion (>60°) had similar outcomes as those repaired at less than 60°, with no increased incidence of stiffness.[11,42]

In the case that stiffness refractory to therapy, splinting, and stretching, radiographs must be obtained to rule out heterotopic ossification.

WEAKNESS

The goal of distal biceps repair is to re-establish the strength and endurance of both elbow flexion and forearm supination. In the absence of frank hardware failure weakness most commonly is a result of poor tendon tensioning and nonanatomic repair of the footprint of the distal biceps tendon.

Results of the original Boyd-Anderson technique showed that when weakness was defined as less than 99% for dominant arm and 80% for nondominant arms, weakness in supination and flexion strength was present in 48% and 15% respectively. Supination endurance was decreased in 38% and elbow flexion in 33%. Modern one- and 2-incision techniques have achieved improved results with most patients regaining greater than 80% of strength and endurance and multiple studies reporting greater than 100% recovery when compared with the contralateral side.[30]

Using modern repair techniques, weakness is caused by poor graft tension or non-anatomic repair. Poor graft tension may lead to weakness by failure to set the muscle at resting tension which may lead to a decrease in flexion efficiency. This weakness may manifest itself in both elbow flexion and supination. Failure to anatomically repair the distal biceps to the posterior/ulnar aspect of the radial tuberosity affects supination due to the decreased moment arm of the biceps. The decreased moment arm decreases the amount of torque that the biceps may impart on the radius which may lead to decreased supination strength.[1–3,32,43,44]

Prevention of elbow flexion weakness and forearm supination weakness centers around anatomic repair of the distal biceps. Nonanatomic repairs such as repairs to the brachialis, anterior/radial aspect of the radius may restore elbow flexion, but supination weakness persists.[44] Cadaveric studies have shown that the insertion of the distal biceps tendon is generally on the posterior and ulnar aspect of the radial tuberosity.[1–3] Further studies have shown that nonanatomic, anterior and radial repair lead to persistent weakness in supination (**Fig. 3**). Some researchers even advocate a 2-incision technique in order to reliably provide an anatomic repair.[32] Regardless of repair technique, the surgeon must reliably be able to perform a strong, anatomic repair, tension the repair appropriately and protect the repair in the early postoperative course to have the most successful outcomes.

HETEROTOPIC OSSIFICATION

HO may be found incidentally on routine radiographs or may lead to severe decrease in elbow and forearm range of motion and even synostosis between the radius and ulna. Early repairs of distal biceps tendon ruptures using the Boyd-Anderson approach were complicated by HO (15%) and synostosis (5%).[30] With the evolution of the modern 2-incision approach and the one-incision approach, the incidence of clinically relevant HO and synostosis has decreased and, in some studies, eliminated. Asymptomatic HO is still reported with rates from 10% to 25%[9,12,14,18,20,34]; however, other researchers claim the complication is underreported and, in one study, may be up to 50%.[45]

In order to prevent heterotopic bone formation and synostosis, some researchers advocate a one-incision approach, whereas others prefer a 2-incision technique that does not violate the interosseous membrane. Careful dissection should be performed through tissue planes, and hemostasis must be maintained. The use of a Kerrison rongeur is recommended in place of power tools to prepare the anterior radial hole to decrease the amount of bone debris. Copious irrigation before wound closure, decreased soft tissue,

and periosteal dissection are also recommended to help prevent HO.

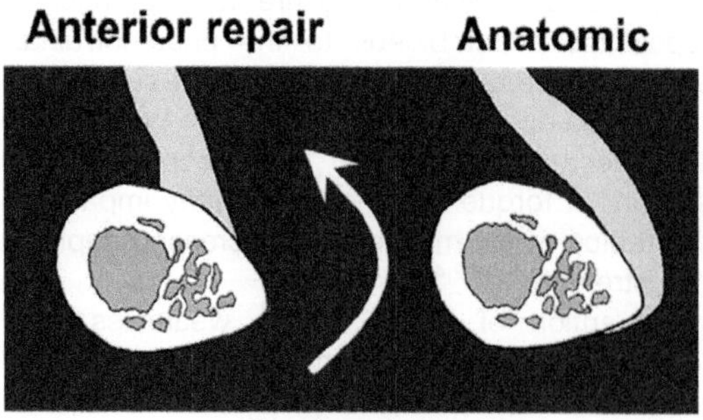

Asymptomatic HO necessitates no intervention, and observation is recommended. Symptomatic HO presents with decreased range of motion of the elbow with a firm end point; in the case of synostosis, the forearm rotation is fixed. In the case of synostosis, radiographically evident HO with flexion less than 130°, or the inability to extend the elbow beyond 30° of flexion, excision of the offending bone is recommended once the bone has matured. At this time no consensus has been established as to when the bone is considered mature; but radiographs, bone scans, and time from surgery have all been used in attempt to identify mature HO. Some surgeons advocate removal of the clinically deleterious bone regardless of maturation as the benefits of early elbow range of motion may outweigh any increase in recurrence of HO in the setting of immature HO. Most researchers agree that regardless of when the clinically evident HO is excised, some sort of prophylaxis should be used perioperatively.

RERUPTURE

Rerupture of the repaired distal biceps tendon is reported to complicate distal biceps repair in 0% to 5.6% of cases.[13,18,31] Most reruptures of the distal biceps tendon occur in the early postoperative period, usually after an accidental or intentional load applied to a flexed and supinated elbow and forearm. Reruptures are also associated with the use of suture anchors and transosseous screws.[33] Rerupture during range-of-motion exercises have not been reported in the literature, when using modern fixation techniques for repair of the distal biceps tendon.[13,18,31]

Appropriate patient education is critical to the postoperative success of a distal biceps tendon repair. In the case of transosseous suture repair, most researchers recommend a period of 2 to 3 weeks of immobilization followed by active-assisted range of motion until 12 weeks when strengthening is started. In the case of cortical button repair, active-assisted range of motion is started immediately, although studies have shown that brief immobilization less than 3 weeks has similar outcomes. The most important factor leading to reruptures of an appropriately repaired distal biceps tendon is the avoidance of an eccentric load applied to the newly repaired tendon.

In the event of rerupture of the repaired distal biceps tendon, it is helpful for both the surgeon and patients to understand the circumstances and likely cause of the reruptured tendon. Before

Fig. 3. An anterior repair can lead to supination weakness. (*From* Schmidt CC, Jarrett CD, Brown BT. The distal biceps tendon. J Hand Surg 2013;38A:814; with permission.)

making any decisions on treatment of the reruptured tendon, patients must understand the increased risk of infection, HO, repair failure, and neurovascular injury, which are all associated with revision surgery. After discussing the risks, benefits, likely outcome, and any possible alterations in perioperative care, such as short-term cast placement, patients must again decide between operative and nonoperative treatment. Nonoperative treatment of reruptured distal biceps tendons is similar to rupture of native tendons, with early range of motion and strengthening as tolerated. In the case of reconstruction of reruptured biceps tendons, the surgeon may have to navigate through scarred tissue planes, poor bone stock, insufficient tendon length, and previously placed hardware. In rare cases, studies have supported repair with elbow flexion greater than 60° and/or allograft.[11,42] Noncompliant patients may benefit from short-term cast application in order to protect the newly repaired distal biceps tendon; however, stiffness may be a problem with extended periods of immobilization.

VASCULAR INJURIES

The vascular anatomy about the elbow is complex and is dominated by the brachial artery and its branches. The radial collateral artery is a branch of the brachial artery; its anastomosis is with the radial recurrent artery, a branch of the posterior interosseous artery. The radial recurrent vessels are commonly ligated in order to provide adequate exposure for repair. The superior ulnar collateral artery communicates with the posterior ulnar recurrent artery, and the inferior ulnar collateral communicates with the anterior ulnar recurrent artery. As the brachial artery enters the forearm, it is medial to the distal biceps tendon and then branches into the radial and ulnar arteries. The ulnar artery gives rise to the common interosseous artery, which ultimately becomes the anterior and posterior interosseous arteries.

Knowledge of complex anatomic relationships, gentle retraction, surgical technique, and timely tendon repair are all essential in prevention of arterial injury. Although small venous branches and the recurrent arteries are commonly ligated, the brachial artery as well as radial and ulnar arteries should be protected throughout the operation. An Allen test should be performed preoperatively in all patients to determine dominance between the radial and ulnar artery and the presence or absence of a complete arch. This determination proves to be instrumental in the event of an arterial injury distal to the brachial artery. Although transection of the brachial, radial, or ulnar arteries

have not been described in the literature, one case of thrombosis and occlusion of the brachial artery has been described during a distal biceps tendon repair. Thrombectomy was performed in this case, which restored the radial pulse. The researchers attributed the thrombosis to aggressive medial retraction, which caused an intimal injury.[13] In the event of embarrassment of the brachial artery, revascularization should be performed emergently to prevent limb loss. In the event of a radial or ulnar artery injury, revascularization is generally recommended; however, if the hand is still perfused after injury, observation is an option.

PROXIMAL RADIAL FRACTURES

Proximal radial fractures after repair of the distal biceps tendon are exceedingly rare with one reported case in the literature. The fracture involved a fall after a revision distal biceps repair using the transosseous suture technique for both the primary and revision surgery. A second set of 2.7 mm bone tunnels were drilled for the revision surgery and the patient fell postoperatively sustaining a fracture through the repair site. The patient was treated with open reduction and internal fixation and had a satisfactory outcome. The authors suggested creating a smaller trough, reducing the size and number of drill holes, reusing drill holes, packing bone graft into unused drill holes and protecting the vulnerable bone with a Muenster cast.[36]

CHRONIC REGIONAL PAIN SYNDROME

CRPS may complicate the postoperative course in about 2% of cases.[33] Treatment of CRPS is multimodal with occupational therapy, pharmacologic therapy, and surgical options all being used.

WOUND COMPLICATIONS

Wound complications may be devastating to patients with a distal biceps tendon repair and are reported in less than 2% of acute repairs and up to 33% in chronic and revision repairs.[11,12,18,33,34] The infection may be superficial in which the skin and subcutaneous tissue is involved or it may be deep involving the tendon, bone, suture, and any hardware implanted. Superficial infections are initially treated with a course of antibiotics with debridement as necessary. In the case of deep infections, intravenous antibiotics, hardware removal, and debridement of bone and tendon may be necessary. Reconstruction after a thorough debridement may be difficult because of inadequate bone stock and soft tissue coverage over the antecubital fossa.

TECHNIQUE-SPECIFIC COMPLICATIONS

Surgeon inexperience has been suggested in the literature as a risk factor for an increased complication rate. The complex anatomy of the antecubital fossa, intricate surgical techniques, and the slim margin of error when repairing distal biceps tendons have likely led to high complication rates.[29] Although there are many approaches to the repair of the distal biceps tendon, a few should be mentioned here for specific complications related to a certain technique.

Although the overall complication rate for the one-versus 2-incision technique is similar, the one-incision technique is associated with LABC palsies, whereas the 2-incision technique is associated with HO and decreased forearm rotation.[18,30] In regard to hardware placement, the cortical button has the strongest load to failure, with suture anchor repair having the highest rerupture rate.[12,18,33] Argument exists in regard to what technique has the highest complication rate, with suture anchor (rerupture in 5%–25%),[12,18,20,33] transosseous screw (LABC palsy in 12%–60%),[12,14,33] and cortical button (10%–20% button displacement and >30% total complication rate)[22] all seeming to have room for improvement. A case report presented a unique complication of incarceration of the PIN between the cortical button and the proximal radius.[46] However, some studies report a low complication rate in repair with a cortical button (<1%),[10,17,24,25,33] whereas transosseous suture repair consistently has a complication rate near 10%.[9,12,18,20,33]

SUMMARY

Repair of the distal biceps tendon can lead to excellent clinical outcomes in active patients; however, common complications, such as nerve injury, HO, stiffness, brachial artery injury, weakness, CRPS, infection, and rerupture, may all complicate the postoperative course. Surgeon experience tends to correlate with complication rates, and patients should be counseled on complications before surgical intervention. Knowledge of anatomic relationships, gentle retraction, sound repair techniques, and postoperative awareness of complications may yield better results and improved patient satisfaction.

REFERENCES

1. Athwal GS, Steinmann SP, Rispoli DM. The distal biceps tendon: footprint and relevant clinical anatomy. J Hand Surg Am 2007;32(8):1225–9.

2. Forthman CL, Zimmerman RM, Sullivan MJ, et al. Cross-sectional anatomy of the bicipital tuberosity and biceps brachii tendon insertion: relevance to anatomic tendon repair. J Shoulder Elbow Surg 2008;17(3):522–6.

3. Hutchinson HL, Gloystein D, Gillespie M. Distal biceps tendon insertion: an anatomic study. J Shoulder Elbow Surg 2008;17(2):342–6.

4. Kelly MP, Perkinson SG, Ablove RH, et al. Distal biceps tendon ruptures: an epidemiological analysis using a large population database. Am J Sports Med 2015;43(8):2012–7.

5. Safran MR, Graham SM. Distal biceps tendon ruptures: incidence, demographics, and the effect of smoking. Clin Orthop Relat Res 2002;(404):275–83.

6. Baker BE, Bierwagen D. Rupture of the distal tendon of the biceps brachii. Operative versus non-operative treatment. J Bone Joint Surg Am 1985;67(3):414–7.

7. Mariani EM, Cofield RH, Askew LJ, et al. Rupture of the tendon of the long head of the biceps brachii. Surgical versus nonsurgical treatment. Clin Orthop Relat Res 1988;(228):233–9.

8. Morrey BF, Askew LJ, An KN, et al. Rupture of the distal tendon of the biceps brachii. A biomechanical study. J Bone Joint Surg Am 1985;67(3):418–21.

9. Hetsroni I, Pilz-Burstein R, Nyska M, et al. Avulsion of the distal biceps brachii tendon in middle-aged population: is surgical repair advisable? A comparative study of 22 patients treated with either nonoperative management or early anatomical repair. Injury 2008;39(7):753–60.

10. Bain GI, Prem H, Heptinstall RJ, et al. Repair of distal biceps tendon rupture: a new technique using the Endobutton. J Shoulder Elbow Surg 2000;9(2):120–6.

11. Bosman HA, Fincher M, Saw N. Anatomic direct repair of chronic distal biceps brachii tendon rupture without interposition graft. J Shoulder Elbow Surg 2012;21(10):1342–7.

12. Citak M, Backhaus M, Seybold D, et al. Surgical repair of the distal biceps brachii tendon: a comparative study of three surgical fixation techniques. Knee Surg Sports Traumatol Arthrosc 2011;19(11):1936–41.

13. Cusick MC, Cottrell BJ, Cain RA, et al. Low incidence of tendon rerupture after distal biceps repair by cortical button and interference screw. J Shoulder Elbow Surg 2014;23(10):1532–6.

14. Eardley WG, Odak S, Adesina TS, et al. Bioabsorbable interference screw fixation of distal biceps ruptures through a single anterior incision: a single-surgeon case series and review of the literature. Arch Orthop Trauma Surg 2010;130(7):875–81.

15. Failla JM, Amadio PC, Morrey BF, et al. Proximal radioulnar synostosis after repair of distal biceps

brachii rupture by the two-incision technique. Report of four cases. Clin Orthop Relat Res 1990;(253):133–6.

16. Greenberg JA. Endobutton repair of distal biceps tendon ruptures. J Hand Surg Am 2009;34(8): 1541–8.

17. Greenberg JA, Fernandez JJ, Wang T, et al. Endo-Button assisted repair of distal biceps tendon ruptures. J Shoulder Elbow Surg 2003;12(5):484–90 [Erratum appears in J Shoulder Elbow Surg 2005; 14(2):231].

18. Grewal R, Athwal GS, MacDermid JC, et al. Single versus double-incision technique for the repair of acute distal biceps tendon ruptures: a randomized clinical trial. J Bone Joint Surg Am 2012;94(13): 1166–74.

19. Grégory T, Roure P, Fontès D. Repair of distal biceps tendon rupture using a suture anchor: description of a new endoscopic procedure. Am J Sports Med 2009;37(3):506–11.

20. Johnson TS, Johnson DC, Shindle MK, et al. One-versus two-incision technique for distal biceps tendon repair. HSS J 2008;4(2):117–22.

21. Kelly EW, Steinmann S, O'Driscoll SW. Surgical treatment of partial distal biceps tendon ruptures through a single posterior incision. J Shoulder Elbow Surg 2003;12(5):456–61.

22. McKee MD, Hirji R, Schemitsch EH, et al. Patient-oriented functional outcome after repair of distal biceps tendon ruptures using a single-incision technique. J Shoulder Elbow Surg 2005;14(3): 302–6.

23. Olsen JR, Shields E, Williams RB, et al. A comparison of cortical button with interference screw versus suture anchor techniques for distal biceps brachii tendon repairs. J Shoulder Elbow Surg 2014; 23(11):1607–11.

24. Patterson RW, Sharma J, Lawton JN, et al. Distal biceps tendon reconstruction with tendoachilles allograft: a modification of the endobutton technique utilizing an ACL reconstruction system. J Hand Surg Am 2009;34(3):545–52.

25. Peeters T, Ching-Soon NG, Jansen N, et al. Functional outcome after repair of distal biceps tendon ruptures using the endobutton technique. J Shoulder Elbow Surg 2009;18(2):283–7.

26. Pereira DS, Kvitne RS, Liang M, et al. Surgical repair of distal biceps tendon ruptures: a biomechanical comparison of two techniques. Am J Sports Med 2002;30(3):432–6.

27. Recordon JA, Misur PN, Isaksson F, et al. Endobutton versus transosseous suture repair of distal biceps rupture using the two-incision technique: a comparison series. J Shoulder Elbow Surg 2015; 24(6):928–33.

28. Sethi P, Obopilwe E, Rincon L, et al. Biomechanical evaluation of distal biceps reconstruction with cortical button and interference screw fixation. J Shoulder Elbow Surg 2010;19(1):53–7.

29. Shields E, Olsen JR, Williams RB, et al. Distal biceps brachii tendon repairs: a single-incision technique using a cortical button with interference screw versus a double-incision technique using suture fixation through bone tunnels. Am J Sports Med 2015; 43(5):1072–6.

30. Karunakar MA, Cha P, Stern PJ. Distal biceps ruptures. A followup of Boyd and Anderson repair. Clin Orthop Relat Res 1999;(363):100–7.

31. Hinchey JW, Aronowitz JG, Sanchez-Sotelo J, et al. Re-rupture rate of primarily repaired distal biceps tendon injuries. J Shoulder Elbow Surg 2014;23(6): 850–4.

32. Hansen G, Smith A, Pollock JW, et al. Anatomic repair of the distal biceps tendon cannot be consistently performed through a classic single-incision suture anchor technique. J Shoulder Elbow Surg 2014;23(12):1898–904.

33. Watson JN, Moretti VM, Schwindel L, et al. Repair techniques for acute distal biceps tendon ruptures: a systematic review. J Bone Joint Surg Am 2014; 96(24):2086–90.

34. Banerjee M, Shafizadeh S, Bouillon B, et al. High complication rate following distal biceps refixation with cortical button. Arch Orthop Trauma Surg 2013;133(10):1361–6.

35. Chavan PR, Duquin TR, Bisson LJ. Repair of the ruptured distal biceps tendon: a systematic review. Am J Sports Med 2008;36(8):1618–24.

36. Badia A, Sambandam SN, Khanchandani P. Proximal radial fracture after revision of distal biceps tendon repair: a case report. J Shoulder Elbow Surg 2007;16(2):e4–6.

37. Thumm N, Hutchinson D, Zhang C, et al. Proximity of the posterior interosseous nerve during cortical button guidewire placement for distal biceps tendon reattachment. J Hand Surg Am 2015;40(3):534–6.

38. Saldua N, Carney J, Dewing C, et al. The effect of drilling angle on posterior interosseous nerve safety during open and endoscopic anterior single-incision repair of the distal biceps tendon. Arthroscopy 2008;24(3):305–10.

39. Lo EY, Li CS, Van den Bogaerde JM. The effect of drill trajectory on proximity to the posterior interosseous nerve during cortical button distal biceps repair. Arthroscopy 2011;27(8):1048–54.

40. Links AC, Graunke KS, Wahl C, et al. Pronation can increase the pressure on the posterior interosseous nerve under the arcade of Frohse: a possible mechanism of palsy after two-incision repair for distal biceps rupture–clinical experience and a cadaveric investigation. J Shoulder Elbow Surg 2009;18(1):64–8.

41. Seiler JG 3rd, Desai MJ, Payne SH. Tendon transfers for radial, median, and ulnar nerve palsy. J Am Acad Orthop Surg 2013;21(11):675–84.

42. Morrey ME, Abdel MP, Sanchez-Sotelo J, et al. Primary repair of retracted distal biceps tendon ruptures in extreme flexion. J Shoulder Elbow Surg 2014;23(5):679–85.

43. Prud'homme-Foster M, Louati H, Pollock JW, et al. Proper placement of the distal biceps tendon during repair improves supination strength–a biomechanical analysis. J Shoulder Elbow Surg 2015;24(4):527–32.

44. De Carli A, Zanzotto E, Vadalà AP, et al. Surgical repair of the distal biceps brachii tendon: clinical and isokinetic long-term follow-up. Knee Surg Sports Traumatol Arthrosc 2009;17(7):850–6.

45. Vidal AF, Koonce RC, Wolcott M, et al. Extensive heterotopic ossification after suspensory cortical fixation of acute distal biceps tendon ruptures. Arthroscopy 2012;28(7):1036–40.

46. Van den Bogaerde J, Shin E. Posterior interosseous nerve incarceration with endobutton repair of distal biceps. Orthopedics 2015;38(1):e68–71.

Complications of Lateral Epicondylar Release

Michael Lucius Pomerantz, MD

KEYWORDS

- Lateral epicondylitis • Tennis elbow • Surgery • Complications • Open • Percutaneous
- Arthroscopic

KEY POINTS

- Overall, there is a low complication rate for lateral epicondylar release, but this complication rate may be underreported.
- Historically, open procedures have had a higher rate and more diverse array of complications.
- Recent, higher-quality studies have not noted these differences in complications.
- Elbow posterolateral rotatory instability (PRLI), permanent nerve injury, and deep infection are possible catastrophic complications.
- Understanding the anatomy is crucial to preventing some complications.

INTRODUCTION

Lateral epicondylitis, also known as tennis elbow, is a common condition affecting an estimated 1% to 3% of adults each year.[1,2] Runge first described it in 1873[3] and in 1883 Major[4] named it "lawn-tennis arm." A single cause of the disease has not yet been elicited, but many think it is associated with the common extensor origin (CEO) at the lateral epicondyle, most specifically the extensor carpi radialis brevis (ECRB). Nirschl and Pettrone[5] described tendinosis of the extensor tendons originating at the lateral epicondyle, predominantly involving the ECRB. They described an angiofibroblastic hyperplastic process consistent with repeated microtrauma with "tendinous non-repair with immature reparative tissue" and noted a lack of true inflammatory cells. These findings have been corroborated in other studies.[6,7] Thus, the term, epicondylitis, is a misnomer in the definition of true inflammation.

Of the many who seek medical treatment of tennis elbow, only approximately 10%[5,8] end up requiring surgical intervention but some studies report greater than 20%.[9,10] Many different surgical procedures have been described and choice of procedure often determined by the surgeon's views on the cause. Wilhelm and Gieseler[11,12] have been proponents of a neurologic cause of the disease and have a published rate of greater than 90% success when pursuing this treatment. Most of the literature regarding treatment of tennis elbow, however, has focused on surgical release of extensor tendon or tendons at the lateral epicondyle. Open, percutaneous, and arthroscopic approaches have all been described with good outcomes and rare complications. The complications are often reported, however, in a manner lacking uniformity and without clear diagnosis. The elbow is an area of complex anatomy with articular, tendinous, ligamentous, and neurologic structures in close proximity that are at risk for injury during surgery. This article illuminates the reported and potential complications associated with tennis elbow surgical procedures.

ANATOMY

A lateral epicondylar release addresses an area of pathology located within the CEO. The extensor carpi radialis longus (ECRL), ECRB, extensor digitorum communis (EDC), extensor digiti minimi, and

Disclosures: No disclosures.
Synergy Specialists Medical Group, Orthopaedic Surgery, Hand/Upper Extremity Sub-specialization, 955 Lane Ave, Suite #200, Chula Vista, CA 91914, USA
E-mail address: LPomerantz@SynergySMG.com

Orthop Clin N Am 47 (2016) 445–469
http://dx.doi.org/10.1016/j.ocl.2015.10.002
0030-5898/16/$ – see front matter © 2016 Elsevier Inc. All rights reserved.

extensor carpi ulnaris (**Fig. 1**A) comprise the CEO. Together, the brachioradialis (BR), ECRL, and ECRB make up the mobile wad compartment of the forearm, which has a septum dividing it from the extensor compartment that contains the remainder of the extensor muscles. The ECRB origin lies deep to the ECRL and EDC on the anterior aspect of the lateral epicondyle. The ECRB may also have additional origin sites, including the intermuscular septum and underlying capsuloligamentous structures.[13] The ECRB tendon coalesces with the tendon of the EDC, making differentiation of their tendinous origins difficult if not impossible.[14,15] The origin of the ECRB lies just lateral and superior to the insertion of the lateral elbow capsular and ligamentous structures. As the ECRB tendon travels distally, its deep fibers are in contact with the superficial aspect of the elbow capsule and lateral ligamentous complex.[14–16]

The radial nerve enters the anterior compartment of the arm approximately 10 cm proximal to the lateral epicondyle (see **Fig. 1**B). The radial nerve exits from between the brachialis and the BR and at the level of the lateral epicondyle (up to 2 cm proximally to 5 cm distally) the radial nerve branches into deep and superficial branches.[13] The deep branch is the posterior interosseous nerve (PIN) that travels through the arcade of Frohse of the supinator muscle and goes on to sequentially innervate dorsal forearm musculature aside from the more proximally innervated ECRL and ECRB. The superficial branch is predominantly sensory and stays beneath the BR muscle until exiting subcutaneously distally in the forearm. The posterior antebrachial cutaneous nerve (PABCN) is a proximal branch of the radial nerve that crosses 1.5 cm anterior to the lateral epicondyle located on the fascia of the lateral part of the BR.[17] Often, it is lying at the junction of the BR and ECRL in a superficial position.

The innervation of the ECRB is either from the PIN or a direct branch from the radial nerve. The mean distance between the radiocapitellar joint and the PIN as it enters the arcade of Frohse is 30 +/−7 mm and the distance from the lateral epicondyle to the PIN is 47 +/−8 mm.[16] Furthermore, Diliberti, and colleagues[18] described the anatomic relationship between the PIN and the radiocapitellar joint depending on whether the arm was in supination or pronation. In supination, the PIN is as close as 22 mm of the radiocapitellar joint, whereas in pronation, that distance increased to at least 38 mm.

The lateral ligamentous complex of the elbow has important anatomic considerations as well. It is made up of 3 components – the annular ligament (AL), radial collateral ligament (RCL), and the lateral ulnar collateral ligament (LUCL)[13,19] (see **Fig. 1**C). The LUCL, confluent with the RCL, originates at the bare area just distal to the lateral epicondyle, dorsal and deep to the ECRB, and fans out distally attaching to the tubercle of the supinator crest on the ulna. Disruption of the LUCL results in PRLI.[19–22]

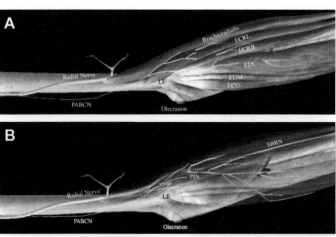

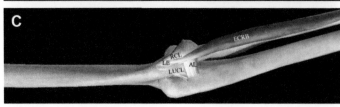

Fig. 1. Representation of anatomy on the lateral aspect of the elbow. (*A*) CEO and location of radial nerve and PABCN. (*B*) Emphasis of radial nerve and its branches. Circle and arrow demonstrate PAL arthroscopic portal and trajectory. (*C*) Lateral ligamentous complex in relation to ECRB. LE, lateral epicondyle; SBRN, superficial branch radial nerve. (*Modified from* Human Anatomy Atlas for iPad, Version 7 by Visible Body®; with permission.)

Anatomic considerations for an arthroscopic approach involve the structures near the proximal anterolateral (PAL) portal, located 2 cm proximal and 1 cm anterior to the lateral epicondyle (see **Fig. 1**B), and the proximal anteromedial (PAM) portal, 2 cm proximal and 1 cm anterior to the medial epicondyle (**Fig. 2**). To increase the distance from arthroscopic instrumentation from neurovascular structures, the joint should be flexed to 90° and distended with saline.[23–28] Unless otherwise stated, the following distances are reported in a flexed and distended elbow joint.

For the PAL portal, the mean distance between the arthroscopic sheath and radial nerve is 14.2 mm (12–17 mm).[29] As the portal site moves distally the distance to the radial nerve decreases, the distances from the midanterolateral and the distal anterolateral portals to the radial nerve are 10.9 mm and 9.1 mm, respectively.[29] Omid and colleagues[30] demonstrate a minimum of 4 mm of brachialis muscle separating the radial nerve from the joint capsule at the level of the radiocapitellar joint and proximally. Over the radial neck, however, the radial nerve is separated from the capsule by only adipose tissue in 50% of the specimens.

For PAM portals, the median nerve is at risk for injury. With the portal located 1 cm anterior and 1 cm proximal to the medial epicondyle and a trajectory toward the center of the joint, the median nerve is located a mean of 22.3 mm from the cannula.[25] A cannula trajectory perpendicular to the median nerve reduces the distance to a mean of 10.7 mm. A different study[27] of the PAM portal shows an average distance of 12.4 mm. The ulnar nerve is not at risk as long as the portal is anterior to the medial intermuscular septum but is a mean distance of 12 mm to 30 mm[24,25,27] from the cannula.

Cutaneous nerves about the elbow are also at risk from arthroscopy portals. They often have variable courses. The PABCN (see **Fig. 1**B) can be touching the anterolateral cannula and the medial antebrachial cutaneous nerve (see **Fig. 2**) can be touching the anteromedial cannula.[24,26,27]

LATERAL EPICONDYLITIS PROCEDURES
Open Approach

The open procedure varies[5,31–45] but the conventional procedure is the one described by Nirschl and Pettrone[5] (**Fig. 3**).

- Historically, distal Z-lengthening of the ECRB tendon, or Garden procedure, at the musculotendinous junction distally[36,46,47] has been also described.
- Alternately, the entire CEO may be released through a transverse incision, which allows the musculotendinous group to retract[34,37,39,45,48] distally as the definitive treatment.

The muscular ECRL origin is anterior to the ECRB tendinous origin, which is often difficult to differentiate from the EDC origin.

- Exploration of the lateral compartment of the elbow can be made by making an opening in the synovial membrane just deep to the ECRB,[5,34,45] which permits possible resection of a portion of the AL.[35,40]

Fibrous and granulation tissue removal may include some of the origin of the EDC and/or ECRL.

- Boyd and McLeod[35] performed a lateral epicondylectomy and most investigators decorticate a portion of the lateral epicondyle with a drill or burr.
- Some investigators argue against decortication.[49,50]
- Transfer of the anconeus muscle to cover the tissue defect after substantial débridement has its proponents,[38,51] whereas other investigators advocate use of suture anchors to repair to the CEO or ECRB.[7,52]

Percutaneous Approach

Baumgard and Schwartz[53] first described the percutaneous procedure where a no. 11 blade was used to make a puncture incision overlying

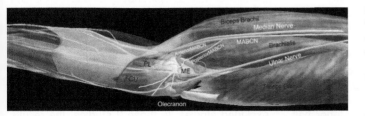

Fig. 2. Representation of anatomy on the medial aspect of the elbow. Circle and arrow represent anteromedial arthroscopic portal and trajectory. FCU, flexor carpi ulnaris; MABCN, medial antebrachial cutaneous nerve; ME, medial epicondyle; PL, palmaris longus. (*Modified from* Human Anatomy Atlas for iPad, Version 7 by Visible Body®; with permission.)

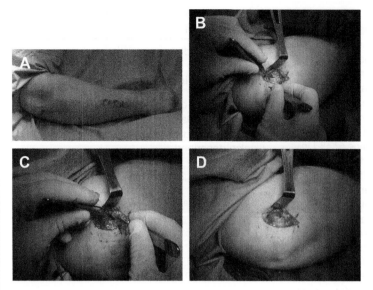

Fig. 3. Operating room photos of a modified Nirschl procedure on a right elbow. (*A*) Right arm prepped and draped. (*B*) Surgical incision revealing CEO, reflecting ECRL upwards to reveal ECRB. (*C*) Excision of pathologic ECRB. (*D*) After removal of pathologic ECRB just before decortication of LE with curette.

the anterior aspect of the lateral epicondyle and the tendinous origin of the CEO released. Similar procedures using a radiofrequency probe[54,55] or ultrasound-guided microresection[56,57] have been described.

Arthroscopic Approach

Arthroscopic surgery as described by Baker and colleagues[58] includes insufflation with 30 mL of sterile normal saline through the soft spot of the lateral epicondyle, radial head, and the olecranon.

- With the forearm in neutral position and the elbow flexed to 90°, the PAM viewing portal located 2 cm proximal and 1 cm anterior to medial epicondyle is established: incise the skin and then use a hemostat to bluntly spread toward the radiocapitellar joint capsule (nick-and-spread).
- The arthroscopic cannula is then introduced, making sure to aim at the center of the joint with avoidance of being too anterior.
- Using an outside-in or inside-out technique, the PAL portal is established in a similar fashion. This portal is 2 cm proximal and 1 cm anterior to the lateral epicondyle.
- The lateral joint capsule is released arthroscopically with shaver or electrothermal device, allowing visualization of the extracapsular ECRB.
- The origin of the ECRB is then débrided from the lateral epicondyle extending proximally from the anterior half of the radial head.
  - Débridement posterior to the anterior half may put the origin of the LUCL at risk.

- Portions of the ECRL and EDC may be débrided as well.
  - There must be caution in going too superficial with the release because it puts the lateral cutaneous tissue at risk.
- The lateral epicondyle can then be decorticated using an arthroscopic shaver, burr, or handheld curette. Any intra-articular pathology can also be addressed arthroscopically.

METHODS

An English literature review in PubMed and Cochrane databases included the MeSH term, "'*Tennis Elbow/complications*'[Mesh] OR '*Tennis Elbow/surgery*'[Mesh]", which included a tree of "Elbow, Tennis", "Elbows, Tennis", "Tennis Elbows", "Epicondylitis, Lateral Humeral", "Epicondylitides, Lateral Humeral", "Humeral Epicondylitides, Lateral", "Humeral Epicondylitis, Lateral", "Lateral Humeral Epicondylitides", and "Lateral Humeral Epicondylitis"; 214 articles, including case reports, were identified and the abstracts reviewed; and 91 articles seemed relevant. The following were excluded: ex vivo studies (3 articles), review articles, or technique guides (8), not studies of lateral epicondylar release (16), and studies with longer-term follow-up on the same cohort of patients (1). This search resulted in 63 articles available for review. Inspection of article references identified 10 additional articles (**Fig. 4**).

Seven studies included medial and lateral epicondyle releases, but only 2 differentiated the results for each.[53,56] See **Table 1** for results of 5 excluded studies. In those 2 studies, the results for only the lateral epicondyle release were used

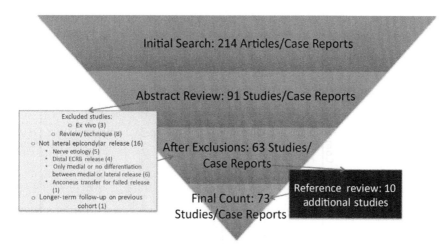

Fig. 4. Flowsheet: details of article search.

in this review. Two other studies compared a studied modality (open, percutaneous, or arthroscopic lateral epicondylar release) to one that is not part of this review.[62,63] In those studies, only the procedures for the studied modality were used in this review. Lastly, a study by Cummins[64] involved an arthroscopic treatment followed by an open treatment to assess the adequacy of arthroscopic débridement. This study is included in both arthroscopic and open procedures review.

Despite only 1 study[9] reporting carpal tunnel syndrome as a late complication, the 2 instances were kept as recorded complication. Residual symptoms, incomplete pain relief, and need for repeat procedures are reported as complications in 2 studies[40,53] totaling 7 complications. Other studies mentioned these complaints as sequelae but not complications.[50,65] The rest of the studies classified these complaints as failures of treatment as opposed to complications. For this reason, they are not included as complications in this review. Residual symptoms, incomplete pain relief, and need for repeat procedures are differentiated from new symptoms at the incision site, which is included as a complication.

RESULTS

There were 67 studies identified and they were divided into open procedures (**Table 2** – 36 studies), percutaneous procedures (**Table 3** – 11 studies), arthroscopic procedures (**Table 4** – 12 studies), and comparative studies (**Table 5** – 9 studies). An additional 6 case reports/studies (**Table 6**) identifying specific complications from lateral epicondylar release were identified. Dates of the studies ranged from 1965 to 2015. Of the 67 articles, 5 were level 1 studies (randomized

controlled trials [RTCs]), 1 level 2 study (prospective cohort study), 8 level 3 studies (retrospective cohorts or case control studies), and 53 studies level 4 studies (case studies). All complications are summarized in **Table 7**.

Total reported complications excluding case reports are 113 and total procedures are 3436, for a complication rate of 3.3%. For all open procedures, the complication rate is 95/2209 (4.3%), percutaneous procedures 11/567 (1.9%), and arthroscopic procedures 7/660 (1.1%).

The comparative studies complication rates were 3/226 (1.3%) for open procedures, 4/332 (1.2%) for arthroscopic procedures, and 0/106 (0%) for percutaneous procedures (**Table 8**). The 3 open procedure complications were 1 suture granuloma, 1 dystrophy, and 1 instance of complex regional pain syndrome (CRPS). The 4 complications in the arthroscopic procedures were 1 superficial infection, 1 deep infection, 1 hematoma, and 1 CRPS.

The rate of complication becomes even smaller by adding all studies with quality level 3 or higher. In the remaining level 3 or higher studies that were not part of comparative studies, there were no additional complications reported, showing a combined complication rate of only 3/388 (0.8%) for open procedures and 4/395 (1.0%) for arthroscopic procedures. No additional procedures were noted for the percutaneous procedures, keeping the rate 0/106 (0%).

Twenty-four distinct complications were identified (see **Table 7**). These were grouped into the following complication categories: wound, infection, loss of range of motion, nerve, elbow instability, ipsilateral arm issues, and ectopic bone. The most common complication was neurologic at 41/113 (36.3%). The second most common

Table 1
Studies with both medial and lateral epicondylar release not differentiating outcomes between the two

Surgery	Author	Study Type	Number of Patients/Procedures — Patients/Procedures at Follow-Up (if Different)	Average Follow-up	Complications	Complications/Operations
CEO release (included medial and lateral epicondylitis)	Spencer & Herndon,[59] 1953	Case series	49 procedures; 43 LE, 6 ME	13.5 mo	2 Hematomas	2/49 (Unclear if ME or LE)
Débridement and repair/medial and lateral epicondylitis	Coonrad & Hooper,[42] 1973	Case series	39 Patients	1–9 y	None	0/39 (Unclear if ME or LE)
Both medial and lateral epicondylitis / Denervation / Open Boyd-McLeod–type procedure	Wittenberg et al,[60] 1992	Retrospective cohort study	86 Procedures; 78 patients/80 procedures; 51 Denervation; 27 Open procedure	—	1 Superficial infection; 2 Hematomas; 3 Severe swelling; 4 Hypertrophic scars	10/80, Not including 1 unstable elbow attributed to prior LE surgery (unclear if ME or LE)
Miniopen Nirschl-type on both medial and lateral epicondylitis	Cho et al,[41] 2009	Case series	41 patients/42 procedures; 32 were LE	13.4 mo	2 Seromas from leakage of joint fluid (managed surgically)	2/42 (Unclear if ME or LE)
Nirschl-type (concurrent medial and lateral epicondylitis)	Schipper et al (Nirschl, senior author),[61] 2011	Case series	92 patients/102 procedures; 48 patients/53 procedures	11.7 y	1 Surgical site infection requiring surgery	1/53 (Unclear of ME or LE)

Data from Refs.[41,42,59–61]

Table 2
Open lateral epicondyle release procedures

Open Lateral Epicondyle Surgery	Author	Study Type	Number of Patients/Procedures at Follow-up — Patients/Procedures (if Different) — Average Follow-up	Complications	Complications/ Procedures
1. Transverse division of CEO	Bosworth,[40] 1965	Case series	16 (Variable follow-up)	None	—
2. (1) + Displacement of orbicular ligament, removal of synovial fringe			2 (11 and 17 y)	None	—
3. (1) + Resection of orbicular ligament			16 (Variable follow-up)	2 Residual pain, 3 weakness of grasp (2 of which had cramping)	5/15
4. Vertical incision of CEO with resection of orbicular ligament and repair of CEO			28 (Variable follow-up)	1 With weakness/cramping	1/28
Modification of Bosworth (AL removed + lateral epicondylectomy)	Boyd & McLeod,[35] 1973	Case series	37 (41 procedures) — Variable follow-up	None	0/41
CEO release (as described by Hohmann in 1933)	Posch et al,[48] 1978	Case series	67 procedures 35/43 8.0 y	2 With sterile wound drainage, recovered without intervention	2/35
ECRB débridement and LE decortication	Nirschl & Pettrone,[5] 1979	Case series	82 — 25 mo	1 Superficial *Staphylococcus aureus* infection treated with antibiotics 1 Deep infection requiring drainage 1 Patient lacked 7° elbow extension	3/82
CEO release	Calvert,[37] 1985	Case series	32/37 — 37 mo	1 Scar sensitivity	1/37

(continued on next page)

Table 2
(continued)

Open Lateral Epicondyle Surgery	Author	Study Type	Number of Patients/Procedures: Patients/Procedures at Follow-up (if Different)	Average Follow-up	Complications	Complications/Procedures
CEO release	Goldberg et al,[66] 1988	Case series	30/37 27/30	48 mo	None	0/30
CEO release + decortication of LE	Doran et al,[6] 1990	Case series[a]	20/22 18/20	2 y	5 With residual tenderness 3 Elbows with limited extension <10°	8/20
Revision open surgery	Morrey,[22] 1992	Case series	13 —	1 y	At time of revision: 3 with PLRI 1 Synovial fistula 1 Adventitial bursa	5/13 Revision cases
CEO release	Verhaar et al,[45] 1993	Case series	62 Available 1 y 57 Available at 5 y	59 mo	— 1 *Staphylococcus aureus* infection treated with antibiotics — —	1/62
CEO release	Newey & Patterson,[67] 1994	Case series	28 —	29.6 mo	1 *Staphylococcus aureus* infection 2 Complaints of weakness	3/28
Limited open débridement Wide débridement with anconeus transfer	Almquist et al,[38] 1998	Retrospective cohort	16 31		None	0/61 Of revisions: 2 with continued 65° flexion contracture
Wide débridement with anconeus transfer in revision setting			14	48 mo	— 18/61 Had rupture of LUCL at time of surgery	

Procedure	Study	Type	Numbers / Follow-up	Complications	Ratio
CEO release	Bankes & Jessop,[39] 1998	Case series	24 / 20 / 16 mo	1 Wound infection treated with antibiotics; 5 With tenderness; 3 With numbness; 7 With loss of forearm rotation <15°	16/20
Variable open procedures	Thurston,[10] 1998	Retrospective cohort study	78 / — / Unclear follow-up	None	0/78
Nirschl release + LE drilling	Khashaba,[49] 2001	RCT	18/23	None	0/23
Nirschl release − LE drilling			— / 6 mo	None	
ECRB V-Y release	Rayan & Coray,[68] 2001	Case series	22/23 / — / 41 mo	Cold intolerance: 5 mild and 1 moderate; 1 Hematoma requiring drainage; 1 With slow resolving elbow stiffness	8/23
Nirschl-type with repair	Rosenberg & Henderson,[69] 2002	Case series	22 / 19 / 2–9 y	None	0/19
CEO release +/− drilling LE	Das & Maffulli,[50] 2002	Case series	111/125 / 87 / 52.8 mo	None	0/125 (Although at 2 wk 30 elbows were tender, 14 stiff, and 1 had instability, all resolved by 6 wk)
ECRB release	Balk et al,[70] 2005	Case series	90/97 / 57/63 / 51 mo	1 PIN palsy requiring subsequent release	1/63
Revision CEO release + anconeus transfer (similar to Almquist et al[38])	Degreef et al,[51] 2005	Case series	10 / — / Minimum of 1 y follow-up	1 Superficial infection	1/10
ECRB débridement and repair with suture anchors	Thornton et al,[52] 2005	Case series	24/26 / 20/22 / 4.1 y	None reported	0/22

(continued on next page)

Table 2
(continued)

Open Lateral Epicondyle Surgery	Author	Study Type	Number of Patients/Procedures		Complications	Complications/Procedures
			Average Follow-up	Patients/Procedures at Follow-up (if Different)		
Arthroscopic LE débridement followed by open procedure to assess débridement	Cummins,[64] 2006	Case series	18 — 21.6 mo		None	0/18
Nirschl-type	Plancher & Bishai,[71] 2006	Case series	38 — Variable follow-up		None reported	0/38
CEO release	Svernlov & Adolfsson,[72] 2006	Case series	53/55 51/53 90 mo		None	0/53
Nirschl-type	Zingg & Schneeberger,[73] 2006	Case Series	22 21 15 mo		1 Hematoma requiring aspiration 1 Frozen shoulder (fibromyalgia patient)	2/21
CEO release	Thomas & Broome,[74] 2007	Case series	18/24 — 6 mo		None	0/24
Nirschl-type	Dunn et al,[75] 2008	Case series	130/139 83/92 12.6 y		None	0/92
Nirschl-type with repair	Pruzansky et al,[7] 2009	Case series	26/28 22/24 64.7 mo		1 Ipsilateral subacromial bursitis treated nonoperatively	1/24
Nirschl-type	Coleman et al,[76] 2010	Case series	158/171 137/149 9.8 y		2 Synovial fistula 4 Loss of elbow extension mean 15°	6/149

Procedure	Author/Year	Study type	No. / Follow-up	Complications	Total
Nirschl-type with repair	Dwyer et al,[77] 2010	Case series	22 21 24 mo	None	0/21
CEO release	Rayan et al,[78] 2010	Case series	40 — 12 mo	None	0/40
ECRB release + PIN release	Bigorre et al,[79] 2011	Case series	28/30 — 21.8 mo	None	0/30
Boyd-McLeod–type procedure	Reddy et al,[33] 2011	Case Series	27/29 — 16 mo	1 Ectopic bone formation and was excised 2 Scar tenderness	3/29
CEO release + decortication of LE	Solheim et al,[34] 2011	Case series	77/80 — 4 y	3 Superficial wound problem/infection 1 Hematoma requiring drainage	4/80
CEO release	Barth et al,[80] 2013	Case series	49/54 44/49 33 mo	1 Hematoma requiring drainage 1 Superficial infection treated without surgery	2/49
CEO release	Cusco et al,[9] 2013	Case series	405 — 6 mo	Early: 1 infection 1 Seroma 10 Cicatrial fibrosis 4 Radial sensory neuritis 2 Reactive dermatitis Late: 1 Frohse arcade syndrome 2 Carpal tunnel syndrome	21/405
CEO + supinator/PIN release	Manon-Matos et al,[44] 2013	Case series	56 — Minimum of 6 mo	None	0/56

[a] Note: prospective cohort study of histology for lateral epicondylar release. Report of clinical results is case series.
Data from Refs.[5–7,9,10,22,33–35,37–40,44,45,48–52,64,66–80]

Table 3
Percutaneous procedures

Percutaneous	Author	Study Type	Number of Patients/Procedures		Complications	Complications/ Operations
			Patients/Procedures at Follow-up (if Different)	Average Follow-up		
Percutaneous release (37 LE and 6 ME cases)	Baumgard & Schwartz,[53] 1982	Case series	32/37 LE — 35 mo		3 With residual band 2 Required repeat procedure (not included in complications for review)	0/37
Percutaneous	Yerger & Turner,[81] 1985	Case series	144/149 — 109 procedures followed up 1–11 y		4 Synovial fistulas, healed without surgery 2 Superficial infections, no surgery	6/149
Percutaneous	Grundberg & Dobson,[82] 2000	Case series	34/38 30/32 26 mo		2 Hematomas (began to leave wound open after these complications and no further hematomas developed)	2/32
Percutaneous	Kaleli et al,[83] 2004	Case series	26 — 32 mo		None	0/26
Microtenotomy with radiofrequency probe	Tasto et al,[54] 2005	Case series	13 — 24 mo		None	0/13

Percutaneous	McShane et al,[84] 2006	Case series	58 55 9 mo	None	0/55
Percutaneous	McShane et al,[85] 2008	Case series	57 52 22 mo	None	0/52
Percutaneous ultrasound radiofrequency lesioning	Lin et al,[55] 2011	Case series	34/35 — 14.3 mo	2 Patients with ecchymosis at 1 wk	2/35
Percutaneous	Nazar et al,[86] 2012	Case series	24/30 26 procedures 36 mo	1 Hematoma	1/30
Percutaneous microresection	Koh et al,[57] 2013	Case series	20 — 12 mo	None	0/20
Percutaneous microresection	Barnes et al,[56] 2015	Case series	19 (12 with LE, 7 ME) 12 mo	None	0/12

Data from Refs.[53–57,81–86]

Table 4
Arthroscopic procedures

Arthroscopic	Author	Study Type	Number of Patients/Procedures Patients/Procedures at Follow-up (if Different) Average Follow-up	Complications	Complications/ Procedures
ECRB débridement +/− decortication	Baker et al,[58] 2000	Case series	40/42 37/39 2.8 y	None	0/42
ECRB débridement and LE decortication	Owens et al,[87] 2001	Case series	16 12 24.1 mo	None	0/16
ECRB débridement	Mullett et al,[88] 2005	Case series	30 — 2 y	None	0/30
ECRB débridement (followed by open assessment)	Cummins,[64] 2006	Case series	18 — 21.6 mo	None	0/18
ECRB débridement and decortication	Jerosch & Schunck,[89] 2006	Case series	20 — 1.8 y	None	0/20
Extra-articular arthroscopic lateral release	Brooks-Hill & Regan,[90] 2008	Case series	20 — Follow-up not defined	None	0/20

Procedure	Study	Design	N / Follow-up	Complications	Incidence
ECRB débridement	Grewal et al,[91] 2009	Case series	48 / 36 / 42 mo	1 Erythema around portals treated with antibiotics	1/36
ECRB débridement	Lattermann et al,[92] 2010	Case series	36 / 32 / 3.5 y	1 Subjective forearm paresthesia resolved after 2 wk	1/36
Arthroscopic ECRB release without decortication	Kim et al,[93] 2011	Retrospective cohort	19 / —	None	0/19
Arthroscopic ECRB release with decortication			19 / 25.2/31.2 mo	None	0/19
Not specified	Marti et al,[94] 2013	Case series	100 / 24 For tennis elbow / Minimum 12 mo	1 Ulnar sensory neuropraxia ×6 mo	1/24
ECRB débridement	Kniesel et al,[95] 2014	Retrospective cohort	40 Total (15 patients with some elbow instability treated with LUCL reconstruction) 25 Just arthroscopically / Minimum of 1 y	None	0/25
ECRB débridement	Oki et al,[96] 2014	Case series	23 / — / 24 mo	None	0/23

Data from Refs.[58,64,87–96]

Table 5
Comparative studies

Comparative	Author	Study Type	Number of Patients/Procedures at Follow-up (if Different) — Follow-up	Complications	Complications/Procedures
PIN neurolysis*	Leppilahti et al,[62] 2001	RCT	13/14	None (6 with local tenderness)	0/14
ECRB release			13/14 — 31 mo	None (8 with local tenderness)	0/14
ECRB débridement with LE drilling	Dunkow et al,[97] 2004	—	24	None	0/24
Percutaneous	—	RCT	23 — 12 mo	None	0/23
Modified Nirschl	Peart et al,[32] 2004	Retrospective cohort	54 procedures 46	None	0/46
Arthroscopic (ECRB + decortication)			33 procedures 29 37 mo	1 Deep infection	1/29
ECRB release	Rubenthaler et al,[98] 2005	Retrospective cohort	13 10	None	0/10
Arthroscopic (ECRB/CEO release)			24 20 92.8 mo	1 Superficial infection 1 Hematoma	2/20

Technique	Author	Study type	N	Follow-up	Complications	Additional surgery
Modified Nirschl	Szabo et al,[65] 2006	Retrospective cohort	41	—	1 CRPS 1 Dystrophy	3/41 (5 Recurred, 2 additional surgery)
Arthroscopic (ECRB + decortication)			44	—	1 Suture granuloma 1 CRPS	1/44 (2 Recurred, 1 additional surgery)
Percutaneous			24	47.8 mo	None	0/24 (3 Additional surgery, performed open)
Nirschl-type	Meknas et al,[99] 2008	RCT	11	—	None	0/11
Radiofrequency microtenotomy			13	10–18 mo	None	0/13
Extracorporeal shockwave therapy*	Radwan et al,[63] 2008	RCT	29	—	1 Temporary paresthesia 2 Temporary myalgias	(3/29)
Percutaneous			27	12 mo	None	0/27
Arthroscopic (CEO release + decortication)	Othman,[100] 2011	Prospective cohort	14	—	None	0/14
Percutaneous			19	12/10 mo	None	0/19
Arthroscopic (ECRB release)	Solheim et al,[101] 2013	Case control series	225	—	None	0/225
CEO release			80	Minimum 3 y	None	0/80
			—		—	

Note: studies with * are of modality not included in this review.
Data from Refs.[32,62,63,65,97–101]

Table 6
Case reports

Study	Report of Complication	Author	Complications
Case report	Lateral epicondylectomy	Cushing et al,[102] 2001	1 Heterotopic ossification
Case report	Lateral osteophyte resection and débridement and reattachment of ECRB with 2 suture anchors	Shapiro & Weiland,[103] 2002	1 Heterotopic ossification
Case series	Open procedures	Dellon et al,[17] 2004	9 Painful neuromas of posterior cutaneous nerve of the forearm Study details treatment with neuroma excision
Case report	Débridement of common extensor tendon	Degreef & De Smet,[20] 2007	Chronic elbow posterolateral dislocation
Case series	Arthroscopic	Carofino et al,[104] 2012	1 Complete injury to PIN 1 Partial median nerve injury (temporary sensory, complete anterior interosseous nerve)
Case report	Open procedure	Iyer,[105] 2014	1 Injury to PABCN

Data from Refs.[17,20,102–105]

was wound related at 34/113 (30.1%). Infections were 16/113 (14.2%) and loss of range of 16/113 (14.2%), making these 4 categories 94.6% of the reported complications.

Percutaneous procedures only had complications involving infection (2 instances) and wound issues (4 synovial fistulas, 3 hematomas, and 2 ecchymosis). There were no complications involving the other categories. Similarly, arthroscopic procedures only had infection issues (3 total), wound issues (1 hematoma), and nerve issues (1 forearm paresthesia, 1 ulnar sensory deficit, and 1 CRPS). Range-of-motion issues, instability, ipsilateral arm complications, and ectopic bone were only reported in open procedures.

In the 6 case reports/studies, the complications were 2 ectopic bone formation, 10 injuries to the PABCN, and 1 chronic posterolateral elbow dislocation after open procedures. There were 2 permanent nerve injuries documented after arthroscopic treatment. These injuries were 1 complete PIN injury and 1 partial median nerve injury.

DISCUSSION

The overall complication rate is low for lateral epicondylar release. Descriptions of complications were diverse and this article placed these complications into 8 broad categories. Complications from percutaneous procedures only involved 2 of these categories, arthroscopic 3 and open all 8.

Open approaches are more invasive and for that reason higher risk for complication would be expected. This impression is not confirmed, however, when looking at more recent, higher-quality studies, which show complication rates of open and arthroscopic essentially the same. In those higher-quality studies, a complication in a percutaneous procedure has yet to be reported, but there are fewer procedures reported. This review article does not take into account success rates of surgery.

The only other review article that described complications rates is the quantitative review article by Karkhanis and colleagues[106] which identified a mean complication rate of 10.6% for open procedures, 6.3% for percutaneous methods, and no reported complications for arthroscopic methods. They had identified 45 articles in their review whereas 67 articles were used in this review.

The types of complications reported fit into known risks of surgery and surgery about the elbow. The vast majority (94.6%) of the complications fell into the categories of nerve injury, wound issues, infection, and loss of range of motion. All surgeries carry the risks of infection, healing problems, and damage to surrounding neurovascular structure, and the elbow is notorious for becoming stiff postsurgically. Unexpected complications include ipsilateral frozen shoulder (in a fibromyalgia patient), subacromial bursitis, and carpal tunnel syndrome. These accounted for 3.5% of total

Table 7
Summary of complications of all studies

Complication	Open	Percutaneous	Arthroscopic	Total	Citation – No. of Instances if Greater Than 1
Nerve (total)	38	0	3	41	
Scar sensitivity	13			13	$5^{6,37}, 5^{39}, 2^{33}$
Dystrophy	1			1	65
Weakness	6			6	$4^{40}, 2^{67}$
Numbness	3			3	3^{39}
Cold intolerance	6			6	6^{68}
Nerve injury/neuritis	8		2	10	$7^{9,70}$, 92,94
CRPS	1		1	2	65,65
Wound (total)	24	9	1	34	
Suture granuloma	1			1	65
Reactive dermatitis	2			2	2^{9}
Synovial fistula	3	4		7	$2^{22,76}, 4^{81}$
Wound drainage	2			2	2^{48}
Seroma	1			1	9
Hematoma	4	3	1	8	$2^{34,68,73,80,82}$ 86,98
Ecchymosis		2		2	2^{55}
Adventitial bursa	1			1	22
Cicatrial fibrosis	10			10	10^{9}
Infection (total)	11	2	3	16	
Superficial	10	2	2	14	$3^{5,34,39,45,51,67}, 2^{9,80,81}$ 91,98
Deep	1		1	2	5,32
Range of motion (total)	16	0	0	16	
Flexion contracture	9			9	$3^{5,6}, 4^{68,76}$
Loss of forearm rotation	7			7	7^{39}
Instability (total)	3	0	0	3	
Posterolateral instability	3			3	3^{22}
Ipsilateral arm (total)	2	0	0	2	
Frozen shoulder	1			1	73
Subacromial bursitis	1			1	7
Ectopic bone (total)	1	0	0	1	
Ectopic bone	1			1	33
All complications	95	11	7	113	
All procedures	2209	567	660	3436	
Complication rate (%)	4.3	1.9	1.1	3.3	
Nerve rate (%)	40.0	0.0	42.9	36.3	
Wound rate (%)	25.3	81.8	14.3	30.1	
Infection rate (%)	11.6	18.2	42.9	14.2	
Range-of-motion rate (%)	16.8	0.0	0.0	14.2	
Instability rate (%)	3.2	0.0	0.0	2.7	
Ipsilateral arm rate (%)	2.1	0.0	0.0	1.8	
Ectopic bone rate (%)	1.1	0.0	0.0	0.9	

Note: orange for open, purple for percutaneous, blue for arthroscopic, and green for total procedures.
Data from Refs.[5–7,9,22,32–34,37,39,40,45,48,51,55,65,67,68,70,73,76,80–82,86,91,92,94,98]

reported complications and, if truly associated with lateral epicondylar release, are rare.

An infection rate of 16/3436 (0.5%) is comparable to similar surgeries, such as shoulder arthroscopy[107] or cubital tunnel release.[108] An infection requiring surgery (deep infection) was reported once for both an open[5] and an arthroscopic procedure.[32] The specific infection rates for open (0.4%), percutaneous (0.4%), and arthroscopic procedures (0.5%) are all low and do not seem to pertain to any increased risk for the specific procedure. Although a specific study regarding prophylactic antibiosis for treatment of tennis elbow has not been performed, it should be considered standard of care. In this review, no specific patient risk factors were identified for increased rates of

Table 8
Summary of complications within comparative studies

Complication	Open	Percutaneous	Arthroscopic	Total	Citation
Nerve (total)	2	0	1	3	
Dystrophy	1			1	63
CRPS	1		1	2	63,63
Wound (total)	1	0	1	2	
Suture granuloma	1			1	63
Ecchymosis			1	1	96
Infection (total)	0	0	2	2	
Superficial			1	1	96
Deep			1	1	30
All complications	3	0	4	7	
All procedures	226	106	332	664	
Complication rate (%)	1.3	0.0	1.2	1.1	
Nerve rate (%)	66.7	0	25	42.9	
Wound rate (%)	33.3	0	25	28.6	
Infection rate (%)	0	0	50	28.6	

Note: orange for open, purple for percutaneous, blue for arthroscopic, and green for total procedures.
Data from Refs.[30,63,96]

infection, but accounting for any may reduce chances of infection.

Wound issues were most frequent in the percutaneous group (9/11 percutaneous complications, 81.8%), but these included inconsequential ecchymoses and hematomas that did not require additional intervention. Open procedures had 24 wound-related complications (24/95, 25.3% of open complications) although 10 of them were from significant scarring or cicatricial fibrosis, all noted in a single large case series.[9] It makes intuitive sense that with more trauma to the surgical area there are more associated complications. When looking at the comparative studies, however, wound issues were recorded only twice – none in percutaneous, 1 in an open (suture granuloma), and 1 in an arthroscopic procedure (hematoma).

The category of neurologic injury had a more admittedly subjective classification as dictated by the subjective nature of the reporting. The reported complications, such as scar sensitivity, dystrophy, weakness, and cold intolerance, are examples likely of neurologic cause but cannot be definitively stated. A likely explanation for scar sensitivity or wound tenderness is cutaneous neuroma. Dellon and colleagues[17] identified 9 patients with painful neuromas of the posterior cutaneous nerve of the forearm within scars for lateral epicondylitis surgery. Iyer[105] also identified this complication in a case report. Cusco and colleagues[9]

did report on 4 instances of "radial sensory neuritis." This is likely an underappreciated source of pain in patients with scar tenderness. The report of dystrophy was not further defined in the article reporting it[65] but resulted in a failure of open surgery. It was categorized along with CRPS as a reason for failure and thus is included in the neurologic complications. Weakness is described as a complication 6 times (6/113, 5.3%) but as a subjective complaint, and no objective measurements of strength were performed in the studies reporting it. Three of these patients were noted to have associated cramping. A possible cause of this complication is an alteration of muscle mechanics after release. A study by Friden and Lieber,[109] however, argued that releasing the ECRB and decreasing its resting tension could actually increase its active force. Furthermore, nearly all studies that objectively measured strength report its near or full return after successful treatment,[110] adding to the evidence that the altered muscle properties, if present, did not contribute to weakness. It could be residual pain limiting strength, which would be a failure of treatment, but was not recorded that way.

Direct nerve injuries were not as prevalent in the reported literature other than the PABCN injuries (discussed previously). Only 1 study[70] reported early injury to the PIN after an open release whereas another reported a late PIN complication.[9] Only 2 nerve injuries were identified in the arthroscopic literature (1 temporary forearm paresthesia[92] and 1 temporary ulnar sensory neuropraxia[94]), although it is likely underreported. A recent survey of American Society for Surgery of the Hand membership who performed elbow arthroscopy received 349 responses reporting 190 nerve injuries, with 67% having limited or no recovery.[111] Carofino and colleagues[104] discuss 2 cases of permanent nerve injury as a result of arthroscopic lateral epicondylar release. These injuries were a complete PIN and a partial median nerve injury with temporary sensory deficits and complete loss of the anterior interosseous nerve function. These case reports doubled the amount of reported nerve injury associated with arthroscopic lateral epicondylar release. To prevent neurologic injury during open procedures, the PABCN should be located immediately after making skin incision[17] and caution should be exercised with dissection anterior and medial to the extensor musculature to avoid injury to the radial nerve or its branches. For arthroscopic procedures, the nick-and-spread technique should be used to avoid cutaneous nerve injuries. Using a proximal lateral portal is the safest lateral portal with respect to the radial nerve, but caution should still be used with trocar placement and use of shavers or cautery avoiding distal and anterior locations.[23,26,92,104] With placement of the anteromedial portal, similar caution must be exercised to prevent injury to the MABCN and median nerve. Placing the portal posterior to the medial intermuscular septum would endanger the ulnar nerve.[24,25,27]

Elbow stiffness or loss of range of motion is often self-limited, although a therapy program may prevent this complication. Less-invasive procedures may decrease stiffness, but other patient factors, including compliance with a home exercise plan and pain tolerance, likely also play a role. A literature search did not reveal any specific studies for postoperative rehabilitation after lateral epicondylar release.

PRLI is only identified as a result of lateral epicondyle release in the study by Morrey,[22] who treated 13 refractory tennis elbow cases, 3 of which he attributed new symptoms to PRLI after their initial surgery. A case report by Degreef and De Smet[20] also identified a chronic posterolateral elbow dislocation after a lateral epicondyle release. Other studies have noted obvious or occult elbow instability associated with tennis elbow, but it was noted either without or prior to lateral epicondylar release.[21,22,38,60,95,112] A study by Almquist and colleagues[38] identified 18 of 61 patients with rupture of the LUCL at the time of surgery. PRLI should be considered in cases of failure of operative or nonoperative treatment of tennis elbow. To prevent PRLI, releasing posterior to the anterior half of the lateral epicondyle (open) or radiocapitellar joint (arthroscopic) must be avoided.

Another complication that is rare in the literature but may also be underreported is the formation of heterotopic bone. Only 1 study reported this complication[33] and it was treated with excision. Two case reports, however, identified the complication.[102,103] The procedures that resulted in the heterotopic bone formation involved open bone drilling or lateral epicondylectomy. Other risk factors could not be specifically noted from these reports. Other interventions such as nonsteroidal anti-inflammatory drugs and their risks, should be weighed against potential patient risk factors.

SUMMARY

Lateral epicondylar release is a procedure that has been documented in literature for more than 80 years.[43] There remains a paucity of quality studies on the topic, but in recent years more quality studies have allowed better comparisons between the various techniques and reporting of outcomes. Heterogeneous outcome reporting and complications described in subjective terms make data extraction for a review difficult. That noted, the success rate in treatment of lateral epicondylitis is approximately 80% to 90% regardless of treatment modality.[106,110] Higher success rates will likely hinge on understanding the true etiology of the disease.

Nerve injury remains the most problematic complication after lateral epicondylitis surgical management. These injuries, especially those resulting in partial or total low radial nerve palsy, are probably more prevalent than the literature suggests. Elbow instability can result from an overly aggressive lateral epicondylar release, and a history of traumatic onset warrants an evaluation for posterolateral elbow instability during the surgical procedure.

Based on this review, it seems that complications make a small contribution to the failure rate. It seems that percutaneous procedures have the lowest rate of complication, but further comparative research is necessary. This review cannot make specific recommendations on superiority of open, percutaneous versus arthroscopic procedures, because all seem to have both low failure and complication rates.

REFERENCES

1. Verhaar JA. Tennis elbow. Anatomical, epidemiological and therapeutic aspects. Int Orthop 1994; 18(5):263–7.

2. De Smedt T, de Jong A, Van Leemput W, et al. Lateral epicondylitis in tennis: update on aetiology, biomechanics and treatment. Br J Sports Med 2007;41(11):816–9.

3. Runge F. Zur genese und behandlung des schreibekrampfes. Berl Klin Wochenschr 1873;10:245–8.

4. Major H. Lawn-tennis elbow. Br Med J 1883;2:557.

5. Nirschl RP, Pettrone FA. Tennis elbow. The surgical treatment of lateral epicondylitis. J Bone Joint Surg Am 1979;61(6A):832–9.

6. Doran A, Gresham GA, Rushton N, et al. Tennis elbow. A clinicopathologic study of 22 cases followed for 2 years. Acta Orthop Scand 1990;61(6):535–8.

7. Pruzansky ME, Gantsoudes GD, Watters N. Late surgical results of reattachment to bone in repair of chronic lateral epicondylitis. Am J Orthop (Belle Mead NJ) 2009;38(6):295–9.

8. Smidt N, Lewis M, VAN DER Windt DA, et al. Lateral epicondylitis in general practice: course and prognostic indicators of outcome. J Rheumatol 2006; 33(10):2053–9.

9. Cusco X, Alsina M, Seijas R, et al. Proximal disinsertion of the common extensor tendon for lateral elbow tendinopathy. J Orthop Surg (Hong Kong) 2013;21(1):100–2.

10. Thurston AJ. Conservative and surgical treatment of tennis elbow: a study of outcome. Aust N Z J Surg 1998;68(8):568–72.

11. Wilhelm A, Gieseler H. Treatment of radiohumeral epicondylitis by denervation. Chirurg 1962;33: 118–22 [in German].

12. Wilhelm A. Tennis elbow: treatment of resistant cases by denervation. J Hand Surg Br 1996; 21(4):523–33.

13. Botte MJ, Doyle JR. Surgical anatomy of the hand and upper extremity. Philadelphia: Lippincott Williams & Wilkins; 2003.

14. Boyer MI, Hastings H 2nd. Lateral tennis elbow: "Is there any science out there?". J Shoulder Elbow Surg 1999;8(5):481–91.

15. Greenbaum B, Itamura J, Vangsness CT, et al. Extensor carpi radialis brevis. An anatomical analysis of its origin. J Bone Joint Surg Br 1999;81(5):926–9.

16. Cohen MS, Romeo AA, Hennigan SP, et al. Lateral epicondylitis: anatomic relationships of the extensor tendon origins and implications for arthroscopic treatment. J Shoulder Elbow Surg 2008; 17(6):954–60.

17. Dellon AL, Kim J, Ducic I. Painful neuroma of the posterior cutaneous nerve of the forearm after surgery for lateral humeral epicondylitis. J Hand Surg Am 2004;29(3):387–90.

18. Diliberti T, Botte MJ, Abrams RA. Anatomical considerations regarding the posterior interosseous nerve during posterolateral approaches to the proximal part of the radius*. J Bone Joint Surg Am 2000;82(6):809–13.

19. Morrey BF, An KN. Functional anatomy of the ligaments of the elbow. Clin Orthop Relat Res 1985;(201):84–90.

20. Degreef I, De Smet L. Chronic elbow dislocation: a rare complication of tennis elbow surgery. Successful treatment by open reduction and external fixator. Chir Main 2007;26(3):150–3.

21. Kalainov DM, Cohen MS. Posterolateral rotatory instability of the elbow in association with lateral epicondylitis. A report of three cases. J Bone Joint Surg Am 2005;87(5):1120–5.

22. Morrey BF. Reoperation for failed surgical treatment of refractory lateral epicondylitis. J Shoulder Elbow Surg 1992;1(1):47–55.

23. Baker CL Jr, Jones GL. Arthroscopy of the elbow. Am J Sports Med 1999;27(2):251–64.

24. Kuklo TR, Taylor KF, Murphy KP, et al. Arthroscopic release for lateral epicondylitis: a cadaveric model. Arthroscopy 1999;15(3):259–64.

25. Lindenfeld TN. Medial approach in elbow arthroscopy. Am J Sports Med 1990;18(4):413–7.

26. Lynch GJ, Meyers JF, Whipple TL, et al. Neurovascular anatomy and elbow arthroscopy: inherent risks. Arthroscopy 1986;2(3):190–7.

27. Stothers K, Day B, Regan WR. Arthroscopy of the elbow: anatomy, portal sites, and a description of the proximal lateral portal. Arthroscopy 1995; 11(4):449–57.

28. Miller CD, Jobe CM, Wright MH. Neuroanatomy in elbow arthroscopy. J Shoulder Elbow Surg 1995; 4(3):168–74.

29. Field LD, Altchek DW, Warren RF, et al. Arthroscopic anatomy of the lateral elbow: a comparison of three portals. Arthroscopy 1994;10(6):602–7.

30. Omid R, Hamid N, Keener JD, et al. Relation of the radial nerve to the anterior capsule of the elbow: anatomy with correlation to arthroscopy. Arthroscopy 2012;28(12):1800–4.

31. Greco S, Nellans KW, Levine WN. Lateral epicondylitis: open versus arthroscopic. Oper Tech Orthop 2009;19(4):228–34.

32. Peart RE, Strickler SS, Schweitzer KM Jr. Lateral epicondylitis: a comparative study of open and arthroscopic lateral release. Am J Orthop (Belle Mead NJ) 2004;33(11):565–7.

33. Reddy VR, Satheesan KS, Bayliss N. Outcome of Boyd-McLeod procedure for recalcitrant lateral epicondylitis of elbow. Rheumatol Int 2011;31(8): 1081–4.

34. Solheim E, Hegna J, Oyen J. Extensor tendon release in tennis elbow: results and prognostic factors in 80 elbows. Knee Surg Sports Traumatol Arthrosc 2011;19(6):1023–7.

35. Boyd HB, McLeod AC Jr. Tennis elbow. J Bone Joint Surg Am 1973;55(6):1183–7.

36. Garden R. Tennis Elbow. J Bone Joint Surg Br 1961;43B(1):100–6.

37. Calvert PT, Allum RL, Macpherson IS, et al. Simple lateral release in treatment of tennis elbow. J R Soc Med 1985;78(11):912–5.

38. Almquist EE, Necking L, Bach AW. Epicondylar resection with anconeus muscle transfer for chronic lateral epicondylitis. J Hand Surg Am 1998;23(4):723–31.

39. Dankes MJ, Jessop JH. Day-case simple extensor origin release for tennis elbow. Arch Orthop Trauma Surg 1998;117(4–5):250–1.

40. Bosworth DM. Surgical treatment of tennis elbow; a follow-up study. J Bone Joint Surg Am 1965;47(8): 1533–6.

41. Cho BK, Kim YM, Kim DS, et al. Mini-open muscle resection procedure under local anesthesia for lateral and medial epicondylitis. Clin Orthop Surg 2009;1(3):123–7.

42. Coonrad RW, Hooper WR. Tennis elbow: its course, natural history, conservative and surgical management. J Bone Joint Surg Am 1973;55(6):1177–82.

43. Hohmann G. Das Wesen und die Behandlung des sogenannten Tennisellbogens. Munch Med Wochenschr 1933;(80):250–2.

44. Manon-Matos Y, Oron A, Wolff TW. Combined common extensor and supinator aponeurotomy for the treatment of lateral epicondylitis. Tech Hand Up Extrem Surg 2013;17(3):179–81.

45. Verhaar J, Walenkamp G, Kester A, et al. Lateral extensor release for tennis elbow. J Bone Joint Surg Am 1993;75(7):1034–43.

46. Kumar VS, Shetty AA, Ravikumar KJ, et al. Tennis elbow–outcome following the Garden procedure: a retrospective study. J Orthop Surg (Hong Kong) 2004;12(2):226–9.

47. Carroll RE, Jorgensen EC. Evaluation of the Garden procedure for lateral epicondylitis. Clin Orthop Relat Res 1968;60:201–4.

48. Posch JN, Goldberg VM, Larrey R. Extensor fasciotomy for tennis elbow: a long-term follow-up study. Clin Orthop Relat Res 1978;(135):179–82.

49. Khashaba A. Nirschl tennis elbow release with or without drilling. Br J Sports Med 2001; 35(3):200–1.

50. Das D, Maffulli N. Surgical management of tennis elbow. J Sports Med Phys Fitness 2002;42(2): 190–7.

51. Degreef I, Van Raebroeckx A, De Smet L. Anconeus muscle transposition for failed surgical treatment of tennis elbow: preliminary results. Acta Orthop Belg 2005;71(2):154–6.

52. Thornton SJ, Rogers JR, Prickett WD, et al. Treatment of recalcitrant lateral epicondylitis with suture anchor repair. Am J Sports Med 2005; 33(10):1558–64.

53. Baumgard SH, Schwartz DR. Percutaneous release of the epicondylar muscles for humeral epicondylitis. Am J Sports Med 1982;10(4):233–6.

54. Tasto JP, Cummings J, Medlock V, et al. Microtenotomy using a radiofrequency probe to treat lateral epicondylitis. Arthroscopy 2005;21(7):851–60.

55. Lin CL, Lee JS, Su WR, et al. Clinical and ultrasonographic results of ultrasonographically guided percutaneous radiofrequency lesioning in the treatment of recalcitrant lateral epicondylitis. Am J Sports Med 2011;39(11):2429–35.

56. Barnes DE, Beckley JM, Smith J. Percutaneous ultrasonic tenotomy for chronic elbow tendinosis: a prospective study. J Shoulder Elbow Surg 2015; 24(1):67–73.

57. Koh JS, Mohan PC, Howe TS, et al. Fasciotomy and surgical tenotomy for recalcitrant lateral elbow tendinopathy: early clinical experience with a novel device for minimally invasive percutaneous microresection. Am J Sports Med 2013;41(3): 636–44.

58. Baker CL Jr, Murphy KP, Gottlob CA, et al. Arthroscopic classification and treatment of lateral epicondylitis: two-year clinical results. J Shoulder Elbow Surg 2000;9(6):475–82.

59. Spencer GE Jr, Herndon CH. Surgical treatment of epicondylitis. J Bone Joint Surg Am 1953;35-A(2): 421–4.

60. Wittenberg RH, Schaal S, Muhr G. Surgical treatment of persistent elbow epicondylitis. Clin Orthop Relat Res 1992;(278):73–80.

61. Schipper ON, Dunn JH, Ochiai DH, et al. Nirschl surgical technique for concomitant lateral and medial elbow tendinosis: a retrospective review of 53 elbows with a mean follow-up of 11.7 years. Am J Sports Med 2011;39(5):972–6.

62. Leppilahti J, Raatikainen T, Pienimaki T, et al. Surgical treatment of resistant tennis elbow. A prospective, randomised study comparing decompression of the posterior interosseous nerve and lengthening of the tendon of the extensor carpi radialis brevis muscle. Arch Orthop Trauma Surg 2001; 121(6):329–32.

63. Radwan YA, ElSobhi G, Badawy WS, et al. Resistant tennis elbow: shock-wave therapy versus percutaneous tenotomy. Int Orthop 2008;32(5):671–7.

64. Cummins CA. Lateral epicondylitis: in vivo assessment of arthroscopic debridement and correlation with patient outcomes. Am J Sports Med 2006; 34(9):1486–91.

65. Szabo SJ, Savoie FH 3rd, Field LD, et al. Tendinosis of the extensor carpi radialis brevis: an evaluation of three methods of operative treatment. J Shoulder Elbow Surg 2006;15(6):721–7.

66. Goldberg EJ, Abraham E, Siegel I. The surgical treatment of chronic lateral humeral epicondylitis by common extensor release. Clin Orthop Relat Res 1988;(233):208–12.

67. Newey ML, Patterson MH. Pain relief following tennis elbow release. J R Coll Surg Edinb 1994;39(1):60–1.

68. Rayan GM, Coray SA. V-Y slide of the common extensor origin for lateral elbow tendonopathy. J Hand Surg Am 2001;26(6):1138–45.

69. Rosenberg N, Henderson I. Surgical treatment of resistant lateral epicondylitis. Follow-up study of 19 patients after excision, release and repair of proximal common extensor tendon origin. Arch Orthop Trauma Surg 2002;122(9–10):514–7.

70. Balk ML, Hagberg WC, Buterbaugh GA, et al. Outcome of surgery for lateral epicondylitis (tennis elbow): effect of worker's compensation. Am J Orthop (Belle Mead NJ) 2005;34(3):122–6 [discussion: 126].

71. Plancher KD, Bishai SK. Open lateral epicondylectomy: a simple technique update for the 21st Century. Tech Orthop 2006;21(4):276–82.

72. Svernlov B, Adolfsson L. Outcome of release of the lateral extensor muscle origin for epicondylitis. Scand J Plast Reconstr Surg Hand Surg 2006; 40(3):161–5.

73. Zingg PO, Schneeberger AG. Debridement of extensors and drilling of the lateral epicondyle for tennis elbow: a retrospective follow-up study. J Shoulder Elbow Surg 2006;15(3):347–50.

74. Thomas S, Broome G. Patient satisfaction after open release of common extensor origin in treating resistant tennis elbow. Acta Orthop Belg 2007; 73(4):443–5.

75. Dunn JH, Kim JJ, Davis L, et al. Ten- to 14-year follow-up of the Nirschl surgical technique for lateral epicondylitis. Am J Sports Med 2008;36(2): 261–6.

76. Coleman B, Quinlan JF, Matheson JA. Surgical treatment for lateral epicondylitis: a long-term follow-up of results. J Shoulder Elbow Surg 2010; 19(3):363–7.

77. Dwyer AJ, Govindaswamy R, Elbouni T, et al. Are "knife and fork" good enough for day case surgery of resistant tennis elbow? Int Orthop 2010;34(1): 57–61.

78. Rayan F, Rao V Sr, Purushothamdas S, et al. Common extensor origin release in recalcitrant lateral epicondylitis - role justified? J Orthop Surg Res 2010;5:31.

79. Bigorre N, Raimbeau G, Fouque PA, et al. Lateral epicondylitis treatment by extensor carpi radialis fasciotomy and radial nerve decompression: is outcome influenced by the occupational disease compensation aspect? Orthop Traumatol Surg Res 2011;97(2):159–63.

80. Barth J, Mahieu P, Hollevoet N. Extensor tendon and fascia sectioning of extensors at the musculotendinous unit in lateral epicondylitis. Acta Orthop Belg 2013;79(3):266–70.

81. Yerger B, Turner T. Percutaneous extensor tenotomy for chronic tennis elbow: an office procedure. Orthopedics 1985;8(10):1261–3.

82. Grundberg AB, Dobson JF. Percutaneous release of the common extensor origin for tennis elbow. Clin Orthop Relat Res 2000;(376):137–40.

83. Kaleli T, Ozturk C, Temiz A, et al. Surgical treatment of tennis elbow: percutaneous release of the common extensor origin. Acta Orthop Belg 2004;70(2):131–3.

84. McShane JM, Nazarian LN, Harwood MI. Sonographically guided percutaneous needle tenotomy for treatment of common extensor tendinosis in the elbow. J Ultrasound Med 2006;25(10):1281–9.

85. McShane JM, Shah VN, Nazarian LN. Sonographically guided percutaneous needle tenotomy for treatment of common extensor tendinosis in the elbow: is a corticosteroid necessary? J Ultrasound Med 2008;27(8):1137–44.

86. Nazar M, Lipscombe S, Morapudi S, et al. Percutaneous tennis elbow release under local anaesthesia. Open Orthop J 2012;6:129–32.

87. Owens BD, Murphy KP, Kuklo TR. Arthroscopic release for lateral epicondylitis. Arthroscopy 2001; 17(6):582–7.

88. Mullett H, Sprague M, Brown G, et al. Arthroscopic treatment of lateral epicondylitis: clinical and cadaveric studies. Clin Orthop Relat Res 2005; 439:123–8.

89. Jerosch J, Schunck J. Arthroscopic treatment of lateral epicondylitis: indication, technique and early results. Knee Surg Sports Traumatol Arthrosc 2006;14(4):379–82.

90. Brooks-Hill AL, Regan WD. Extra-articular arthroscopic lateral elbow release. Arthroscopy 2008; 24(4):483–5.

91. Grewal R, MacDermid JC, Shah P, et al. Functional outcome of arthroscopic extensor carpi radialis brevis tendon release in chronic lateral epicondylitis. J Hand Surg Am 2009;34(5):849–57.

92. Lattermann C, Romeo AA, Anbari A, et al. Arthroscopic debridement of the extensor carpi radialis brevis for recalcitrant lateral epicondylitis. J Shoulder Elbow Surg 2010;19(5):651–6.

93. Kim JW, Chun CH, Shim DM, et al. Arthroscopic treatment of lateral epicondylitis: comparison of the outcome of ECRB release with and without decortication. Knee Surg Sports Traumatol Arthrosc 2011;19(7):1178–83.

94. Marti D, Spross C, Jost B. The first 100 elbow arthroscopies of one surgeon: analysis of complications. J Shoulder Elbow Surg 2013;22(4):567–73.

95. Kniesel B, Huth J, Bauer G, et al. Systematic diagnosis and therapy of lateral elbow pain with emphasis on elbow instability. Arch Orthop Trauma Surg 2014;134(12):1641–7.

96. Oki G, Iba K, Sasaki K, et al. Time to functional recovery after arthroscopic surgery for tennis elbow. J Shoulder Elbow Surg 2014;23(10):1527–31.

97. Dunkow PD, Jatti M, Muddu BN. A comparison of open and percutaneous techniques in the surgical

treatment of tennis elbow. J Bone Joint Surg Br 2004;86(5):701–4.

98. Rubenthaler F, Wiese M, Senge A, et al. Long-term follow-up of open and endoscopic Hohmann procedures for lateral epicondylitis. Arthroscopy 2005;21(6):684–90.

99. Meknas K, Odden-Miland A, Mercer JB, et al. Radiofrequency microtenotomy. a promising method for treatment of recalcitrant lateral epicondylitis. Am J Sports Med 2008;36(10):1960–5.

100. Othman AM. Arthroscopic versus percutaneous release of common extensor origin for treatment of chronic tennis elbow. Arch Orthop Trauma Surg 2011;131(3):383–8.

101. Solheim E, Hegna J, Oyen J. Arthroscopic versus open tennis elbow release: 3- to 6-year results of a case-control series of 305 elbows. Arthroscopy 2013;29(5):854–9.

102. Cushing M, Lourie GM, Miller DV, et al. Heterotopic ossification after lateral epicondylectomy. J South Orthop Assoc 2001;10(1):53–6.

103. Shapiro GS, Weiland AJ. Reactive bone formation after surgery for lateral epicondylitis. J Shoulder Elbow Surg 2002;11(4):383–5.

104. Carofino BC, Bishop AT, Spinner RJ, et al. Nerve injuries resulting from arthroscopic treatment of lateral epicondylitis: report of 2 cases. J Hand Surg Am 2012;37(6):1208–10.

105. Iyer VG. Iatrogenic injury to posterior antebrachial cutaneous nerve. Muscle Nerve 2014; 50(6):1024–5.

106. Karkhanis S, Frost A, Maffulli N. Operative management of tennis elbow: a quantitative review. Br Med Bull 2008;88(1):171–88.

107. Randelli P, Castagna A, Cabitza F, et al. Infectious and thromboembolic complications of arthroscopic shoulder surgery. J Shoulder Elbow Surg 2010; 19(1):97–101.

108. Bartels RH, Menovsky T, Van Overbeeke JJ, et al. Surgical management of ulnar nerve compression at the elbow: an analysis of the literature. J Neurosurg 1998;89(5):722–7.

109. Friden J, Lieber RL. Physiologic consequences of surgical lengthening of extensor carpi radialis brevis muscle-tendon junction for tennis elbow. J Hand Surg Am 1994;19(2):269–74.

110. Lo MY, Safran MR. Surgical treatment of lateral epicondylitis: a systematic review. Clin Orthop Relat Res 2007;463:98–106.

111. Lodha S, Mithani SK, Srinivasan RC, et al. Nerve Injuries Following Elbow Arthroscopy. J Hand Surg 2013;38(10):e14–5.

112. Dzugan SS, Savoie FH 3rd, Field LD, et al. Acute radial ulno-humeral ligament injury in patients with chronic lateral epicondylitis: an observational report. J Shoulder Elbow Surg 2012; 21(12):1651–5.

Foot and Ankle

Deep Vein Thrombosis in Foot and Ankle Surgery

John Chao, MD

KEYWORDS

- Foot and ankle • Venous thromboembolism • DVT • Pulmonary embolism

KEY POINTS

- The incidence of venous thromboembolism is reported to be low regarding elective and traumatic foot and ankle procedures.
- There is scarce literature offering high-level recommendations for or against venous thromboembolism prophylaxis.
- Although venous thromboembolism can be a devastating complication of treatment of foot and ankle conditions, there are also significant risk factors associated with chemical prophylaxis.
- Most articles suggest considering a chemical prophylaxis in high-risk individuals.
- The ultimate decision of using chemical prophylaxis must be a discussion between the physician and the patient.

INTRODUCTION

Deep vein thrombosis (DVT) is a frequent complication after elective orthopedic surgery and can be a significant cause of morbidity and mortality. Although the incidence of DVT after foot and ankle surgery is low, a DVT leading to pulmonary embolism (PE) can be a cause of mortality. Commonly used DVT prophylaxis includes early mobilization, foot pumps, compression stockings, and chemical prophylaxis.[1] Many of the recommendations for DVT prophylaxis after foot and ankle surgery have been extrapolated from the total joint arthroplasty literature. The incidence of DVT after hip and knee surgery can be more than 60%, with up to 13% subsequently having pulmonary emboli.[2] Despite the benefits of chemical prophylaxis, chemical prophylaxis can be costly and cause wound healing complications.[3] Risk factors should be taken into consideration when discussing potential chemical prophylaxis. Unfortunately, there are several risk factors that make preoperative screening for venous thromboembolism (VTE) more difficult. Some risk factors include family or personal history, older age, immobilization, stroke, cancer, lengthy surgical procedure, air travel, cigarette smoking, and oral contraceptives.[4–11] The decision for DVT prophylaxis should be individualized for each patient after foot and ankle surgery.

VENOUS THROMBOEMBOLISM PROPHYLAXIS

The 2 main categories of VTE prophylaxis are mechanical and chemical. Mechanical prophylaxis includes compression stockings, ambulation, and intermittent pneumatic compression devices. Even if a patient is casted postoperatively, a weight-bearing cast may allow for muscle contraction and decrease the risk of DVT. Chemical prophylaxis includes aspirin, warfarin, low-molecular-weight heparins (LMWH, ie, Enoxaparin), and direct Xa inhibitors (ie, rivaroxaban). Although the use of direct Xa inhibitors is increasing in joint replacement patients, limited literature exists for the direct Xa inhibitors, especially in foot and ankle surgery.

The author has no disclosures.

Department of Orthopaedic Surgery, Peachtree Orthopaedic Clinic, 5505 Peachtree Dunwoody Road, Suite 600, Atlanta, GA 30342, USA

E-mail address: jchao@pocatlanta.com

Orthop Clin N Am 47 (2016) 471–475

http://dx.doi.org/10.1016/j.ocl.2015.10.001

Because the literature is poor regarding DVT prophylaxis in foot and ankle surgery, extrapolations have been used from joint replacement literature. Newer literature has suggested that aspirin is an appropriate agent for chemical DVT prophylaxis in total joint patients. In patients undergoing total joint arthroplasty, symptomatic thromboembolic events were lower in patients receiving 325 mg aspirin twice a day versus patients receiving warfarin.[12] Pulmonary embolism rates were 0.14% in the aspirin group versus 1.07% in the warfarin group (P<.001). The aspirin group also had significantly fewer symptomatic DVTs, less wound related problems, and shorter related hospital stays.

Aspirin has also been studied in foot and ankle patients. However, the dosage and frequency of aspirin was much lower than what is recommended for a postoperative arthroplasty patient. In a study of VTE in foot and ankle surgery, placebo was compared with 75 mg of aspirin a day.[13] The overall incidence of VTE was 0.42%, but there was no protective mechanism by this aspirin dose. The authors concluded that incidence of VTE is low, and chemical prophylaxis does not seem to be necessary if the patient is not high risk.

RISKS OF THROMBOPROPHYLAXIS

It is important to understand that mechanical and chemical DVT prophylaxis may decrease the incidence of VTE but does not make the risk zero. Risks of VTE prophylaxis, albeit low, sometimes outweigh the benefit of prophylaxis. In multiple studies, warfarin and LMWH have increased wound complications and superficial and deep infections.[12,14] Warfarin has many food and drug interactions, requiring frequent monitoring and dose adjustments. In patients who do not adhere to a strict diet, international normalized ratio levels may fluctuate significantly.

Heparin-induced thrombocytopenia (HIT) is also a serious complication with absolute risk in orthopedic surgery of 0.2% for LMWH and 2.6% for unfractionated heparin.[15] HIT often manifests 1 to 2 weeks after initiation of therapy but may occur as early as 1 to 2 days.[16,17] It is identified by significant decrease in platelet count and positive HIT panel, and treatment involves cessation of heparin products and consultation with a specialist.

RISKS FOR VENOUS THROMBOEMBOLISM

Any factors increasing hypercoagulation, venous stasis, or endothelial vessel damage increase the risk for thrombosis. The preoperative evaluation of each patient should consist of an evaluation of postoperative VTE risk. Previous history of DVT, obesity, increasing age, cigarette use, oral contraceptive use, and tourniquet use have been reported as risk factors in differing articles.[4–11] It is also important to ask if there is a family history of DVT and, if there is, whether there was ever a history of hypercoagulation workup.

TOURNIQUET

In foot and ankle surgery, tourniquets are helpful for maintaining a bloodless surgical field and increasing the ease of surgery. However, the literature is not conclusive about the correlation of DVT and tourniquet use in the foot and ankle. Maffulli and colleagues[7] noted that thrombosis was more common with the use of a tourniquet in operatively treated ankle fractures compared with a control group, but the statistical significance of this increase was not calculated between the 2 groups. Conversely, in a prospective study, Simon and colleagues[18] did not show an increased rate of thrombosis with the use of a thigh tourniquet in 117 patients undergoing forefoot surgery.

CHEST Guidelines

The American College of Chest Physicians produce recommendations on venous thromboprophylaxis in orthopedic surgery.[19]

- Thirty-five days of chemical prophylaxis should be used in patients undergoing total hip or knee arthroplasty.
  - Includes LMWH, fondaparinux, apixaban, dabigatran, rivaroxaban, unfractionated heparin, vitamin K antagonists, aspirin, or intermittent pneumatic compression device.
- Chemical prophylaxis should start 12 hours or more postoperatively.
- Recommend against Doppler ultrasound screening for asymptomatic patients.
- Inferior vena cava filter may be used for primary prevention in patients with increased bleeding risk or contraindications to chemical/mechanical thromboprophylaxis.
- No prophylaxis for isolated lower leg injury requiring immobilization.

Foot and Ankle Surgery

Studies evaluating heterogeneous populations after foot and ankle surgery concluded that the risk is low for a thromboembolic event. Each study identified its own risk factors (**Table 1**).

Surveys of Practice

Two surveys evaluating the use of DVT prophylaxis after foot and ankle surgery found that most

Table 1
Studies evaluating heterogeneous populations after foot and ankle surgery

Study	Rate	Risk Factors	Conclusion
Solis & Saxby,[20] 2002	Asymptomatic DVT 7/210 (3.5%)	n/a	Rate and progression of DVT after foot and ankle surgery is low and does not require routine prophylaxis.
Mizel et al,[8] 1998	Symptomatic DVT 6/2733 (0.22%) Symptomatic PE 4/2733 (0.15%)	Non–weight bearing and cast immobilization	Incidence low
Hanslow et al,[4] 2006	Symptomatic DVT 24/602 (4%) Symptomatic PE 8/602 (1.3%)	Rheumatoid arthritis, recent air travel, history of thromboembolic event, limb immobilization	No association with the type of surgery, or the use of tourniquet
Jameson et al,[5] 2011	Symptomatic DVT 58/88,241 (0.07%) Symptomatic PE 93/88,241 (0.11%)	Patients undergoing ankle ORIF and aged >50 y or a Charlson score >2 at increased risk	VTE after foot and ankle surgery is extremely rare and do not recommend widespread use of prophylaxis
Wukich & Waters,[11] 2008	Symptomatic DVT 4/1000 (0.4%) Symptomatic PE 3/1000 (0.3%) 10% received LMWH × 14 d due to high-risk factors	Age >40, non–weight bearing, or obesity	Incidence low

Data from Refs.[4,5,8,11,20]

orthopedic surgeons did not routinely use chemical prophylaxis (**Table 2**).[1,21]

TRAUMA

Trauma patients are a cohort of foot and ankle patients that may be at higher risk for VTE. However, the incidence of DVT and PE in foot and ankle

trauma patients in a national trauma databank was low. Of 160 patients with isolated foot and ankle trauma, the incidence of DVT and PE was 0.28 and 0.21, respectively.[10] This low rate of VTE is in agreement with the recommendations of the American College of Chest Physicians that no prophylaxis is necessary for isolated lower leg injury requiring immobilization.[19]

Table 2
Surveys evaluating the use of DVT prophylaxis after foot and ankle surgery

Study	Routine Usage (%)	Prophylaxis Methods	Surgeons' Viewpoints
Wolf & DiGiovanni,[21] 2004	44	Most commonly used sequential compression device and LMWH.	<50% used prophylaxis, but 70% believed it was sometimes necessary
Gadgil & Thomas,[1] 2007	19	Wide variety in thromboembolic prophylaxis	Lack of published evidence and low rate of VTE were most common reasons for not using prophylaxis

Data from Gadgil A, Thomas RH. Current trends in thromboprophylaxis in surgery of the foot and ankle. Foot Ankle Int 2007;28(10):1069–73; and Wolf JM, DiGiovanni CW. A survey of orthopedic surgeons regarding DVT prophylaxis in foot and ankle trauma surgery. Orthopedics 2004;27(5):504–8.

ANKLE FRACTURES

Ankle fractures are some of the most common injuries treated by orthopedic surgeons. Despite this, there are few studies investigating VTE and ankle fractures. In a prospective cohort, Selby and colleagues[22] evaluated symptomatic VTE in patients with a tibial, fibular, or ankle fracture (treated nonoperatively) or a patellar or foot fracture (treated operatively or conservatively). There was no chemical DVT prophylaxis, and only 7 of the 1179 patients (0.7%) had a thromboembolic event. The authors concluded that symptomatic VTE is an infrequent complication in lower limb fractures, and these fractures can be managed without thromboprophylaxis.

In a larger retrospective review, the incidence of thromboembolic event was 3% in 1540 patients who underwent ankle open reduction and internal fixation (ORIF). The authors noted that the VTE rate was not affected by the use of chemical prophylaxis.[23]

In a prospective, randomized, control trial, 272 patients undergoing ankle ORIF were randomly assigned to dalteparin or placebo for DVT prophylaxis. There was no difference in the rate of DVTs, and no PEs occurred in either group.[24]

METATARSAL FRACTURES

Most patients with nonoperative metatarsal fractures are allowed to weight bear in a protective device. The spectrum of metatarsal fractures requiring operative intervention is wide, and the number of patients required to have an appropriately powered study would be difficult. There was only one study investigating PE and surgical fixation of a metatarsal fracture. In this retrospective review of 1477 patients, there were 4 patients (0.27%) who were diagnosed with a symptomatic PE within 90 days of the initial procedure.[25] Because of this low rate in this heterogenous population, the authors concluded routine thromboprophylaxis may not be necessary for isolated metatarsal fractures.

HALLUX VALGUS

In the elective setting, there are even fewer articles about VTE. There was only one study identified regarding hallux valgus. This was a prospective study in which patients were screened for venous thrombosis after chevron bunionectomy, even in the absence of symptoms.[26] None of the 100 patients received chemical prophylaxis, and only 4 patients had a venous thrombosis. The average age of the DVT group was significantly higher than the non-DVT group. Because of these results,

the authors concluded that patients are at low risk for venous thrombosis after surgical treatment for hallux valgus, but routine prophylaxis may be justified for patients older than 60 years.

Achilles Tendon Rupture

Achilles tendon ruptures are also a common injury that is treated by all orthopedic surgeons. The literature on Achilles tendon VTE is more comprehensive than other foot and ankle conditions but still does not compare in thoroughness to joint replacement data. Lapidus and colleagues[27] prospectively evaluated 91 patients surgically treated for Achilles tendon ruptures. The patients were randomly divided into 2 groups (dalteparin vs placebo) and were evaluated at 3 and 6 weeks after surgery for DVT regardless of symptoms. Both groups showed a high rate of DVT (34% in dalteparin group and 36% in placebo group), and no significant difference existed between the 2 groups.

Patel and colleagues[9] reached a similar conclusion on their retrospectively study of 1172 patients who had an Achilles tendon rupture diagnosed. The rates for symptomatic DVT and PE after an Achilles tendon rupture were 5 of 1172 (0.43%) and 4 of 1172 (0.34%), respectively. The investigators noted that body mass index, age, and surgical repair did not significantly influence the rates of thrombosis.

It is common practice to temporarily immobilize the limb after an acute Achilles injury. Even with aggressive functional rehabilitation, a period of 1 to 2 weeks of immobilization is common. Healy and colleagues[28] retrospectively evaluated 208 patients with an Achilles tendon injury that was treated with cast immobilization for at least 1 week. They reported a 6.3% rate of symptomatic DVT and 1.4% rate of PE. Despite this higher incidence of VTE, it is difficult to conclude that the cast immobilization was the cause of the VTE, as proximal retraction of the rupture has been theorized to increase pressures on the deep calf veins.

SUMMARY/DISCUSSION

The approach to chemical DVT prophylaxis should be individualized in each patient. The literature is not conclusive with strong recommendations for or against DVT prophylaxis. More high-quality studies must be done before strong recommendations can be made. The presence of risk factors should be strongly considered when making the determination of whether to place patients on chemical prophylaxis. The discussion of DVT prophylaxis as well as nonoperative treatment of

Achilles tendon ruptures should be made with each patient before any surgical treatment.

REFERENCES

1. Gadgil A, Thomas RH. Current trends in thromboprophylaxis in surgery of the foot and ankle. Foot Ankle Int 2007;28(10):1069–73.

2. Gillespie W, Murray D, Gregg PJ, et al. Risks and benefits of prophylaxis against venous thromboembolism in orthopaedic surgery. J Bone Joint Surg Br 2000;82(4):475–9.

3. Patel VP, Walsh M, Sehgal B, et al. Factors associated with prolonged wound drainage after primary total hip and knee arthroplasty. J Bone Joint Surg Am 2007;89(1):33–8.

4. Hanslow S, Grujic L, Slater HK, et al. Thromboembolic disease after foot and ankle surgery. Foot Ankle Int 2006;27(9):693–5.

5. Jameson S, Augustine A, James P, et al. Venous thromboembolic events following foot and ankle surgery in the English National Health Service. J Bone Joint Surg Br 2011;93(4):490–7.

6. Kock H, Schmit-Neuerburg KP, Hanke J, et al. Thromboprophylaxis with low-molecular-weight heparin in outpatients with plaster-cast immobilisation of the leg. Lancet 1995;346(8973):459–61.

7. Maffulli N, Testa V, Capasso G. Use of a tourniquet in the internal fixation of fractures of the distal part of the fibula. A prospective, randomized trial. J Bone Joint Surg Am 1993;75(5):700–3.

8. Mizel M, Temple HT, Michelson JD, et al. Thromboembolism after foot and ankle surgery. A multicenter study. Clin Orthop Relat Res 1998;348:180–5.

9. Patel A, Ogawa B, Charlton T, et al. Incidence of deep vein thrombosis and pulmonary embolism after Achilles tendon rupture. Clin Orthop Relat Res 2012;470(1):270–4.

10. Shibuya N, Frost CH, Campbell JD, et al. Incidence of acute deep vein thrombosis and pulmonary embolism in foot and ankle trauma: analysis of the National Trauma Data Bank. J Foot Ankle Surg 2012; 51(1):63–8.

11. Wukich DK, Waters DH. Thromboembolism following foot and ankle surgery: a case series and literature review. J Foot Ankle Surg 2008;47(3):243–9.

12. Raphael IJ, Tischler EH, Huang R, et al. Aspirin: an alternative for pulmonary embolism prophylaxis after arthroplasty? Clin Orthop Relat Res 2014;472(2): 482–8.

13. Griffiths JT, Matthews L, Pearce CJ, et al. Incidence of venous thromboembolism in elective foot and ankle surgery with and without aspirin prophylaxis. J Bone Joint Surg Br 2012;94(2):210–4.

14. Sachs R, Smith JH, Kuney M, et al. Does anticoagulation do more harm than good?: a comparison of patients treated without prophylaxis and patients treated with low-dose warfarin after total knee arthroplasty. J Arthroplasty 2003;18(4):389–95.

15. Martel N, Lee J, Wells PS. Risk for heparin-induced thrombocytopenia with unfractionated and low-molecular-weight heparin thromboprophylaxis: a meta-analysis. Blood 2005;106(8):2710–5.

16. Kibbe MR, Rhee RY. Heparin-induced thrombocytopenia: pathophysiology. Semin Vasc Surg 1996;9(4): 284–91.

17. Ramakrishna R, Manoharan A, Kwan YL, et al. Heparin-induced thrombocytopenia: cross-reactivity between standard heparin, low molecular weight heparin, dalteparin (Fragmin) and heparinoid, danaparoid (Orgaran). Br J Haematol 1995;91(3):736–8.

18. Simon MA, Mass DP, Zarins CK, et al. The effect of a thigh tourniquet on the incidence of deep venous thrombosis after operations on the fore part of the foot. J Bone Joint Surg Am 1982;64(2):188–91.

19. Falck-Ytter Y, Francis CW, Johanson NA, et al. Prevention of VTE in orthopedic surgery patients: antithrombotic therapy and prevention of thrombosis, 9th ed: American College of Chest Physicians evidence-based clinical practice guidelines. Chest 2012;141(2 Suppl):e278S–325S.

20. Solis G, Saxby T. Incidence of DVT following surgery of the foot and ankle. Foot Ankle Int 2002;23(5):411–4.

21. Wolf JM, DiGiovanni CW. A survey of orthopedic surgeons regarding DVT prophylaxis in foot and ankle trauma surgery. Orthopedics 2004;27(5):504–8.

22. Selby R, Geerts WH, Kreder HJ, et al. Symptomatic venous thromboembolism uncommon without thromboprophylaxis after isolated lower-limb fracture: the knee-to-ankle fracture (KAF) cohort study. J Bone Joint Surg Am 2014;96(10):e83.

23. Pelet S, Roger ME, Belzile EL, et al. The incidence of thromboembolic events in surgically treated ankle fracture. J Bone Joint Surg Am 2012;94(6):502–6.

24. Lapidus L, Ponzer S, Elvin A, et al. Prolonged thromboprophylaxis with Dalteparin during immobilization after ankle fracture surgery: a randomized placebo-controlled, double-blind study. Acta Orthop 2007; 78(4):528–35.

25. Soohoo N, Farng E, Zingmond DS. Incidence of pulmonary embolism following surgical treatment of metatarsal fractures. Foot Ankle Int 2010;31(7):600–3.

26. Radl R, Kastner N, Aigner C, et al. Venous thrombosis after hallux valgus surgery. J Bone Joint Surg Am 2003;85-A(7):1204–8.

27. Lapidus L, Rosfors S, Ponzer S, et al. Prolonged thromboprophylaxis with dalteparin after surgical treatment of achilles tendon rupture: a randomized, placebo-controlled study. J Orthop Trauma 2007; 21(1):52–7.

28. Healy B, Beasley R, Weatherall M. Venous thromboembolism following prolonged cast immobilisation for injury to the tendo Achillis. J Bone Joint Surg Br 2010;92(5):646–50.

Index

Note: Page numbers of article titles are in **boldface** type.

Orthop Clin N Am 47 (2016) 477–483
http://dx.doi.org/10.1016/S0030-5898(15)00281-3
0030-5898/16/$ – see front matter © 2016 Elsevier Inc. All rights reserved.

Moving?

Make sure your subscription moves with you!

To notify us of your new address, find your **Clinics Account Number** (located on your mailing label above your name), and contact customer service at:

Email: journalscustomerservice-usa@elsevier.com

800-654-2452 (subscribers in the U.S. & Canada)
314-447-8871 (subscribers outside of the U.S. & Canada)

Fax number: 314-447-8029

Elsevier Health Sciences Division
Subscription Customer Service
3251 Riverport Lane
Maryland Heights, MO 63043

ELSEVIER

Printed and bound by CPI Group (UK) Ltd, Croydon, CR0 4YY

08/05/2025

01865194-0002